Praise for *Paleo for Life*

"It makes perfect sense to eat the 'native' human diet, the one on which we evolved millions of years ago. To start, we ate a plant-based diet, but we also added moderate amounts of animal foods that filled important nutrient gaps, especially for women. *Paleo for Life* provides everything you need to know to live a long and happy life. No one knows this subject better than Loren Cordain."

—Dr. Jennie Brand-Miller, PhD, *New York Times* bestselling author of *The New Glucose Revolution* and *The Low GI Diet Revolution* and emeritus professor of nutrition at the University of Sydney

"*Paleo for Life* distills the latest nutritional science into easy-to-follow guidelines and delicious recipes. The science continues to grow, and it shows that adoption of the Paleo diet is one of the most health-supportive steps for anyone with a chronic health problem. I conduct dietary research studies, and the Paleo dietary intervention consistently improves health outcomes across multiple disease states. If you want to thrive well into your nineties, this book is for you."

—Dr. Terry Wahls, MD, FACP, author of *The Wahls Protocol: A Radical New Way to Treat All Chronic Autoimmune Conditions Using Paleo Principles* and clinical professor of medicine at the University of Iowa

"Dr. Loren Cordain's knowledge of nutrition is exceptional. In this book, you will learn about the effects of nutrition on healthspan and lifespan—and it will change you."

—Joe Friel, coauthor of *The Paleo Diet for Athletes* and author of *The Triathlete's Training Bible*

"Loren Cordain is one of the true pioneers in Paleonutrition. In his new book, *Paleo for Life*, he dispels myths about what a Paleo diet is and isn't, sheds light on what foods in our ancestral pantry provide us the best chance for long and healthy lives, and gives us a blueprint of meal plans and recipes for implementing this way of eating to our greatest benefit. This important book arrives at a time when our nation's health is in decline. It couldn't have come at a better time."

—Mary Dan Eades, MD, and Michael R. Eades, MD, authors of the *New York Times* bestselling *Protein Power* and *The Protein Power LifePlan*

"An easily read and intelligent review of Dr. Cordain's work on the mismatch between our physiology and what we eat. Helpful to anyone interested in improving their health by improving their diet."

—Lynda Frassetto, MD, emeritus professor of medicine and nephrology at the University of California, San Francisco

"A comprehensive blend of nutritional and longevity science, *Paleo for Life* offers a nuanced survey of superfoods and dietary habits that will set you up for a vibrant, active lifestyle as you grow older. Equally valuable from your thirties to your nineties, Dr. Cordain's approach offers a long-lasting boost to energy, mental acuity, and overall health."

—**Paul Laursen, PhD, cofounder of Athletica and HIIT Science and adjunct professor at Auckland University of Technology and the University of Agder**

"This extraordinary resource is an essential, life-changing road map to optimal health that will serve you for decades to come. Masterfully balancing scientific rigor with accessibility, it illuminates how whole-food eating patterns and interventions like the addition of superfoods into your diet can revolutionize your well-being. Inspiring real-life success stories provide motivation and invaluable insights, while the exceptional recipes make implementation effortless."

—**Kiira Heymann, director of strategic partnerships, learning, and community at the Non-GMO Project**

"Loren Cordain's *Paleo for Life* rises above the noise. It combines state-of-the-art knowledge from nutritional, health, and biomedical sciences with a deep understanding of the diets, foodways, and health of both living and prehistoric humans the world over. This wonderful book draws its insights and builds its recommendations through the careful integration of knowledge from the full scope of human experience. To me, that's what makes *Paleo for Life* such a fundamental baseline for anyone thinking about how to improve their well-being through healthy eating."

—**John D. Speth, PhD, emeritus professor of anthropology at the University of Michigan–Ann Arbor**

"*Paleo for Life* builds a robust foundation for health, performance, and longevity."

—**Dr. Marc Bubbs, performance and clinical nutritionist and chief nutrition officer at ProBio Nutrition**

"I love how this book empowers people to understand their own health. It's inspiring to see such a clear, science-backed path toward vitality and longevity—rooted in the kinds of whole, nutrient-dense foods our bodies were designed to thrive on. As someone deeply involved in the regenerative movement, it's exciting to see the early threads being drawn between the health of our food and the health of our soil. *Paleo for Life* helps advance a deeper awareness that what's good for our bodies can also be good for the planet—and that's a story well worth telling."

—**Finian Makepeace, cofounder of Kiss the Ground and producer of the Netflix documentaries *Kiss the Ground* and *Common Ground***

"In 2001, Dr. Cordain gifted us with his first book, *The Paleo Diet*, which changed my life and that of countless others. His teachings about the most authentic, health-promoting diet for humans have transformed the way we think about what foods will make us thrive. In *Paleo for Life*, Dr. Cordain builds upon how to eat to be healthy now with how to live an optimally healthy life for the long term."

—**Nell Stephenson, coauthor of *The Paleo Diet Cookbook***

PALEO
FOR LIFE

Other books by Loren Cordain, PhD

The Paleo Diet

The Paleo Diet Cookbook
(with Nell Stephenson and Lorrie Cordain)

The Paleo Answer

The Paleo Diet for Athletes (with Joe Friel)

The Real Paleo Diet Cookbook

Real Paleo Fast & Easy

PALEO
FOR LIFE

Superfoods to Slow Aging,
Boost Longevity, and
Enhance Your Well-Being

LOREN CORDAIN, PhD

with Trevor Connor and Mark J. Smith, PhD

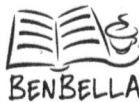

BENBELLA

BenBella Books, Inc.
Dallas, TX

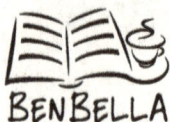

BENBELLA

BenBella Books, Inc.
8080 N. Central Expressway
Suite 1700
Dallas, TX 75206
benbellabooks.com
Send feedback to feedback@benbellabooks.com

BenBella is a federally registered trademark.

Printed in the United States of America
10 9 8 7 6 5 4 3 2 1

Library of Congress Control Number: 2025018951
ISBN 9781637747490 (hardcover)
ISBN 9781637747506 (electronic)

Editing by Holly Robinson, Joe Rhatigan, and Claire Schulz
Copyediting by Karen Wise
Proofreading by Marissa Wold Urhina and Jenny Bridges
Indexing by WordCo Indexing Services, Inc.
Text design and composition by PerfecType, Nashville, TN
Cover design by Morgan Carr
Printed by Lake Book Manufacturing

Special discounts for bulk sales are available. Please contact bulkorders@benbellabooks.com.

For Lorrie, Kyle, Kevin, and Kenny, whose love, support, and dedication have made this book possible. I am eternally grateful.

—Loren Cordain

CONTENTS

PART III
Add Animal Foods to Promote Longevity

PART IV
Your Paleo Journey

INTRODUCTION

Y ou had a good reason to pick up this book. Maybe your knees ached walking upstairs today, your doctor just put you on blood thinners, or you can't seem to remember things the way you did when you were younger. It feels like your whole body is starting to fall apart, and you're worried your health will keep going downhill as you get older.

You can't turn back the hands of time, but you *can* take simple steps right now to live a longer, healthier life. We've written this book to show you how.

In 2001, Loren Cordain published his first book, *The Paleo Diet*, introducing the public to the benefits of eating like our hunter-gatherer ancestors. Since then, we—Dr. Cordain and us, two of his former graduate students, Trevor Connor, MS, and Mark J. Smith, PhD—have continued our research to learn even more about the benefits of eating Paleo as we age.

Longevity statistics tell us that the average age of mortality, or the age at death, is 76 years old in the United States and on the decline for the first time in generations. But here's an even more important marker to consider: the age of morbidity. That's the age at which chronic illnesses such as arthritis, cancer, cardiovascular disease, diabetes, and neurological conditions like Alzheimer's begin having negative impacts on our lives. Too often, that starts happening as early as our 30s and 40s, which means many people face decades of ill health. According to the National Council on Aging, nearly 95 percent of Americans will have at least one chronic illness by the time they reach age 60, and almost 80 percent will battle two. The rest will remain blessedly healthy enough to enjoy travel, social activities, and an active retirement without chronic illness.

So what's the secret? Why do certain people enjoy not only longer lives, but healthier ones as well? Genetics can certainly play a part. People with longer-lived parents have a better shot at living longer themselves, according to researchers. Otherwise, the one thing scientists agree on is that a poor diet can damage our health and lower our quality of life as we age. During the 20th century, the top killer in terms of disease shifted from viruses and pathogens to chronic inflammatory conditions. That's due in part to modern medicine dramatically reducing deaths from infectious diseases in the last century.

It is widely agreed in scientific circles that the rise of inflammatory conditions, or what are commonly known as the diseases of civilization, is largely the result of what we eat. Many processed foods Americans consume today have a high glycemic load, which abnormally elevates blood sugar levels. That's why so many of us experience *metabolic syndrome* as we age, an umbrella term for many conditions, including increased blood pressure, high blood sugar, excess body fat around the waist, and abnormal blood lipid profiles. Together, these conditions increase the risk of heart disease, stroke, and type 2 diabetes. While we're all aware of the issues with high blood sugar, that's only one of many concerns caused by a highly processed diet, which we'll address later in the book.

Almost all of us hope to become healthy centenarians. Getting to that point in our lives takes a certain amount of luck plus the right roll of the genetic dice. Beyond that, it's up to you. Dietary changes can have an immediate impact on both how good you feel and on slowing the aging process.

That's where The Paleo Diet® comes in.

It's the Human Way to Eat

While Dr. Cordain is considered to be the original "father of the Paleo Diet," he likes to emphasize that he didn't create it. That job belonged to nature. Over the past three decades, Dr. Cordain and his colleagues from the fields of medicine, nutrition, and anthropology simply did the research and uncovered the science that stands as the foundation of the diet to this day.

Many of our most problematic foods have been introduced only within the past 200 years. In *The Paleo Diet*, Dr. Cordain's first book, he explained the benefits of eating the way people did over the course of over a million years, right up until the rise of agriculture 12,000 years ago. His argument was simple: By eating more like hunter-gatherer populations and eliminating foods introduced after humans began farming—such as grains, dairy, legumes, simple carbohydrates, and added salt—we can live healthier, longer lives. When you eat Paleo, you're consuming the optimal nutrients for your body, literally programmed into your DNA.

The modern Paleo Diet mimics the foods we would have consumed in our historic past. It's true that many of the foods we evolved around no longer exist. For instance, our ancestors ate fruits and vegetables that tended to be smaller, had less sugar, and had more nutrient density—with a high mineral and vitamin content relative to their weight—compared to what's available now.

When we compare the Paleo Diet to a modern Western diet, the differences are stark. Up to 70 percent of the foods typical of a Western diet have been available for only a few generations. These foods include vegetable oils, refined sugar, and processed foods. Because of how recently those changes have taken place, our bodies haven't had ample time to adapt to consuming these foods.

By returning to the diet we evolved eating, it's possible to live both a longer and healthier life.

How Does the Paleo Diet Boost Healthy Aging?

As the science of nutrition advances, so does our understanding of the long-term health benefits of the Paleo Diet. For instance, one of the first large-scale meta-analyses on diet and chronic disease showing the benefits of the Paleo Diet was published in the journal *Nutrients* in December 2022. A peer-reviewed meta-analysis is considered the gold standard for generating scientific consensus because it gathers all the prior research on a topic, discards poorly controlled or biased studies, and then reconciles the results of the remaining reliable studies into a consensus of findings.

The researchers conducting this meta-analysis study demonstrated how much the scientific body of evidence supporting the Paleo Diet has grown over the past 20 years. In considering 4,008 different studies, 68 articles were ultimately used to compare the health impacts of many of the most popular diets, including the Mediterranean diet, the Paleo Diet, the DASH (Dietary Approaches to Stop Hypertension) diet, a plant-based diet, a low-carbohydrate diet, a high-fat (ketogenic) diet, a typical Western diet, and a diet based on government guidelines.

Guess what? The Paleo Diet ranked highest when it comes to fighting inflammation, improving lipid panels, and lowering blood sugar—factors that contribute to the chronic conditions we associate with aging. Specifically, the *Nutrients* study highlighted these two key discoveries:

1. The Paleo Diet performed best at improving the markers of chronic disease and proved to be the healthiest diet overall, with a score of 67 percent. DASH came in at 62 percent, followed by the Mediterranean at 57 percent. Not surprisingly, the traditional Western diet ranked lowest, at 36 percent. The government guidelines and plant-based diets also performed poorly, at 48.5 percent and 49.3 percent, respectively.

2. The researchers concluded that the specific foods you choose to eat are the most important factor for improving chronic disease markers. Focusing on macronutrients alone, like following a low-fat or low-carb diet, isn't an effective way to improve health.

Why This Book Now?

Now, nearly a quarter century after Dr. Cordain's first book came out, we have written *Paleo for Life* to build on the scientifically sound themes of the original Paleo Diet to chronicle new advances in science, zeroing in on specific Paleo superfoods that confer longevity-boosting effects, including reduced inflammation and greater resistance to age-related chronic illnesses. You'll come away with a deeper understanding of our typical Western diet's flaws and how individual foods can work as anti-aging catalysts. You'll also discover the cultural history of some of these foods.

For instance, our entire food industry is based on engineering foods to be so highly addictive that people don't want to give them up. Two of the most addictive ingredients are salt and sugar. In this book, you'll discover why we advocate for a lower-salt diet than is typically consumed and why it's so essential to focus on "nutrient density," a measure of the amount of nutrients (such as vitamins, minerals, and essential fatty acids) in a food relative to its calories.

Another key principle of the Paleo Diet is finding the optimal ratios of certain nutrients. We'll show you how to do that as well. There is no such thing as one perfect food, but there is a perfect mix of foods that will help you reach that centenarian milestone while still celebrating good health.

This book is full of news about individual foods and food groups that are specifically associated with longevity. You may have heard before that some of these foods, such as olive oil and chocolate, are healthy. What you'll learn here is how, exactly, to choose the best foods to thwart the aging process. For example, which herbs and spices give you the biggest health-boosting bang for your buck? What fruits should consistently rank high on your grocery list? What's more, you'll become familiar with lesser-known longevity nutrients that deserve to be in the spotlight, such as taurine, ergothioneine, PQQ, and berberine, which we'll discuss later in the book.

Finally, we'll give you some tips for getting started on your Paleo journey and share a collection of more than 50 new recipes using the specific longevity superfoods we discuss in this book, along with a 14-day meal planner and autoimmune protocol (AIP) diet substitutes. You'll be surprised by how easy—and how delicious—these meals are, and how much better you'll feel after only a few weeks of adjusting your food choices to support a longer, healthier life.

PART I

The Power of Paleo
to Boost Longevity

CHAPTER ONE

The Paleo Diet 2.0: Eating for Longevity

Kim was in her mid-40s and juggling a teaching job with raising two children when she noticed her energy slipping. When a nutritionist suggested she try eating Paleo, she was skeptical at first, wondering if it was sustainable.

"I'd never tried eliminating anything from my diet because I always thought of myself as a healthy eater," she says. "You know, just a regular meat and potatoes diet. All the good stuff."

The first thing she cut out of her diet was gluten. Then she started eating Paleo regularly and began noticing profound changes within a couple of weeks. She was not only more energetic, she says, "but cognitively my mind was very sharp. I had this clarity of thinking and recall I didn't have before."

Her sister and various friends commented on her complexion, saying her skin was "glowing" on the Paleo Diet, and she lost 12 pounds. The biggest surprise of all, though, was Kim's annual physical, where her doctor did a blood lipid panel that was significantly improved from the tests she'd had the year before. "I was pretty surprised," she says, "but I guess this happened because I was eating really natural foods that we evolved to eat."

If you're new to the Paleo Diet concept or could use a refresher, you might be like Kim and wonder if it's worth trying. We'll discuss how the Paleo Diet improves health and energy in this chapter, while also shattering some popular misconceptions and showing you the foods you can eat when you're on the Paleo Diet.

How Does the Paleo Diet Improve Health and Energy?

While the focus of this book is on longevity, a key part of longevity is improved health and energy. We've covered in previous books how a Paleo lifestyle improves your vitality, but here is a summary of Paleo Diet benefits:

Paleo improves nutrient density

On the Paleo Diet, you won't focus on macronutrient ratios (like how much protein versus carbohydrate you consume). Consider the range of foods our ancestors ate: Hunter-gatherer societies living near the equator consumed higher levels of carbohydrates, while those farther north enjoyed higher volumes of protein and fat. Likewise, our ancestral diet changed seasonally, so macronutrient ratios fluctuated throughout the year. Plus, while our hunter-gatherer ancestors naturally ate healthy diets, not one of them knew what a carbohydrate was. They just knew which foods to eat and which to avoid. On the Paleo Diet, you'll forget about the ratio of carbs to fat to protein and instead eat the most nutrient-dense foods, such as leafy green vegetables, blueberries, salmon, and grass-fed beef. (We discuss the importance of nutrient density in greater detail on page 8.)

Paleo stops cravings, helps you maintain a healthy weight, and makes you feel more energetic

On the Paleo Diet, you will consume a lower overall calorie count because your body will get the nutrients it needs. The benefits of eating nutrient-dense foods are threefold:

1. You will feel more consistently energetic.
2. You'll eliminate daily cravings.
3. You will more easily control your weight by eating foods that are lower in calories and higher in nutrients.

Paleo reduces dips in energy

You will eat foods with a lower *glycemic load* on the Paleo Diet. Glycemic load is similar to the more commonly known *glycemic index* in that they both measure the impact of foods on your blood sugar levels, but glycemic load is more realistic. A food's glycemic index is a score between 0 and 100 based on how drastically its carbohydrate makes your blood sugar rise. But that tells just part of the story.

The problem with the glycemic index is that it doesn't consider how much of the food you're actually eating. Glycemic load, on the other hand, takes into account both the glycemic index of a food and how much carbohydrate you're getting from the serving you're eating. Watermelon, for example, has a high glycemic index (80), but a serving of watermelon has so little carbohydrate that its glycemic load is only 5. By eating low glycemic–load meals and lowering your sugar intake, your blood sugar levels should be reduced and stabilized. This means you'll experience fewer energy crashes and have more energy. In case you're interested in measuring it, there are now many apps available on your phone that will help you determine the glycemic loads of the foods and meals you eat.

Paleo will help you improve key nutrient ratios

We all know that we need vitamins and minerals to stay healthy, but there's often a more-is-better approach in our culture that doesn't always lead to better health. What's more important and almost never covered in the media is that eating key nutrients in the right ratios is extremely important to our health. The Paleo Diet brings those ratios—such as calcium-to-magnesium, and sodium-to-potassium—back into the best balance for our bodies. For example, the optimal calcium-to-magnesium ratio is 2:1. Too high *and* too low a ratio are both associated with heart disease.

Paleo helps you eat the right ratios of fatty acids

For years, the USDA and nutritionists alike promoted a low-fat diet as healthy. Researchers believed that consuming fat—any fat—led to elevated cholesterol and, ultimately, heart disease. This belief has been mostly debunked. What's more important is eating the right ratios of fats—for example, consuming similar amounts of omega-3 and omega-6 fatty acids. The Paleo Diet is based on fish, fresh lean meats, and healthy fruits and vegetables, so it naturally provides an optimal ratio of these essential fatty acids.

Paleo improves your acid–base balance

A typical Western diet is acidic. This is again why our ratios are so important—a high sodium-to-potassium ratio is a key contributor to increasing the acidity of our blood. Consuming foods and drinks with a healthy sodium-to-potassium ratio is critical for reducing the acidic effects of our diet. In a Western diet, this ratio typically sits at 2:1 or higher, while the optimal ratio should be 1:5 and even as much as 1:10. An acidic diet is problematic because it can lead to inflammation and can also be a major contributor to osteoporosis. When our bodies need to address a high acid load, they leach calcium from our bones, which is our best source of base in the body. (It's like popping a Tums when you have stomach acid.) Over time, this leaching leads to osteoporosis.

Few studies support the idea that calcium supplementation can help osteoporosis. If you have this condition, or think you're at risk for it, you should be very concerned about your sodium and potassium consumption and less worried about your calcium consumption. As we've already mentioned and will discuss in detail later, consuming too much calcium can contribute to heart disease. Bottom line: Increasing potassium consumption by eating highly nutritious vegetables is one of the best ways to prevent osteoporosis.

Paleo decreases antinutrient consumption

We'll examine antinutrients closely in more detail in chapter 4, but for now, let's take a look at grains such as wheat and pseudo-grains such as quinoa. These grains contain saponins, lectins, and many other antinutrients. These tiny molecules are extremely effective at evading your intestinal defense mechanisms, opening the tight junctions in your gut, and making you sick if you consume them raw. Cooking grains eliminates many, but not all, of these antinutrients. Cooked wheat might even be worse for you than eating it raw, because if you ate wheat raw, you'd likely become ill and never want to touch it again.

By cooking most of the antinutrients out, we convince ourselves that these grain products are safe. Over time, however, the small quantities of antinutrients we consume can cause chronic inflammation and lead to autoimmune diseases and even cancer. The Paleo Diet eliminates foods high in these antinutrients.

Trevor's Story: Nutrient Density and Obvious Foods of Destruction

I was first introduced to the concept of nutrient density while training at the National Cycling Centre in Canada. Each month, we did a five-day training camp, with five- to six-hour daily rides. I loved these rides, but at one particular camp, I was struggling. When the group stopped at rest stops to grab food, my usual Gatorade and several bags of candy didn't seem very appealing. (Yes, that's what sports nutrition told athletes to eat back then.) Instead, I couldn't get enough turkey jerky.

When I asked my sports nutrition instructor if he had any idea what was going on, we were both left scratching our heads for the first few days of the camp. Then a new symptom appeared: I developed cracks at the corners of my lips.

One of the causes of lips cracking at the corners is riboflavin deficiency. What is turkey jerky high in? Riboflavin. That's when I realized that my body knew what I needed and was using hunger signals to try to make me eat it.

Nutrient density is a measure of the amount of essential nutrients (like vitamins, minerals, and essential fatty acids) in a food relative to its calorie content. Or, to put it another way, foods that have a high nutrient density provide a lot of essential nutrients per calorie, while foods with a low nutrient density offer relatively few. Nutrient-dense foods feature prominently in the Paleo Diet and pack such a powerful longevity punch that they can help you avoid many conditions of aging.

While the concept of nutrient density may seem obvious now, it wasn't even recognized until 2005, when epidemiologist Dr. Adam Drewnowski of the University of Washington's School of Public Health published his seminal paper on the topic. He has conducted extensive research on the role of nutrient density in health outcomes, including the relationship between nutrient density and obesity, and the impact of nutrient density on food choices and dietary patterns. His nutrient profiling systems, like the Nutrient Rich Foods (NRF) index, are widely used to assess the nutrient density of foods and inform public health policy.

Dr. Drewnowski's work, and that of many researchers who have followed his lead, shows that nutrient density can play an important role in the development and prevention of obesity. When you eat foods low in nutrient density, such as processed snacks and sugary beverages, you're apt to consume more calories to meet your nutrient needs. This leads to weight gain over time. On the other hand, eating foods that are high in nutrient density, like fruits, vegetables, mushrooms, meats, and seafood, can help your body feel satisfied with fewer calories. This reduces the risk of overeating.

Think about it this way: Hunger is not an on-off switch. When you feel hungry, your hunger isn't simply satisfied by eating whatever is readily available. Normally, you are hungry for nutrients your body needs. This is a familiar experience during pregnancy. It creates "strange" food cravings because of deficiencies in specific nutrients, and the foods that are craved are often very high in those nutrients.

The problem is that if you treat your hunger like an on-off switch and try to satisfy it with a processed hamburger and fries—which are very low in nutrient density—your body will tell you, "Thanks for the calories! I'm going to store those as fat, but you didn't give me the B vitamins or potassium I needed, so I'm not going to shut off the hunger signals. Keep eating!"

A diet rich in nutrient-dense foods is not only an important factor in preventing and managing obesity, but also a great way to maintain your long-term health because nutrient-dense foods also tend to be anti-inflammatory, while ultra-processed foods, which are generally very low in nutrient density, are often the most inflammatory foods we can eat.

Breaking Down Popular Paleo Diet Myths

When the Paleo Diet was first introduced, it was criticized by the nutrition community and called a fad diet because there weren't yet any randomized clinical trials to support its many benefits. Dr. Cordain's first book sparked hundreds of research papers and set off an industry of Paleo Diet–friendly foods, as well as our own company and food-certification program. The Paleo Diet also reinvigorated and accelerated related nutrition movements, including low-carb, gluten-free, ketogenic, autoimmune, anti-inflammatory, and organic/non-GMO diets. Today, our program impacts the lives of over 30 million people who are eating Paleo.

Still, some people hesitate to try a diet of primarily Paleo nutrition because there are so many misconceptions about it. Let's take a moment to break down some lingering Paleo Diet myths.

Paleo is a salt-heavy diet

While we recognize that some in the Paleo community are touting high-salt diets, we argue this doesn't fit with nature or nutrition science. You'll read more about this in chapter 8. For now, we'll just point out that because salt contributes to inflammation and many other chronic conditions that can compromise healthy aging, a diet without added salt is an important component of the Paleo Diet. Although sodium is an extremely important element, any you consume should be done so naturally through the Paleo foods on your plate.

Paleo is a meat-centric diet

While we do encourage you to eat animal protein (see part III), you might eat more fruits and vegetables by volume when you embrace a Paleo lifestyle. We don't recommend a particular ratio of plant and animal food. Our ancestors' diets varied pretty dramatically. You should eat the ratio that feels right to you.

You won't get enough calcium because people who eat Paleo don't eat dairy

Americans tend to overconsume calcium and underconsume magnesium. This is an issue because the science shows that the ratio of calcium to magnesium is far more important to your long-term health than how much calcium you consume. Science has even shown that bone density can be increased by upping magnesium consumption *without* increasing calcium. Whereas the typical Western diet gives us a ratio of calcium to magnesium at 3:1 or higher, the optimal ratio is between 1.7:1 and 2.6:1. Green leafy vegetables are a great addition to your diet because they can help you get that ratio back in balance.

You have to cut carbs

While we encourage you to stay away from simple carbohydrates like bread and pasta, you'll get plenty of complex carbs from sweet potatoes, squash, and other fruits and vegetables.

You must count calories

We've challenged people to try to overeat on the Paleo Diet, and they can't do it. Think of it this way: One slice of pizza is 450 calories—as many calories as six apples! The fiber and nutrients in natural foods are going to fill you up long before your calorie count gets out of control as it can with heavily processed foods.

You have to say goodbye to your favorite foods

Actually, unless you're choosing Paleo to treat an autoimmune disease or other medical condition, we typically advise people to eat Paleo about 85 percent of the time. We'll give you some examples of how you can do that in part IV, where we also include delicious, easy Paleo recipes for you to try as you take your first steps toward better health. For now, though, we'll just say that most people don't have to eat Paleo 100 percent of the time. That's because many researchers believe in the value of nutritional hormesis—the process by which a low dose of a nutritionally stressful stimulant activates the body to increase resistance to that stress through different mechanisms, including gene repair and cellular death. In other words, it's beneficial to challenge the body's digestive and immune systems with minor irritants from time to time to help keep systems regulated, primed, and functioning at their best. Nutritional hormesis has even been suggested by some researchers as a strategy for slowing down the aging process.

In fact, one popular theory to explain autoimmune disease is called the "hygiene hypothesis," which basically states that our immune systems are designed to work optimally with some constant level of viruses and bacteria in our bodies. In countries with highly developed healthcare systems like ours, the relative lack of viruses and bacteria means our immune systems might be "over-revved" without an invader to address. In some people, this can lead their immune systems to ultimately start attacking their own bodies. That means a few treats now and again might be good for you.

Also, trying to stay 100 percent Paleo in today's fast-paced Western culture is just too challenging for most people and will likely cause frustration and failure. That's not how we want you to feel about food, eating, and health. In our collective experience, starting slowly by replacing certain foods with Paleo choices and eventually eating Paleo about 85 percent of the time is enough to offer significant health benefits to most people.

What Foods Can You Eat on a Paleo Diet?

The biggest challenge for many people is to find the "right" healthy diet. What science considers healthy foods often conflicts with media reports, making it even tougher. One minute, you might read about a study showing that eating eggs is the fast track to heart disease. The next minute, there's a report that eggs will keep your heart healthy for decades. (We cover this hot debate in chapter 12.) In both cases, the media is misrepresenting science. That's why we work so hard to keep up with the latest research and offer you the healthiest options out there on the Paleo Diet.

While the Paleo Diet may exclude some foods you might be used to eating daily, like beans, grains, and dairy products, there are countless nutritious whole foods you can eat to satisfy your appetite instead, including:

- avocado
- beef (unprocessed and preferably grass-fed)
- chicken (pasture-raised and free of preservatives)
- cacao, cocoa, and cocoa butter
- chocolate, dark (at least 80 percent cacao)
- coconut
- coffee
- eggs
- fruit (emphasizing berries, citrus, and other lower-sugar fruits)
- game meat (such as bison, moose, venison, and rabbit)
- healthy oils (avocado oil, coconut oil, nut oils, and extra-virgin olive oil)
- honey (raw and in relatively small amounts)
- nut butter (in relatively small amounts)
- nuts (in relatively small amounts)
- organ meats
- pork (unprocessed and naturally raised)
- seeds (in small amounts)
- turkey (pasture-raised and free of preservatives)
- seafood (wild-caught or sustainably farm-raised)
- tea
- vegetables

The Paleo Diet mimics the eating habits of our ancient ancestors and can help you increase energy levels, prevent disease, and lose weight. In the next chapter, we'll look at the most recent longevity research examining how and why our bodies age the way they do. By understanding that research, you'll discover the science showing how a Paleo Diet can help slow the aging process, increasing your odds of enjoying a longer, healthier life.

CHAPTER TWO

The Science of Paleo Longevity

By the time he was 65 and decided to retire, Jim was in "bad, bad shape," he says. "I could hardly take a step because my knees were in such severe pain."

Jim worked as a home builder and contractor all his life. While some people said his joint pain must have resulted from working such a physically demanding job, he suspected it had more to do with the junk food he'd been consuming all his life. Retirement brought more free time, so he decided to devote himself to getting in shape by working out regularly. He also began reading books on health and wellness. That's how he came across *The Paleo Diet* and decided to change his eating habits.

"I would say about a year into eating Paleo, all the pain in my knees was gone," says Jim, who began going to a local butcher for grass-fed meat. He also started buying organic vegetables, he explains, "because if you're eating vegetables that have been sprayed to control pests, you're also eating the junk that's killing the pests." Although eating this way costs more, he adds, "It's more expensive to have the health problems you get when you don't eat that way."

His new eating habits have paid off. Now 77, Jim is free of joint pain and still working out six days a week. He has lost 85 pounds and has been able to stop all six of the medications his doctor had put him on to control his high blood pressure and poor lipid profile.

"Sick care" is not the same thing as "healthcare," he notes, adding that he wishes Americans could see fewer commercials about Big Pharma products on television and more ads showcasing foods that serve as proper fuel for health and well-being. "How I feed my cells has given me a new life," Jim says. "I have more energy now than I did at age 50."

Like Jim, we believe that eating Paleo will help you dodge, or at least lessen, those aching joints and other chronic conditions of aging that are considered unavoidable by many. First, though, it's important to understand the science of aging.

What Happens to Our Bodies as We Age?

Some effects of aging are easily visible on the outside, like wrinkles and gray hair. Other mechanisms of the aging process are invisible until they negatively impact things like our sleep patterns, energy, and overall health. While we can't avoid growing older, many of the effects we think of as part of the "natural aging process" can be delayed and reduced with better diet and exercise.

There's a common belief that "cavemen" died of old age at 40, but that couldn't be further from the truth. Yes, the average age of death for our hunter-gatherer ancestors was around 40, but that was because of injuries, infectious diseases (they didn't have our modern medical system), and high infant mortality. They were exposed daily to the dangers of nature in ways we're not used to in modern society. Those who escaped these dangers lived about as long as we do today (maybe longer!) and didn't experience what we've come to think of as "natural aging." Even the eldest in their tribes were robust, agile, and active. It was only in the last few months of their lives that age took its toll.

So, why do we age so differently now? There are many factors at play, but perhaps none as crucial as diet. And, while we addressed this in previous books, there was a key piece to the aging puzzle that we missed: a concept called "longevity vitamins."

The Triage Theory: A Key Evolutionary Concept

In 2006, Dr. Bruce N. Ames, a well-known professor of biochemistry at the University of California, Berkeley, introduced the Triage Theory of Aging. We should add that this is a man who knows a lot about healthy aging: He's still teaching and wrote his most recent paper on the subject at age 93.

Like the Paleo Diet, the Triage Theory is grounded in evolutionary biology. It's a concept we didn't discuss in our earlier books, but we now believe this theory helps explain why a Western diet accelerates aging and how adding even a few Paleo choices to your routine may help you age better.

We all know that vitamins and minerals are essential nutrients we need to consume to survive. Scientists identified many of these essential nutrients a century ago, including vitamins C, E, and B and minerals like magnesium and calcium. These nutrients are relatively easy to identify because people and animals quickly become sick if they don't get enough of them in their diets. According to Dr. Ames, these are *survival vitamins* because we need them for short-term survival. However, there is a second category of nutrients he calls *longevity vitamins*. We are less familiar with these nutrients because deficiencies don't show up immediately but can lead to chronic disease and rapid aging over decades.

The Triage Theory suggests that many nutrients serve as both survival and longevity vitamins. Evolution has ensured that when we are deficient in one of these nutrients, our bodies prioritize their survival role over their longevity role. So, we may get enough of a certain nutrient to serve its survival role, but not enough to support its longevity role.

The problem is that the recommended intakes—called the RDA (recommended dietary allowance) or EAR (estimated average requirement) by the US government—are based on the survival role. In other words, even if we're meeting our EARs, we may not be getting enough of these nutrients to ensure healthy longevity.

A sad fact is that many North Americans aren't even meeting the EARs, let alone meeting their longevity needs. Some of the most common deficiencies include vitamin D, vitamin E, magnesium, vitamin K, and folate.

While many survival vitamins also serve a longevity role, many more nutrients serve *only* a longevity role. Because the government hasn't yet identified them as vitamins, there aren't any specific dietary recommendations for them to date. These important longevity nutrients include taurine, ergothioneine, pyrroloquinoline quinone (PQQ), berberine, and a host of carotenoids and flavonoids (which are a large group of natural plant substances recognized for their beneficial impact on human health).

This may be why multivitamins have consistently been shown to be ineffective in supporting long-term health. A recent meta-analysis showed that taking multivitamins was actually associated with a greater risk of all-cause mortality. No, this isn't an error in our text. The researchers really did report that people who consume the most multivitamins don't live as long as those who take fewer! Our explanation for this is that people who take a lot of multivitamins also tend to eat nutrient-poor diets and rely on multivitamins to compensate. Sadly, they're only meeting their survival needs and missing out on what they need for longevity.

In this book, we're going to tell you how several of these recently identified, exciting longevity nutrients help extend both your life and health, and how to ensure you include them in your diet. Keep in mind, though, that many more longevity vitamins will likely be identified over the decades to come. Ultimately, the only way to ensure you're getting all of the survival and longevity vitamins you need is to eat a nutrient-dense diet—which, of course, is a central tenet of the Paleo Diet.

Four Powerful Longevity Nutrients

These antioxidants deserve to be in the spotlight:

- Taurine—Shown to improve strength, coordination, vision, and memory while lowering blood pressure and improving blood lipids.
- Ergothioneine—Associated with scavenging a particularly potent type of free radical, protecting telomere length (protective caps on the ends of chromosomes), and lowering the incidence of cardiovascular disease and chronic inflammatory conditions.
- PQQ (pyrroloquinoline quinone)—Found to enhance cognitive function in older adults and critical for its role in reducing inflammation and maintaining adequate blood flow.
- Berberine—Proven to be promising in improving blood lipids and regulating blood pressure.

Longevity vitamins impact the various processes in our bodies that determine how well we age. The full list of aging factors is beyond the scope of this book, but here are five of the most important that we'll be discussing in the coming chapters:

Oxidative stress: How unstable oxygen molecules wreak havoc on healthy cells

Millions of years before the Paleolithic era, life on Earth was limited to single-cell organisms. These cells could only produce energy anaerobically (without oxygen). While this way of producing energy sustained single-cell life, it wasn't very efficient and couldn't support multicellular organisms. Then an extraordinary event happened. Called the Great

Oxidation Event by scientists, this was a period when there was such a dramatic increase in oxygen that it became a major component of the Earth's atmosphere.

Using this now readily available oxygen, cells could produce energy more efficiently and in a far greater capacity. Oxygen allowed cells to break down fats for fuel, which released 20 to 30 times more energy than anaerobic energy production and ultimately allowed multicell organisms to exist. This had many advantages, but it came at a substantial cost. While anaerobic organisms could die from mutations or changes in their environments, they could otherwise live extremely long lives; in essence, they were immortal. In 2005, for instance, scientists found viable 35,000-year-old protozoa in the Russian tundra.

We could argue that aging was the price of aerobic metabolism, since oxygen is highly damaging to cells. You probably have not heard of "reactive oxygen species" (ROS). You've surely heard of antioxidants, which are so valuable partly because they address the damaging ROS in our bodies, and "free radicals," which are not the same as ROS. There are many types of ROS, but the one thing they have in common is unstable oxygen molecules. This means the oxygen has an unpaired electron, so the oxygen "steals" electrons from the molecules that make up DNA, proteins, and other components of the body, potentially causing damage to healthy cells and accelerating aging through oxidative stress. Our ability to manage this oxidative stress is a key factor in our aging.

Much of the ROS in our bodies is produced by our own mitochondria, the organelles found inside almost every cell of the human body where aerobic metabolism occurs. Mitochondria produce a lot of ROS, but luckily, the mitochondria have multiple membranes that help contain them. As we age, however, mitochondria can stop functioning as effectively, allowing more ROS to spill out into our systems and contributing to conditions like inflammation. While our mitochondria are the major natural source of ROS, toxins like cigarette smoke, medication, and radiation can also contribute to oxidative stress.

This free radical theory of aging was originally proposed by Denham Harman in 1956. There have been many challenges and revisions to the theory since, but the collective evidence indicates that the leakage of ROS by mitochondrial membranes represents a major player, if not *the* major player, in the pathophysiology of aging. Luckily, many foods featured in the Paleo Diet—which we'll highlight throughout the book—are full of particularly potent antioxidants that can reduce the potential harm oxidative stress can do to our bodies.

Telomere length: One of your most important biomarkers of aging

Another important factor in aging is the shortening of our telomeres, the loop-shaped DNA protein structures found at the end of every chromosome in our DNA. This extra material is designed to protect our DNA by preventing our chromosomes from degrading. It's like putting tape at the end of a rope to keep it from fraying. But if telomeres become damaged or shortened, the protective loops can open and activate a DNA damage response that leads to cell death and age-related disease.

Your telomeres shorten naturally with aging. Every time a cell reproduces, the chromosomes split and duplicate. The problem is that it's not a perfect process. Some of the material at the ends of the chromosomes can be lost each time they split. That's fine if it's the telomeres that are lost, just like it's OK if the tape is damaged as long as the rope remains intact. However, if the telomeres continue to shorten as cells replicate again and again through the decades, eventually there will be no telomeres left, and critical genetic material will start to erode. This process prevents our cells from effectively performing their functions, leading to age-related conditions like inflammation, mitochondrial dysfunction, and serious diseases like cancer.

Telomere length has become such an important theory to explain why we age that scientists often measure the telomere length in human blood lymphocytes as a biomarker of aging and mortality. For instance, older people with shorter telomeres are at three times the risk of dying from heart disease and up to eight times the risk of dying from infectious diseases.

There are many ways to maintain healthy telomere lengths, including exercise, consuming certain foods, and reducing salt. We'll discuss specific dietary choices to promote your telomere health later in the book.

Nutrient sensing: The life cycle of your cells impacts your longevity

A steady supply of glucose is essential to our bodies. This may seem surprising if you think about how our hunter-gatherer ancestors didn't always have a lot of carbohydrates available to them, especially if they lived in colder climates where they could forage plant foods only in warmer months and were otherwise limited to mostly animal foods. However, evolution has created various important mechanisms in our bodies to regulate our glucose levels and ensure that we have an adequate glucose supply even when we can't get it from our diets.

You're probably familiar with the protein insulin, which regulates glucose after a meal. It is just one of several proteins in our bodies that respond to glucose levels in our blood. These other glucose-sensing proteins instigate a host of processes in our bodies depending on how much glucose is available to us. This helps our bodies manage times of low and high carbohydrate availability. One of the most important processes controlled by the glucose level in our bodies is the life cycle of our cells. When glucose levels are high, cells proliferate. When glucose levels drop, cells stop proliferating. It's the body's way of saying, "There isn't enough fuel right now, so stop growing." And if glucose levels get very low, cells can enter programmed cell death. That sounds bad, but for optimal health, our cells actually need to go through all three of these stages regularly.

To emphasize this point, let's look at what happens when cells get stuck for too long in any of these phases. It's important for cells to have periods when they stop proliferating because that's when they perform

DNA repair and other critical functions. But, if levels stay low for a long time, cells become "senescent," meaning they can start to deteriorate. Excess *cellular senescence* is a hallmark of poor aging. So, does this mean that we should try to keep our cells in a constant state of proliferation to avoid senescence? Absolutely not. Constant proliferation is a feature of cancer cells, which are also known as "immortal cells" because they never stop reproducing or enter programmed cell death.

For over 100 years, we've been aware of a phenomenon in cancer cells called the Warburg Effect. It's a complex process, but what it boils down to is that cancer cells mostly lose their ability to use fat for fuel and rely almost exclusively on glucose. As a result, cancer cells maintain a constant high-glucose environment around them. In fact, it's often not the cancer cells that directly kill the patient, but cachexia—the wasting of the body as its fuel (glucose) is stolen from the rest of the body by these very hungry cancer cells. By maintaining a constant high-glucose environment, cancer cells stay in a constant state of proliferation. That's clearly detrimental to our health.

Does this mean that we should focus on a ketogenic diet and keep our glucose levels very low at all times? Ketosis has been shown to help protect against cancer and neurodegeneration in the short run, but its promotion of senescence and cell death can speed aging in the long run. That's why we don't recommend eating keto long-term.

Many nutritionists talk about the benefits of metabolic flexibility, which is just a fancy term for letting your body fluctuate between high and low glucose states to encourage the full cell cycle. Like our ancestors, we should have periods when we eat a higher carbohydrate diet and periods when we eat fewer carbohydrates. We recommend intermittent periods of higher carbohydrate intake and short periods where you're eating ketogenic, or almost ketogenic. This way, you'll promote all stages of the cell cycle, which in turn supports cellular and mitochondrial health, and ultimately better aging. Being metabolically flexible promotes a healthy cell cycle, and science backs that up.

Chronic inflammation: A nearly invisible but powerful contributor to disease

Dee Ann was visiting her parents for the Christmas holidays in 2004 when her life changed literally overnight. At 42, she was active and fit from running, weightlifting, and biking. She'd gone out for her regular run on December 26, but woke up on December 27 "feeling like I had rocks in my feet."

She saw her doctor when she returned home, who suggested that she "exercise more." Dee Ann knew she was already exercising far more than most women her age, so she sought a second opinion. The next doctor said, "I think you have rheumatoid arthritis," a chronic inflammatory disease that causes joint pain, stiffness, and decreased movement over time.

When blood tests confirmed the diagnosis, the first rheumatologist Dee Ann saw was blunt about her prognosis. "He said my condition was so severe that I'd probably be in a wheelchair in five years and could be dead in ten."

Dee Ann immediately began researching her condition to see what treatments were available. In exploring foods that might alleviate the pain and swelling in her joints, she discovered the Paleo Diet.

"I went cold turkey Paleo twenty years ago," she says. "The results have been astonishing. I don't have any of the fatigue or brain fog you can get with autoimmune diseases, and I have much less inflammation than most people with this condition."

So much less inflammation, in fact, that today, at 61, Dee Ann continues to enjoy an active life, from refinishing doors for her farmhouse to volunteering with the Red Cross and working with a raptor rehabilitation group to rescue and rehabilitate injured owls, hawks, and other birds of prey.

"Paleo is all about eating what nourishes my mind and body," she says. "It's the best thing I could have done for myself."

While scientists haven't yet described one clear pathway linking chronic inflammation to aging the way they have with telomere length and the cell cycle, as Dee Ann discovered firsthand, chronic inflammation may be the sneakiest contributor to aging because of the many mechanisms through which it negatively affects our bodies. Reducing inflammation is perhaps one of the most beneficial impacts that diet can have on helping us age well.

Let's start by defining the difference between inflammation and chronic inflammation. We all know what inflammation looks like on the outside: If you stub your toe or bang your knee, the area will swell and turn red. That's a sign that your body is sending immune cells to clean up the damage. *Inflammation* is the word we use to describe the process where our immune systems ramp up to fight a virus or bacterial infection, or to repair damage. When our bodies are healthy, it is a temporary condition that addresses the issue and then fades away.

On the other hand, chronic inflammation—which is often caused by poor diet and lack of exercise—is invisible, but it's linked to almost every chronic disease of aging, including autoimmune conditions like rheumatoid arthritis, cancer, cardiovascular disease, diabetes, and neurodegeneration. Chronic inflammation has also been closely linked to oxidative stress, telomere shortening, and the other factors we've discussed here that are involved in the aging process.

Chronic inflammation is the result of your immune system acting as if the body is under attack when it isn't. In response to a variety of issues, the immune system releases small proteins called *cytokines*. Some cytokines attract immune cells and activate key inflammatory processes, while others calm the immune system down. Cytokines are essential messengers that direct our immune systems, but chronically elevated inflammatory cytokines can lead to damage to healthy cells. When cytokines are released in response to a viral or bacterial invader, they attract immune cells, which kill the invaders. Collateral damage to nearby cells is an unfortunate but accepted sacrifice. It's critical that the immune system is activated to deal with a threat and then stand down after the threat has passed. In a healthy body, inflammatory cytokines then give way to the anti-inflammatory cytokines and the immune system calms down.

Bad things happen when the immune system remains activated. In fact, it's been shown that chronic elevation of a particularly damaging immune cell called T_H17 precedes almost every autoimmune disease. Some of the foods in our modern diet are remarkably effective at promoting highly inflammatory cytokines and keeping them elevated. Wheat, and particularly gluten, has multiple mechanisms to activate T_H17 cells. Of the over 100 known autoimmune diseases in humans, the trigger has been identified for only two. In both cases it was gluten.

Inflammation can also be caused by senescent cells—those cells that stop multiplying but never die or get washed out of your body. As we age, our immune systems begin deteriorating, and other bodily systems may become weakened, which means these junk cells can accumulate and damage otherwise healthy cells, causing chronic inflammation.

In that large-scale meta-analysis on diet and chronic disease that we mentioned in the introduction, the Paleo Diet was by far the most effective diet at reducing biomarkers of inflammation with a SUCRA score of 87 percent, reinforcing existing science that shows the Paleo Diet is a strongly anti-inflammatory diet. (SUCRA—"surface under the cumulative ranking curve"—is a well-known research tool used in meta-analysis studies. The SUCRA number is a score from 0 to 100 percent that compares all the treatments included in a study or analysis. Higher SUCRA scores indicate that a treatment is more likely to be effective than lower-scored treatments.)

The DASH diet, which is designed to lower blood pressure through foods lower in sodium and higher in potassium, magnesium, and calcium, came in second to the Paleo Diet, at 71.3 percent. The Mediterranean diet, which includes foods associated with inflammation like processed grains and legumes, earned a SUCRA score of 58.1 percent, showing that it is significantly less effective than the Paleo Diet at addressing inflammation.

Besides highlighting the power of the Paleo Diet, this meta-analysis had one other important revelation: The US government's nutritional guidelines aren't very good for you. The government-recommended dietary guidelines scored just 48.5 percent on the SUCRA scale. In other words, if you eat according to the "official" recommendations of the US government, you'll be more at risk for chronic disease as you age. Likewise, as stated earlier, the plant-based diet was ranked almost as low, coming in at just 49.3 percent.

Epigenetic Changes

A biology text might illustrate our DNA as nice Xs and Ys, but in actuality, our DNA looks more like a giant ball of string with only a small part of each chromosome exposed at the surface. Which parts of the chromosomes are exposed can greatly impact how our cells function. Scientists believe that how the balls of DNA are wound up changes as we age to emphasize some genes in our youth and others as we grow older. For example, the genes that allow us to digest milk are exposed when we are infants but are buried deep in the ball later in life and effectively turned off. What this means is that epigenetic changes—or changing how the chromosomes are bunched up—may be a key factor in how we age.

The most important takeaway from this chapter is this: Your chronological age really is just a number. Your body will react to the foods you eat, so if you eat the clean, healthy, whole foods of the Paleo Diet and continue engaging in activities that exercise your mind and body, you'll increase your chances of living a healthier, happier, more energetic life. As we'll discuss in part II, plant foods play an essential role in helping you age not only gracefully, but energetically, because plants contain some of our most important longevity nutrients.

Plant Foods for Power
and Healthy Aging

PART II

Plant Foods for Power
and Healthy Aging

Trevor's Paleo Story

I don't blame anyone for being skeptical about the benefits of the Paleo Diet. I was once a skeptic, too.

I was first introduced to the Paleo Diet in 2009 when I became a graduate student at Colorado State University. As a teaching assistant (TA), I was marched into the TA office on my first day, where a group of TAs were sitting around talking about how the "Paleo guy" was actually a teacher at CSU. I had no idea who they were talking about.

"You haven't heard of the cereal killer?" they asked.

I hadn't, but I quickly discovered that a graduate course on the Paleo Diet, taught by the cereal killer himself, Dr. Loren Cordain, was a requirement for me that spring. I looked forward to it. I loved studying sports nutrition and thought his ancestral perspective would be interesting. Of course, as an athlete—I'm a competitive cyclist—I also assumed the course would confirm what I already knew about how to best fuel the body for endurance sports.

Just three weeks into the class, however, I was convinced that everything Dr. Cordain said was wrong. "This guy's full of it," I frequently thought to myself.

What Dr. Cordain taught flew in the face of everything I had learned in sports nutrition, where I had lost count of the studies I'd read showing

the importance of consuming as many simple carbohydrates as possible
to support a top competitive performance. That's what all endurance athletes did. Eating a couple pounds of pasta the night before a race was just
good practice. So how could it be bad for you?

I was so angry about the class that when the semester ended, I decided
to dedicate part of my summer to proving Dr. Cordain wrong. I started
with cereal. He had to be wrong about that—cereal was consistently
touted as one of the healthiest things we could eat. I personally ate two
bowls of cereal every morning and I had been a high-performing athlete
for years. But, as I went through the research, I reluctantly admitted he
had a point. As it turned out, most cereal was low in nutrient density,
spiked our insulin, and was very high in calories—I was eating over 1,000
kcal at breakfast. Fine, cereal's out, but he has to be wrong about . . .

One by one, I dug into the science about the things he had to be
wrong about but begrudgingly kept proving him right. As I did, I started
changing my own diet without even being fully aware of it. By December of that year, I was pretty much Paleo.

Then something very interesting happened. Just before starting my
graduate studies at CSU, I had retired as a full-time athlete. I had been
training out of the Canadian National Cycling Centre in British Colum-
bia and loved being a competitive athlete, but in my final year, I'd started
to struggle because I frequently came down with unidentified, low-grade
viruses that would last weeks. I could mostly function throughout the
day, but being sick impacted my training. I finally chalked it up to being
in my late thirties and came to terms with the fact that my professional
cycling career was behind me.

That winter, after going Paleo, I didn't get sick once. Not only that,
but I was also able to train as hard as I ever had, all while being a full-
time student and running a coaching business. Even when I was at my
best back at the Centre, constant fatigue had prevented me from doing
much beyond my training. Now, the fatigue was still there, but it just
wasn't the same. I could do a six-hour ride and then work at the library
until midnight and not pay for it the next day.

The training went so well, that summer I jumped back into a few professional races and flew up to compete in the Canadian Nationals, which happened to be on my 39th birthday. I raced in the professional race, where I broke away for half the race, dropping a guy who rode for Garmin-Slipstream, a Tour de France squad. By the time I reached the final kilometer, I was still solo in third place. Painfully, a small group caught me literally on the line, ultimately landing me in 12th place, but all I could think was, "missed a podium by a hair—not bad for a 39-year-old."

Convinced that my performance was linked to my Paleo Diet, I asked Dr. Cordain to take me on as his graduate student. The next year, I joined a semi-professional team in Colorado called Team Rio Grande and raced a full professional calendar in the US while being a full-time student. The year I turned 40, I had one of my strongest years as a cyclist: I finished fifth at one of the biggest races in the country, was briefly ranked in the top 20 in the US, earned the title as the top-ranked 35+ rider in the country, and dropped a guy who had finished third in the Tour de France after he and I had dropped the entire professional peloton.

At the races, my teammates would have the usual "cyclist's pasta party" for dinner while I'd have a piece of salmon and vegetables. On the way to races, they'd suck down energy gels and I'd snack on some low-sodium beef jerky. They'd tell me I was eating wrong but couldn't explain how this old guy was beating them. For years, I had eaten just like them—the way traditional sports nutrition had told me was best. But I had switched to the Paleo Diet and was better for it.

At 47, when I took over the Paleo Diet business from Dr. Cordain, I was still eating Paleo and regularly competing in professional races. More importantly, I was still getting results.

One of the most common questions I'm asked by other endurance athletes is how I can train and race without eating carbohydrates, since it's a common misconception among athletes that the only source of carbohydrates is pasta, bread, and gels. I always respond that I get lots of carbohydrates—I eat tons of fruits and vegetables.

CHAPTER THREE

The Longevity Power of Plant Foods

About three years ago, Tom's health reached "a point where I knew something had to change," he says. "There were days when I was in so much pain that getting out of bed was something I didn't want to do."

Tom's pain was due to several factors. When he was only 28 years old, he was struck by a truck in a work-related highway accident. That accident led to spinal surgeries and two decades of pain medications. He started experiencing an inflamed gut, and then suffered a case of chronic Lyme disease and encephalitis. Still, he was determined to kick the pain medication he'd been on since his first spinal surgery. One year later, he just stopped taking the pills of his own accord.

"My gut and brain were both on fire," he says. "Whenever my brain was inflamed, it was like a cluster of migraines that lasted for three days. I'd have pain, dizziness, vertigo, and ringing ears."

When one of Tom's adult daughters moved in with him and started the Paleo Diet for her own health issues, she encouraged him to try it. He'd always eaten foods that most of the world would have considered "healthy," like steak burritos with flour taco shells, rice, beans, chicken noodle soup with peas, yogurt, and Mediterranean pizza. Then he went Paleo and realized that everything he'd been taught was healthy was a lie. That was his big "aha" moment. After Tom switched to healthy foods like grass-fed beef, wild-caught salmon, and organic vegetables, he began gradually feeling better. Now 50 years old, he says that eating Paleo "has made a huge difference in my life."

These days, whenever Tom's digestive system acts up, "I'll try to eat some fish that day, and I'll make up a simple smoothie of avocado, kale, spinach, and other microgreens we grow in the house. The Paleo Diet has improved my gut microbiome, which has led to reduced inflammation throughout my body and improved mobility. Lowering my brain/brain stem/spinal cord inflammation has comprehensively lessened my neuropathy."

Tom realizes now that taking opioids, muscle relaxers, and anti-inflammatory medications ultimately exacerbated his conditions. "For example, anti-inflammatory medications and opioids damage your organs, and muscle relaxers lead to rigidity of muscles from long-term use," he explains. "That's why the Paleo Diet is so important: It helps you kick these damaging medications and allows your body to naturally heal itself, leading to sustainable, long-term health."

When it comes to longevity, there is abundant scientific evidence demonstrating that consuming particular vegetables and fruits has a hugely protective effect in helping us fight disease and prevent chronic illnesses as we age. In this section, we'll zero in on the best mix of vegetables for combating oxidative stress, reducing inflammation, lowering blood pressure, promoting better lipids, and decreasing the risk of diseases—from diabetes to heart disease, from Alzheimer's to cancer—that can cut life short or make the years we have left a challenge to enjoy.

The Surprising Longevity Power of Plant Foods

As we noted, when debunking the myths surrounding the Paleo Diet, it isn't only meat-based. In fact, by volume, the diet can be primarily plant-based. We pack our menus with healthy, unprocessed plant foods not only because they're low in calories, but because these foods are dense with health-boosting nutrients. We've seen a host of studies, reviews, and meta-analyses demonstrating that when you eat plant foods, you're consuming vitamins, minerals, and other healthy bioactive compounds. Three of the most important are plant polyphenols, dietary nitrate, and folate. Plant food is also critical for elevating Nrf2 (see page 38).

Put simply, polyphenols are bioactive plant compounds that may be your top-secret ingredient to healthier aging. Scientists have so far identified about 8,000 of these compounds. Named for the multiple (poly) phenolic rings that make up their chemical structures, plants produce polyphenols as a defense against ultraviolet radiation and pathogens. When you eat plant foods, you're incorporating these helpful compounds into your body's tissues; in your body, polyphenols act as antioxidants, battling oxidative stress on your cells to help protect brain health, fight inflammation, and lower your risk of cardiovascular disease, cancer, and other diseases of aging. These compounds include a diverse group of nutrients, with about 60 percent classified as flavonoids, like quercetin, kaempferol, catechins, and anthocyanins.

Adding vegetables to your Paleo lifestyle will also help ensure that you consume important vitamins like folate, or B9, which your body needs to make genetic material like DNA. Studies have demonstrated that plant foods are also rich in dietary nitrate, which can act as a substrate for your body's production of nitric oxide. Nitric oxide is important because this short-lived gas molecule can quickly scavenge reactive oxygen species, acting as a powerful antioxidant to keep your cells healthy. Nitric oxide can also signal other antioxidants to spring into action.

Just keep in mind that there are many "plant-based foods" on the shelves that are actually ultra-processed. These foods have been stripped of most of their nutrient density and benefits. For the sake of your longevity and health, try to stick to unprocessed, organic plant foods.

Nrf2: The Gatekeeper of Longevity

One of the most important reasons why the Paleo Diet is not solely meat-based is because of a very important protein in our bodies that you've likely never encountered: nuclear factor erythroid-2-related factor 2, or Nrf2 for short. In a relatively recent study, researchers referred to Nrf2 in the title as "a guardian of health span and gatekeeper of species longevity." We couldn't agree more, since Nrf2 regulates more than 500 genes. We explained some of the mechanisms that control aging on page 19, and these 500 genes are related to almost every one of them. This has led many scientists to claim that Nrf2 is a key, if not *the* key, regulator of longevity.

The best-known function of Nrf2 is as a master regulator of our bodies' natural antioxidant defense mechanisms, but it also has many anti-inflammatory functions. This protein appears to be an essential player in maintaining healthy mitochondria. Nrf2 also helps detoxify our bodies from toxins such as heavy metals.

Considering its anti-inflammatory and antioxidant roles, it shouldn't be surprising that Nrf2 is also protective against a host of chronic diseases, including cardiovascular disease, neurodegeneration, cancer, kidney disease, diabetes, autoimmune illness, depression, macular degeneration, cataracts, and even altitude sickness. In short, Nrf2 is a longevity powerhouse.

The reason we're spotlighting Nrf2 is that scientists have identified 10 factors that raise the level of Nrf2 in our bodies. One of them is exercise, but eight are dietary. Of the eight dietary factors, two are related to seafood: omega-3s from fish oil and taurine, both of which we cover in chapter 13. The rest of those dietary factors come from plants high in at least one longevity nutrient.

For instance, Nrf2 is elevated by phenolic compounds found in many vegetables and in olive oil. It's also elevated by isothiocyanates from cruciferous vegetables, triterpenoids found in spinach, sulfur compounds in garlic and onions, and the carotenoids that give carrots, peppers, and green leafy vegetables their rich colors.

Sirtuins: A Second Gatekeeper

When we addressed nutrient sensing earlier in this chapter as a key part of healthy aging, we stated that excess cellular senescence is a hallmark of poor aging. Consequently, preventing, slowing, or even reversing cellular senescence has become a key target for increasing longevity.

Sirtuins, often called "longevity proteins," are a family of seven nicotine adenine dinucleotide (NAD+)-dependent signaling proteins. They are involved in metabolic regulation and are essential factors in delaying cellular senescence primarily through DNA damage repair, maintaining genome integrity, and delaying telomere attrition. They also interact with several lifespan-regulating signaling pathways, including changes to your DNA, otherwise known as epigenetic modifications. This has led researchers to examine how sirtuins are activated as a way of improving longevity. Both caloric restriction and exercise are two avenues for increasing sirtuin activation, via an increase in the ratio of NAD+ to NADH, which are key proteins themselves in our metabolic processes. Because of the importance of NAD+ to our metabolic health, several other methods of increasing NAD+ in our cells have also become extremely popular, such as several forms of vitamin B3 that demonstrate significant increases.

Following the initial excitement around sirtuins and their ability to prolong longevity, there has been some controversy. For instance, one review published in 2022 strongly criticized the "over-hype" of sirtuins by researchers and the media as a longevity gene. While it is likely that the trend to do anything to raise sirtuin levels for longevity has been overblown—including some extreme supplementation—there is evidence that sirtuins, at the very least, promote our metabolic health. Eating healthy foods that promote sirtuin expression is likely going to help you stay healthy long-term.

This brings us back to plant foods, which have been shown to directly activate sirtuins. Two particularly effective nutrients for doing so are resveratrol and curcumin.

The foods highest in resveratrol all happen to be Paleo foods, with fruits constituting the primary source for most people. While red grapes (and the resultant red wine) have a reputation as a great source of resveratrol, they have significantly less (79 µg/100 g) than the highest-containing foods. Beating grapes are walnuts (1,585 µg/100 g), tangerines (1,061 µg/100 g), sweet potatoes (952 µg/100 g), peaches (461 µg/100 g), oranges (155 µg/100 g), and grapefruits (82 µg/100 g). While resveratrol can be consumed as a supplement, we would urge you to obtain it from foods, because in that way you will also acquire important complementary nutrients. In addition, resveratrol can be unstable once extracted because it is sensitive to light, pH, and high temperatures. Of further significance, all non-Paleo plant foods have low or very low resveratrol concentrations.

CHAPTER FOUR

Top-Tier Longevity Vegetables

When she was in her 30s, Megan started having digestive issues serious enough to ask her doctor to test her for celiac disease, a chronic immune disorder caused by an allergy to wheat. When the test came up negative, her doctor encouraged her to "keep eating wheat and any other grains I wanted," she reports.

Around 2001, however, things started to really go south when Megan was diagnosed with Graves' disease, an autoimmune condition that involves an overactive thyroid; with fibromyalgia, which causes chronic inflammation and pain; and with Sjogren's syndrome, an immune disorder that manifests as a persistently dry mouth and dry eyes. "Sometimes the pain was so bad that I had to leave work and go out to my car to lie down," she says.

That's when Megan, who works in the nonprofit sector, decided to step away from Western medicine and see a naturopath. When tests showed that Megan had a strong reaction not only to gluten, but to all grains, the naturopath encouraged her to try an elimination diet that was "really restrictive" to detox her system. Megan gave up grains, dairy, and sugar completely. Shortly after that, she discovered the Paleo Diet and started using only Paleo cookbooks.

The result? Her pain and inflammation subsided almost immediately, and within a few weeks, her blood tests were back to normal. Perhaps most exciting was the fact that her ANA (antinuclear antibody) test, which checks to see if you have an autoimmune disorder, was now negative.

"I feel so much better," she says. "It breaks my heart that none of the doctors I saw before that ever suggested excluding inflammatory foods to treat my autoimmune diseases."

Now, after over 20 years of eating mostly Paleo, Megan feels good enough to cheat now and then on her diet, though never with gluten. "If I do eat gluten, the next day my hands are swollen when I wake up and I feel like I'm coming down with the flu. Everything aches and I have a foggy brain. The thing is, we have a lot of really awful food in this country," she adds. "I choose not eat processed grains or other unhealthy foods because I want to live the best version of myself and feel as good as possible."

These days, Megan sticks mostly to a Paleo lifestyle. Along with fresh vegetables and fruits, she relies on naturally raised animal proteins. She's "about 90 percent dairy-free," but makes up for that by treating herself to coconut cream in her coffee and using it as the base for a delicious clam chowder. "Coconut is a great alternative to dairy," she says, "especially because it gives you other health benefits as well."

What About Calcium?

Humanity's original carbohydrate sources weren't high-glycemic, starchy grains and potatoes, but wild fruits and vegetables with low glycemic indices. Our hunter-gatherer ancestors did eat higher glycemic load carbohydrates from honey, but it was a treat, not a staple. The nonstarchy carbohydrates that served as their dietary mainstay can help normalize your blood glucose and insulin levels so you can maintain a healthy weight, keep your blood sugar levels low, and feel more energetic.

You already know from chapter 2 that vegetables are rich in vitamins and *phytochemicals*—the biologically active chemicals produced by plants, including carotenoids and polyphenols, that can serve as powerful allies when it comes to helping us reduce oxidative stress and fight inflammation, which adds up to preventing or lessening the typical diseases of aging. Perhaps more surprisingly, consuming vegetables can slow or prevent the loss of bone density that can lead to osteoporosis.

How can this be true, when most of us grow up being told that we need to drink milk and take vitamin D to have healthy bones by maintaining healthy calcium levels? First, vegetables can be one of our richest dietary sources of calcium. Second, while we tend to focus on how much calcium we consume, what's more important is how much calcium our bodies retain in our bones. The main factor that affects calcium loss is your body's acid-base balance.

If you eat an acidic diet, you'll leach calcium from your bones to de-acidify your blood. But if you eat a more alkalizing diet, you'll protect your bones and reduce your dietary calcium requirements. Salty processed foods, cereals, most dairy products, legumes, meat, fish, and eggs produce net acid loads in the body. Even worse are hard cheeses, which are high in calcium but in fact can promote bone loss and osteoporosis if you don't eat enough alkalizing foods to offset their acidifying effect.

And guess what? Nearly all vegetables and fruits are powerful alkalizers because they are low in sodium and high in potassium, which has been shown to be far more effective than calcium supplements in preventing osteoporosis. By adopting the Paleo Diet, you'll be getting more of your daily calories as healthful alkalizing foods that will neutralize the mildly acidic loads you get from meat and seafood, and you'll lower your risk of osteoporosis.

Allium Vegetables: Not Always Pretty, but Potent

Admittedly, some veggies are prettier on the plate than others. Who doesn't want to load up on those bright orange carrots and deep green broccoli florets instead of reaching for a white onion? But don't overlook the paler vegetables in the *Allium* genus, which has more than 1,000 accepted species, including onions, garlic, leeks, and chives. These nutritional powerhouses provide so many health benefits that they've been used in traditional medicines around the world for centuries. For instance, the use of garlic is documented in Sanskrit texts dating back 5,000 years; it has been featured in so many curative treatments worldwide that it would be impossible to list them all in this space. Here's just a sample of the conditions treated by garlic: heart disease, asthma, pain, respiratory diseases, hair loss, diabetes, cough, and even paralysis.

Onions, too, have been incorporated into traditional medicine for centuries to treat common diseases like asthma. In ancient Greece, Hippocrates prescribed onions for pneumonia and healing wounds, while medieval care providers relied on onions to treat everything from headaches, fever, and flatulence to rheumatism and high blood pressure. Leeks, too, have their place in human history: *The Compendium of Materia Medica* by Shizhen Li, written in 16th-century China, describes how cooked leek roots can help treat abdominal pain, stop bleeding pus, and be used as a medicine to treat rabies, snake bite, scorpion stings, and more.

As so often happens, we can learn a lot from our ancestors. Today's researchers are exploring the potential of alliums to keep us living longer, healthier lives, and they've made some important discoveries. Garlic, onion, leeks, and other vegetables in this plant genus contain important phytochemicals and other nutritional constituents, like potassium, phosphorus zinc, sulfur, calcium, magnesium, manganese, iron, and vitamins A, C, and B-complex, that all support our health.

Among the most potent bioactive compounds in *Allium* vegetables are organic sulfides like allyl cysteines, thiosulfates, and polyphenols like flavonoids and phenolic acids. Many of these nutrients help raise Nrf2, which, as we explained earlier (see page 38), is a potent regulator of our longevity. In garlic, probably the most beneficial are the sulfur-containing compounds like allicin, which gives garlic its distinctive smell. Onions and leeks are especially rich sources of health-boosting flavonoid compounds like quercetin, one of the most powerful antioxidants in plants, as well as other organosulfur and phenolic compounds that support health and promote longevity.

A variety of laboratory and clinical studies have shown that consuming *Allium* vegetables may have anticarcinogenic, antidiabetic, anti-inflammatory, and antioxidant effects, while also powering up the immune system and protecting cardiovascular health. When it comes to living a longer, healthier life, adding alliums to your diet has many benefits. They can help with the following longevity contributors.

Alliums protect against oxidative stress

As you know from chapter 2, oxidative stress is one of the primary causes of aging. Adding garlic, onion, and other *Allium* vegetables to your menu is a terrific way to incorporate more antioxidants into your daily diet since they're loaded with phenolic and organosulfur compounds. For instance, aged garlic extract has been shown to decrease reactive oxygen species produced through chronic inflammation or increased metabolism. Many studies have also demonstrated onions' powerful potential as an antioxidant, including its ability to upregulate Nrf2, the protein that controls the body's natural antioxidant defense mechanisms (see page 38).

Alliums reduce inflammation

We've discussed how many diseases of aging are associated with chronic inflammation, so it's good news that researchers are highlighting garlic's potential to exert anti-inflammatory effects. Cytokines—substances excreted by immune cells—can be divided into anti-inflammatory and pro-inflammatory; eating *Allium* vegetables increases anti-inflammatory cytokines while helping to suppress anti-inflammatory cytokines. Leeks have also demonstrated anti-inflammatory activities in many studies.

Alliums lower blood pressure

In a study where people with moderately elevated cholesterol were given garlic extract or dried garlic powder every day for four weeks, they saw a decrease in both systolic and diastolic blood pressure by 5.5 percent. Studies have also shown that supplementing your diet with onion may significantly reduce systolic blood pressure.

Alliums maintain heart health

Risk factors for cardiovascular disease include high blood pressure and elevated LDL cholesterol levels; consuming garlic powder is linked to lowering those factors and protecting heart health. In one double-blind study, obese patients given 400 mg of garlic extract daily for three months showed an enhanced antioxidant status, reducing their risk of inflammation and cardiovascular risk. Various studies have also shown that garlic can significantly reduce the risk of atherosclerosis, hypertension, ischemic stroke, and myocardial infarction. In addition, research using laboratory animals has shown that animals fed high-cholesterol or high-fat diets experience decreased levels of total cholesterol, triglyceride, and LDL cholesterol when fed onion extracts, while leek roots have proven effective in promoting blood circulation.

Alliums protect against cancer

Garlic can help prevent cancer. It has been shown to reduce cancerous lesions and cancer mortality in multiple studies, and today's researchers are examining the association between consuming alliums and a lower risk of breast, colorectal, and liver cancer. Recent studies have also highlighted the potential of the sulfur-containing compounds in garlic to inhibit the growth of cancer cells in the gastrointestinal tract, lungs, urinary tract, and more. In addition, in vitro studies have linked garlic's sulfur-containing compounds with protection against cancer-causing substances. Studies show that onion-derived quercetin and diosgenin also help fight cancer, with onion extract and its bioactive compounds demonstrating the potential to kill off cancer cells and keep them from proliferating in colon, laryngeal, liver, pancreatic, and other types of cancer. Fresh onion consumption has been associated with improving insulin sensitivity and fasting blood glucose in breast cancer patients treated with doxorubicin. Human breast cancer cells treated with leek extract for 24 hours in another study demonstrated slower cell proliferation and an uptick in cell death, which is a good thing when you're dealing with cancer cells.

Alliums fight metabolic syndrome

Metabolic syndrome (see page xii) is associated with cardiovascular disease and other diseases of aging. Fortunately, *Allium* vegetables can help protect us against metabolic syndrome. For instance, people consuming 100 mg of raw crushed garlic twice a day for a month significantly reduced a number of the key risk factors that help define metabolic syndrome, including high blood pressure, triglycerides, and glucose levels. Many studies have also demonstrated that onions and their bioactive compounds, like the flavonoids quercetin and kaempferol, act as powerful antioxidants that can help lower metabolic risk factors like high blood glucose, hypertension, and hyperlipidemia.

Alliums boost bone health

As we age, many of us experience extensive degeneration of our joints and chronic pain. In a study where overweight or obese women with knee osteoarthritis were given 1,000 mg daily of a garlic supplement, they experienced symptom relief. Another similar study showed over-weight women with knee osteoarthritis also experienced less pain after taking 500 mg garlic tablets twice a day.

Alliums manage diabetes

Researchers found that diabetic patients were better able to regulate their serum cholesterol and triglyceride levels by taking a combination of olive oil and garlic. In addition, people with type 2 diabetes were able to reduce their blood glucose and improve their lipid panels by consuming garlic cloves for 30 days. Studies have also shown that garlic prevented pancreatic cell damage caused by diabetes and reduced diabetes-linked retinopathy. In addition, various researchers conducting both in vitro and animal studies have highlighted how onions can treat diabetic complications as well as help manage the disease. For instance, in one such study, scientists demonstrated that blood glucose levels declined in diabetic rats fed a diet supplemented with onion powder or onion peel extract.

Alliums protect your brain

Garlic may also prove to be a useful ally in protecting our brains as we age. Research with rats has shown that a garlic ethanol extract had an important neuroprotective effect, reducing the loss of important neurons and increasing levels of chemicals that play an important role in enhancing memory. Likewise, onions seem to boost brain health; several studies have demonstrated the neuroprotective effects of onion consumption against brain issues like cerebral injury, memory issues, and Parkinson's disease.

You may find it surprising how many positive ways onions and other alliums can impact our health. But it's important to remember that like many of the plant foods in this section, they also contain longevity nutrients that have a positive impact on key regulators of health and longevity, like Nrf2 and sirtuins. Getting more of these longevity nutrients through natural sources can have vast positive impacts on your body.

Cruciferous Vegetables: Good Stuff in the Crunch

When it comes to promoting longevity, there are few foods better than cruciferous vegetables, such as arugula, broccoli, collard greens, and cabbage (see full list on the next page). Cruciferous vegetables are part of the *Brassicaceae* family, whose alternate name, *cruciferae*, means "cross-bearing" and comes from the cross-shaped flowers of these plants. Like beets, they're rich in beneficial bioactive compounds like ascorbic acid, essential minerals, and polyphenols.

What puts cruciferous vegetables at the top of the Paleo Diet longevity list is that they're an especially rich source of sulfur-containing compounds called *sulforaphanes* (*glucosinolates*). When cruciferous vegetables are chewed, chopped, boiled, or otherwise disrupted, a plant enzyme called *myrosinase* converts the molecule *glucoraphanin* into sulforaphane. Our own bodies do this anytime we eat vegetables because we have bacteria in our guts that produce myrosinase, making it easy for us to absorb. This is exciting news, because a slew of recent studies has shown that sulforaphane can prevent cancer cells from growing and even kill them. The bottom line is that taking care of the microflora in your gut is one of the best things you can do to support your overall long-term health. Eating cruciferous vegetables is one way to do that.

Plant-derived substances have been used to fight various diseases throughout human history, but the effects of their phytochemicals are often limited due to their bioavailability. Sulforaphane, on the other hand, has an 80 percent bioavailability. It is 14 times more powerful when it comes to inducing detoxifying enzymes than other phytochemicals and exhibits much greater bioavailability than other popular antioxidant phytochemicals like curcumin and quercetin. Sulforaphane is also a very potent promoter of Nrf2, which, as you know (see page 38), plays a critical role in the ability of our bodies to fight most inflammatory diseases—including cancer, heart disease, diabetes, and autoimmune conditions.

Various epidemiological studies have demonstrated that eating broccoli, Brussels sprouts, cabbage, and other cruciferous vegetables not only lessens the incidence of many types of cancer, but helps protects against gastric ulcers, has a renal protective effect in kidney disease, and helps regulate glucose in people with type 2 diabetes. Animal studies have also highlighted how this humble compound has the potential to lower uric acid in the human body by improving the microbial ecosystem and function of the gut—good news for the 20 percent of Americans suffering from gout (hyperuricemia). Studies even suggest that sulforaphane may prolong overall lifespan through its impact on Nrf2 and sirtuins.

Cruciferous Vegetables

Arugula (also known as rocket)	Horseradish
	Kale
Bok choy (also known as pak choi)	Kohlrabi
	Mustard greens
Broccoli	Radishes
Broccoli rabe (also known as rapini)	Rutabagas
	Shepherd's purse
Brussels sprouts	Swiss chard
Cabbage (all types)	Tatsoi
Cauliflower	Turnips
Collard greens	Watercress
Daikon	

Are Canned or Frozen Vegetables as Good as Fresh?

Your best option is always to buy local produce at a farmers' market, but if you can't get what you want that way, frozen fruits and vegetables might be a better choice than what you find in the produce section of your grocery store. That's because plant foods in the produce section often must go through an extended transport to get to your supermarket, so they're more likely to be picked before they're ripe and then chemically ripened when they arrive at the destination. High-quality frozen fruits and vegetables are typically grown until they're ready to eat, then flash-frozen, which can avoid chemical ripening agents and increase their nutrient density.

However, beware of canned plant foods. Canned fruit is often packed with sugar, and canned vegetables might also be preserved with ingredients that contain antinutrients that can reduce the health benefits of the vegetables. Be sure to read labels carefully.

Beets: One of Our Top Functional Foods

Beets, with their rich, deep red and yellow colors, are among the most aesthetically pleasing vegetables you can add to your Paleo Diet plate. Beets are also one of our top functional foods because of their marvelous longevity benefits.

Growing up, you might have only eaten beets as those red circles that came in a can, but the truth is that beets can be white, yellow, or red. Both beet leaves and roots are not only edible but also deliciously healthy. In addition to providing minerals and vitamins, red beets are a rich source of antioxidants. Probably the most important of these are the *betalains*, which give red beets their color and are made up of water-soluble pigments that contain nitrogen. The betalain in red beets, known as *betanin*, is the most beneficial because they are the most easily absorbed.

The most important longevity action of betanin is its ability to scavenge reactive oxygen species, which reduces oxidative stress and helps reverse tissue damage. Other studies have shown that betanin can help reduce the risk of some cancers by keeping tumor cells from proliferating, as well as by regulating liver and glucose metabolism pathways. For instance, in one animal study, the results showed that giving betanin extract helped stop skin and lung tumors in mice; in lung tumors, the reduction rate was a whopping 60 percent.

Consuming beets also means you'll be adding to your body's store of nitrate, which researchers have reported can enhance performance in athletes as well as conferring a number of other health benefits. Ongoing studies have shown that when nitrate comes from food sources, it triggers the body to produce nitric oxide, a powerful antioxidant.

Here are some of the overall potential health benefits of beets in your diet.

Beets lower blood pressure

Like most plants, beets are rich in organic acids, which can help protect your cells against pathogens, toxins, and nutrient deficiencies. This may sound confusing since we warned you about the dangers of an acidic diet (see page 43). Well, here's where it gets even more confusing: Consuming acidic foods doesn't necessarily mean they are acidifying. All food you eat goes right into a pool of hydrochloric acid in your stomach, which is far more acidic than any food you eat. It's not the acidity of the original food that matters; it's the acidity of the final nutrients that are absorbed in the digestive tract, and many of those healthful organic acids don't add to the body's acid load once they're absorbed. So, beets are alkalizing. In fact, many vegetables contain acids that are generally healthy for you.

Beets, for instance, have a high percentage of citric acid and ascorbic acid (vitamin C), which both act as antioxidants. Ascorbic acid has also been shown to regulate collagen synthesis in blood vessels and help

improve cardiovascular function. The dietary nitrate in beets also supports healthy vascular function. Studies have shown that beetroot nitrate
can lead to improved blood flow and decreased blood pressure.

Beets reduce inflammation and control glucose levels

The most abundant polyphenol in beets is gallic acid, which serves a
number of biological functions in humans, like fighting inflammation
and controlling glucose metabolism. In addition, animal models show
that the betanin in beets has an antidiabetic role.

Beets support heart and organ health

Scientists have shown that beets have the potential to keep your organs
healthier. In one study, mice were fed long-term with beet juice, then
injected with *dimethylnitrosamine*, which can induce liver damage. The
scientists discovered that the beet juice increased enzyme activity and
prevented systemic liver damage. And, in a clinical study with nonsmoking adults diagnosed with coronary artery disease, a two-week regime of
betalin-rich extract brought down their total levels of blood cholesterol
and triglycerides.

Beets protect your memory

Scientists concur that one cause of cognitive impairment is a deficiency
in nitric oxide, so today's researchers are especially excited about the
potential of beets to generate nitric oxide in the body. In one wide-
ranging review of studies supporting the impact of beet consumption on
cognitive health, the authors cited one study in which researchers found
that supplementing with beets could increase cerebral blood flow and
improve cognition, and another study demonstrating that patients with
type 2 diabetes had quicker reaction times after beet intake.

Beets support your aerobic system

Beet juice is one of only a handful of supplements that has been con-
clusively proven to enhance performance in endurance athletes. It does
this by supporting our aerobic systems. You may not care about performance, but the more important message here is that beets help support
the health and function of our mitochondria—the aerobic machinery of
our bodies—which is critical to longevity.

Seaweed: A Storied History of Health Benefits

Seaweed is the name we typically use for the huge variety of plants that
grow in water, whether that water is a salty ocean, a rushing river, or a
freshwater lake. Some seaweeds are microscopic, while others grow in
huge underwater forests on the ocean floor. Seaweed has a long history
of serving not only as human food, but as medicine. People have been
consuming seaweed in East Asia for thousands of years. In China, books
from the Qin and Han dynasties reveal that seaweed was used to help
treat cancer, gas, and goiters caused by iodine deficiency.

There are about 25,000 different species of seaweed, and they're classified into three basic groups based on color: brown (*Phaeophyceae*), green
(*Clorophyta*), and red (*Rhodophyta*). All three groups are rich sources of
valuable nutrients and bioactive compounds, with *polysaccharides* (the scientific term for what we commonly call complex carbohydrates, which
are composed of chains of monosaccharide units, or simple carbohydrates) making up about three-quarters of their biomass. If you don't yet
recognize seaweed as one of the most valuable vegetables to add to your
Paleo Diet, we promise you will soon: Analysts predict that seaweed
products will grow to be a booming $85 billion business worldwide by
2026 due to an increased worldwide recognition of their importance as
nutritional foods rich in dietary fiber, minerals, protein, and vitamins.

Today's researchers are perhaps most excited by the potential of
seaweed polysaccharides to have therapeutic effects on the metastasis

of various cancers, including breast, cervical, liver, and lung. There are ongoing scientific explorations in other arenas of human health as well. For example, the world has seen new epidemic or pandemic respiratory illnesses since the beginning of the 21st century, and recent studies have shown that the polysaccharides in seaweeds may have powerful antiviral potential against these infections.

Meanwhile, the polyphenols and proteins from all seaweed varieties are being widely studied for their antibacterial, antifungal, and antioxidant properties. For instance, researchers have shown that seaweeds are a rich source of carotenoids that act as antioxidants. These include beta-carotene (which your body converts to vitamin A), lutein, astaxanthin, and fucoxanthin, all of which can help fight inflammation and support cell health. Carotenoids also help elevate Nrf2.

From brown seaweed, scientists are especially focused on extracting and studying *fucoidans*, a family of molecules derived from *sulfated polysaccharides* with demonstrated anticancer, antidiabetic, anti-inflammatory, and antiviral activities, among others. *Alginate*, another polysaccharide in brown seaweeds, has shown promise in studies focused on wound healing, drug delivery, and tissue engineering. Recently, alginate has also received attention for its potential to decrease the risk of inflammation and heart disease and support gut health. Finally, brown seaweed is a great source of omega-3 polyunsaturated fatty acids, which can help protect brain health. The human body can't really use the forms of omega-3s found in most plant foods, but seaweed is the exception. It contains the forms of omega-3s we can use, namely DHA (docosahexaenoic acid) and EPA (eicosapentaenoic acid). We discuss DHA and EPA in more detail on page 184.

From red seaweed, scientists have been studying agar, a polysaccharide that demonstrates anti-pathogenic activity and the ability to help maintain the ionic equilibrium of cells. Researchers are also examining the potential therapeutic effects of rhamnan sulfate in green algae, which has been shown to protect against metabolic syndrome as well as the SARS and delta variants of the COVID virus.

Additionally, scientists have discovered in recent years that the poly-saccharides in algae have wonderful potential as therapeutic agents for treating IBD (inflammatory bowel disease) and other intestinal inflammatory diseases because they're resistant to gastric juice and enzymes. This means they can serve as a fermentation substrate that allows healthy microbes to grow. Other studies are exploring how specific nutrients in seaweed, especially fucoidan, alginate, and other polysaccharides, have the potential to act as prebiotics, boosting gut health by promoting the growth of beneficial bacteria while inhibiting the growth of pathogenic bacteria, leading to better metabolic and overall health.

Spinach: Popeye Was Right

Eating your spinach can indeed make you stronger. It's one of the most nutritious foods you can add to your Paleo shopping list because it's packed with vitamins, iron, and antioxidants like beta-carotene and lutein that will boost everything from your immune system to your vision. In addition, the high potassium levels in spinach can help lower blood pressure.

But what really sets spinach apart is its high levels of folate. Folate—also known as vitamin B9—plays a crucial role in your body's ability to grow and repair tissues, as well as in the formation of red and white blood cells. Folate, along with vitamins B6 and B12, is also critical to the folate cycle, one of the most important metabolic pathways in the body. We'll discuss the folate cycle again in chapter 12, but what you need to know right here is that the folate cycle is essential for your body's overall maintenance of cellular functions.

Doctors often recommend folate supplements during pregnancy because a folate deficiency can increase the risk of neural tube defects in the developing fetus, but getting enough folate as we age is important as well. Studies have suggested that low folate levels may be linked to the cognitive decline associated with aging as well as with a higher risk of developing cancer. Researchers believe this is partly because the primary role of the folate cycle is in *methylation*, a process that regulates gene expression and helps maintain proper cellular function. Methylation patterns can change as we age, and this contributes to age-related diseases and a decline in overall health.

Because of how important folate is to our health, many people who aren't pregnant take supplements, too. However, it's important to know that almost all supplements are folic acid and not folate. Folic acid was created in a lab and doesn't exist in nature. More concerning is that it has been associated with an increased risk of some forms of cancer. Fortunately, by eating Paleo, you'll be consuming plenty of green vegetables, fruits, and even liver, which contain all the folate you need for healthy aging.

It's important to point out that spinach has one of the highest concentrations of an antinutrient (explained on page 58) called *oxalate*. The only food with a higher concentration is chocolate (see chapter 9). Oxalate can cause several health problems, including cardiovascular disease and sudden cardiac death. It can also bind with calcium to form very painful kidney stones. This has caused some nutrition experts to recommend against any plant foods containing oxalate.

But it's also important to note that our bodies produce oxalate, so we don't believe it should be completely eliminated. What may be more important here is our magnesium-to-calcium ratio. There is evidence that when we get sufficient magnesium in the diet compared to calcium, many of the negative effects of oxalate are mediated.

Having said that, however, if oxalate is truly an issue for you—for example, if you suffer from kidney stones—then try cooking your spinach (which reduces oxalates) or simply avoid eating it. You'll still be able to obtain all of the nutrients spinach offers from eating a balanced Paleo Diet.

Vegetables and Weight Loss

We don't recommend counting calories on the Paleo Diet. It isn't an enjoyable (or, often, even a healthy) way to lose weight. However, we love to issue this challenge: If you're not down to the weight you'd like to be, try to eat as many vegetables as you can and not lose weight. It's surprisingly hard to do! Because of their nutrient density, the vegetables we discuss in this chapter are highly satiating. If you are eating vegetables often throughout the day, you're going to feel full long before you've consumed too many calories. A slice of pizza is nearly 400 kcal and leaves you wanting more, but you'd have to eat over 50 cups of kale or spinach to get the same number of calories. Now *that's* a challenge!

Antinutrients in Vegetables

In his book *The Paleo Answer*, Dr. Cordain discussed many of the antinutrients found in non-Paleo foods, such as grains (including rice, though it's a staple around the world), pseudo-grains (also known as grain-like seeds), legumes, white potatoes, cassava, and any foods that contain non-Paleo additives. The reason for antinutrients in many of these foods is simple. All living things want to defend themselves from being eaten. Animals can fight or run away, but plants don't have that option. So, one key defense mechanism they've developed is antinutrients. This is especially true of most grains and legumes. If you ate raw wheat, you'd get violently sick and never try to eat it again. Likewise, that's why we have to soak beans in water for hours before they can be cooked and eaten.

So why don't we get sick when we eat fresh fruit? Fruit plants have a different mechanism. They put an indigestible seed inside a very tasty fruit. Animals enjoy the fruit, and then they deposit the intact seed elsewhere with a natural fertilizer. It's a symbiotic relationship.

Antinutrients can exert their negative influence via several mechanisms, including blocking the absorption or assimilation of important nutrients, changing a normal physiological process in the body, or breaking down the defenses in the gut.

If you're wondering, yes, some plant foods that we consider Paleo do also contain antinutrients. For instance, let's look at sweet potatoes, which are included in the Paleo Diet, and white potatoes, which we exclude. Sweet potatoes and white potatoes both contain antinutrients such as saponins, which may increase your intestinal permeability. However, white potatoes are nightshade vegetables, which may contribute to lowgrade chronic inflammation in those who have a nightshade sensitivity. Sweet potatoes, on the other hand, have a lower glycemic index than white potatoes, are packed with nutrients, and are anti-inflammatory. (While they are called potatoes, they're not actually in the same family as white potatoes.) So although sweet potatoes also contain antinutrients, their benefits outweigh the antinutrient risk.

To eliminate all antinutrients, we'd have to stop eating a number of vegetables and pretty much all nuts and seeds. However, we don't feel most people need to be that strict. As a general guideline, if you can eat the raw form of the plant without getting sick, the antinutrient content shouldn't be a concern except for people with an autoimmune condition.

The prevalence of autoimmune diseases has increased significantly over recent decades. Antinutrients in plant foods appear to play a key role in many autoimmune conditions. As a result, both research and clinical observations have further identified several foods considered Paleo that, while likely not the cause of the autoimmune condition, can be problematic for individuals who currently have an autoimmune disease. This has led to what is commonly now called the autoimmune protocol (AIP) and is essentially a stricter version of the Paleo Diet to further eliminate potentially problematic antinutrients from the diet of autoimmune disease patients.

Table 1 in the Appendix (page 271) contains a list of the commonly identified foods that should be avoided on the AIP. In addition to the list, some general "Paleo" food categories should also be eliminated, including all nuts and seeds, all spices made from nuts and seeds, and all nightshade plants, the most common of which are included in the list. Notice that the list only has one fruit, banana (which is not problematic for most on an AIP). However, fruits and vegetables that contain very small seeds, such as cucumbers, can be problematic for a small percentage of people who need to follow the AIP, and may also need to be avoided. If you do have an autoimmune condition, you won't have to be concerned about our recipe section at the end of the book, as we have suggested substitutions for any noncompliant AIP ingredient.

Ultimately, an individual with an autoimmune issue needs to understand that any food has the potential to be problematic. For some people, this includes the consumption of vegetables, which do contain some antinutrients. In chapter 5 on fruits, you'll read about some research that shows a health benefit from consuming fruits but not vegetables for some of the reasons explained above—evolution chose a symbiotic relationship with mammals for most fruits.

You might be asking yourself, "Wait, you've just been sharing all of the amazing longevity nutrients found in vegetables, and now you're saying vegetables can be a problem?" That's correct, they can be problematic, and to make things even more confusing, the flip side is that these antinutrients can be beneficial for some people, depending on their genetics and the food's culinary treatment. Nutrition is nuanced, and an individual approach will often yield the best results. That being said, we are confident the Paleo Diet is your best starting point, but if you need to avoid antinutrients, some tweaking here and there could provide better benefits to you as an individual. Clinically, a diet of animal protein and fruits has often been very effective as an elimination diet for autoimmune patients who often present with a simultaneous leaky gut. However, once the gut has healed, most people can reintroduce vegetables first, then nuts and seeds. It is prudent to reintroduce foods one at a time, waiting a few days before adding another to see if the new food causes any issues.

CHAPTER FIVE

The Best Fruits to Boost
Healthy Aging

When Jamie was diagnosed with Hashimoto's disease after her thyroid levels kept dropping, she cut back on alcohol and caffeine
to ease her symptoms, specifically the fatigue, joint pain, and weight
loss resistance. She also researched her condition and "discovered actual
studies showing Paleo works well with Hashimoto's," she says.

Now 48, Jamie decided to give the Paleo Diet a try as part of an
autoimmune protocol (AIP) elimination diet and began seeing the benefits within a week. "I had been on WeightWatchers since the start of
the year and lost 15 pounds, but in the past few months, I'd plateaued.
Within the first month on Paleo, I lost another 12 pounds. My fatigue
improved and, most notably, my joint pain was greatly reduced."

Even more surprising to Jamie was that her new Paleo lifestyle
reduced sciatica pain. "I've taken loved ones to the ER four times in the
last month. Normally a long day sitting in a plastic chair would result in
bad sciatica pain, but I've had no pain at all."

Probably the best feature of the Paleo Diet for Jamie is that "there's a great variety of food, and that makes the lifestyle easier to follow." She suggests that people new to a Paleo lifestyle do "pantry prep" by going to the grocery store and making sure they have the right healthy foods at home. "Once you get through the first week of Paleo, it's easy after that. Even in restaurants, you can always order a meal of salad, vegetables, and protein," she says, adding, "Before you start, take a couple of weeks to wean yourself off sugar, so you can be more appreciative of what fruit tastes like."

For many people trying to maintain a healthy weight, fruit is often struck off the list as being too high in sugar. But, as Jamie has discovered, fruit—with its rich variety of colors, flavors, and surprising textures—is one of nature's sweetest delights. More importantly, a diet rich in fruit can protect us against inflammation, cognitive issues, and many diseases of aging, including arthritis, diabetes, heart disease, hypertension, and cancer.

The Lifelong Power of Fruit

Why is fruit such a crucial longevity and health ally? You already know that fruit is a terrific source of vitamins and minerals, but more importantly, fruit contains alkaloids, carotenoids, glucosinolates, and polyphenols. As we explained earlier, polyphenols are a diverse group of powerful organic chemical compounds. We'll highlight and explain the longevity benefits of polyphenols in more detail below. After that, we'll discuss some of the most nutrient-dense fruits that have clear anti-aging properties. Some may surprise you—like coconuts. Other top longevity fruits—like avocados, bananas, berries, and pomegranates—may be more familiar, but it's worth highlighting the latest scientific studies linking the consumption of those fruits to longevity.

For example, in one recent cross-sectional study involving 1,346 participants (ages 25 to 79; 47 percent men, 53 percent women), researchers found that a higher intake of both alpha-carotene and beta-carotene was associated with a reduced overall risk of metabolic syndrome. Drilling down to specifics in their 2024 paper, these researchers discovered that a higher intake of alpha-carotene correlated with healthier fasting glucose and triglyceride levels, and beta-carotene was associated with better triglyceride levels.

Our best sources of carotenoids are fruits and vegetables—carotenoids give fruits and vegetables their yellow, orange, and red colors. So it's no surprise that greater consumption of fruit and vegetables is linked to a lower risk of chronic diseases associated with aging, inflammation, and oxidative stress. On the flip side, without an adequate intake of fruit and vegetables, you're more likely to suffer from disease.

Interestingly, scientists have even linked the consumption of more fruit in midlife with a lower incidence of depression among older adults. In a 2024 Chinese study of 13,738 adults, the researchers followed up with them some 19 years later and found that 3,180 of those participants suffered from depressive symptoms. Delving more deeply into their eating habits, the researchers concluded that those who ate more fruit were less apt to be among those exhibiting depression—especially if the adults regularly ate tangerines, oranges, bananas, papaya, and watermelon. The same researchers found no similar protective benefits against depression from consuming vegetables.

Eat the Rainbow

During childhood, you probably heard a parent or teacher say, "Eat the rainbow" when it came to selecting fruits and vegetables. As silly as it sounds, there is wisdom in this advice. About 78 percent of adults around the world suffer a nutrient gap because they fail to eat not only adequate amounts of fruit and vegetables, but also enough variety. In other words, they're not eating the rainbow.

Why does it matter whether your fruits and vegetables are green, red, yellow, orange, or purple? It's because those different colors correspond to different naturally occurring phytonutrients (otherwise called *bioactive pigments*), and each of those phytonutrients acts in a slightly different way to help your body combat the diseases of aging.

Orange plant foods, for instance, are typically rich in carotenoids like beta-carotene (associated with a lower risk of cardiovascular disease) and lutein (known to improve the risk of stroke), while blue and purple fruits boost the anthocyanins in your diet, which are associated with lower inflammatory markers. In a 2022 meta-analysis published in *Molecules*, researchers synthesized data from 2,847 research studies and found that people who consumed at least three different bioactive pigments daily were often healthier, with better lipid profiles, lower inflammatory markers, and a decreased risk of multiple cancers.

Anthocyanins: A Top-Secret Ingredient to a Longer, Healthier Life

Polyphenols (as discussed on page 37) are abundant in certain fruits. About 60 percent of the 8,000 polyphenols identified to date are classified as flavonoids. Like carotenoids, flavonoids give many fruits their rich colors—particularly one of the most important, *anthocyanins*, which bestow that gorgeous red, purple, blue, or black coloring on certain fruits, such as blackberries and cherries. But anthocyanins do more than give your fruit a pretty face.

Lately, researchers have focused on anthocyanins' health benefits and longevity properties, which include reducing inflammation and lowering the risk of chronic diseases such as heart disease, cancer, and neurodegeneration. The benefits of anthocyanins appear to be linked in part to their involvement in promoting a healthy cell cycle and aiding mitochondrial biogenesis. They promote both sirtuins and Nrf2, which we discussed in chapter 3 as being central to healthy longevity.

Anthocyanins have also been attributed to reducing obesity-induced inflammation, the cause of so many chronic noncommunicable diseases. This is accomplished by the anthocyanins eliminating reactive oxygen species, decreasing pro-inflammatory mediators, and improving gut dysbiosis.

What About the High Sugar Content in Fruit?

A lot of people ask the Paleo Diet team if they should worry about the sugar in the fruit they eat. If you're not diabetic, generally the answer is no, because fruit contains a good amount of fiber and seeds that lower the glycemic load from the sugars contained in fruit. As a result, eating whole fruit can actually help keep your blood sugar normalized.

Another important factor with sugars is whether they are *bound* or *free*. A free sugar is one that has been processed and then added to the food, such as sugar-sweetened drinks. Free sugars are associated with a host of medical conditions like cardiovascular disease, stroke, and neuro-degeneration. Because the sugar in fruit is still bound, it doesn't have the same negative health impacts. In fact, a diet including fruits is associated with a reduced risk of cardiovascular disease.

However, it's important to note that the common fruits we eat today have little resemblance to their wild ancestors. Domesticated fruits are almost always larger and sweeter and contain less fiber than their wild counterparts. Compare a Golden Delicious apple to a crab apple, and you get the idea. We recommend that most people eat fresh fruit as their appetite dictates. Note that some fruits, like avocados, lemons, and limes, are very low in total sugar and don't need to be restricted. (See the table on page 66.) But if you're currently over-weight or insulin-resistant, limit your consumption of high-sugar fruits like grapes, bananas, mangoes, sweet cherries, apples, pineapples, and pears. Instead, choose the low-sugar fruits mentioned above or per-haps more vegetables, since vegetables offer many of the same longevity health benefits with less simple sugar.

You'll also want to be wary of the high sugar levels in many dried fruits. In the drying process, dehydration concentrates the sugar. In

addition, the sugars can degrade during this process and become effectively unbound. As you can see from the table, some dried fruits more
closely resemble commercial candy than fresh, whole fruit. For example,
a serving of Zante currants has 70 grams of sugar, while a serving of
Milk Duds contains only 50 grams. Luckily, most fresh fruits fall far
below those numbers.

Fruit and Sugar Content

Fruit	Portion Size	Sugar Content
Pears, dried, sulfured, uncooked	1 cup, halves	111.96 g
Dates, deglet noor	1 cup, chopped	93.12 g
Figs, dried, uncooked	1 cup	71.40 g
Apricots, dried, sulfured, uncooked	1 cup, halves	69.47 g
Strawberries, frozen, sweetened	1 cup	61.23 g
Peaches, frozen, sweetened	1 cup	55.45 g
Peaches, dried	1 cup	43.83 g
Apples, dried	1 cup	33.97 g
Cranberries, dried, sweetened	¼ cup	29.02 g
Bananas	1 cup, mashed	27.52 g
Raisins, golden seedless	¼ cup, packed	27.10 g
Blueberries, dried, sweetened	¼ cup	27.00 g
Passion fruit	1 cup	26.43 g
Grapes, red or green	1 cup	23.37 g
Mangoes	1 cup, chunks	22.54 g
Plums	1 cup, slices	16.37 g
Pineapple	1 cup, chunks	16.25 g
Grapefruit	1 cup, sections with juice	15.85 g
Oranges, navel	1 cup, sections	14.03 g
Melons, cantaloupe	1 cup, balls	13.91 g
Melons, honeydew	1 cup, diced	13.80 g

Fruit	Portion Size	Sugar Content
Pears, Bartlett	1 cup, slices	13.57 g
Cherries, sour, red	1 cup, pitted	13.16 g
Blueberries, frozen, unsweetened	1 cup	13.10 g
Apples, Fuji, with skin	1 cup, sliced	12.80 g
Pears, red Anjou	1 small	12.02 g
Papaya	1 cup, chunks	11.34 g
Apples, Gala, with skin	1 cup, slices	11.30 g
Apples, Golden Delicious, with skin	1 cup, slices	10.94 g
Apples, Granny Smith, with skin	1 cup, slices	10.45 g
Strawberries, frozen, unsweetened	1 cup	10.08 g
Watermelon	1 cup, chunks	9.55 g
Raspberries, frozen, unsweetened	1 cup	9.16 g
Strawberries	1 cup	7.43 g
Blackberries	1 cup	7.03 g
Clementines	1	6.79 g
Raspberries	1 cup	5.44 g
Cranberries, raw	1 cup	4.70 g

Does Juicing Offer the Same Benefits as Unprocessed Fruit and Vegetables?

Walk through any US city, and you'll probably see a juice bar and people wandering around with giant plastic cups filled with thick, colorful shakes made of fruits and veggies. While this seems like a new health trend, it isn't new, nor is juicing necessarily healthy, either.

Juicing has been around for millennia, with humans mashing fruit into liquids as early as 150 BC and none other than the Dead Sea Scrolls reporting that a tribe in Israel had made juice from mashed pomegranates and figs. Then, in the 1930s, Dr. Norman Walker invented the first juicing machine with a hydraulic press to extract juice. This machine made juicing more feasible to the public, and by the 1950s there were masticating juicers, centrifugal juicers, and juicers to use at home. In California, always a hotbed of health trends, pioneer juicers like Dave Otto, who opened the Beverly Hills Juice Club in 1975, began cashing in on the hype, and by the 1990s juice chains like Jamba Juice were appearing in malls.

While juicing extracts liquid from vegetables and fruit to make tasty, portable drinks, it isn't any healthier than consuming the raw, unprocessed foods you use to make the juice. In fact, juicing usually removes the fiber that helps your body regulate sugar spikes, and some people who do prolonged juicing to lose weight or "cleanse" their bodies of toxins are at risk for nutrient deficiencies. We typically recommend juicing as part of a healthy Paleo Diet, not as a substitute for food. And, if you do choose to juice, make your smoothies with a blender, not a juicing machine, because that will give you a healthier drink with more fiber and plant nutrients.

Why Coconuts Aren't Just Any Fruit

Despite its name, a coconut isn't a nut, but a fruit—a one-seeded *drupe*, in botanical terms. This drops the coconut into the category of stone fruits, which includes peaches, cherries, mangoes, olives, and dates, all of which are characterized by a hard, stony covering around the seed embryo.

The coconut has been foraged, eaten, and revered around the world throughout human history. The *Cocos nucifera*—the only type of palm tree that produces coconuts—originated in India and Southeast Asia. Coconuts float, so this fruit was able to travel easily on ocean currents to different parts of the world. Coconuts were also carried overland and by sea to different lands by traders and travelers.

In parts of India, the *Cocos nucifera* is called *Kalpavriksha*, or "the tree that provides all the necessities of life," while to the Malays it's *Pokok seribu guna*, the "tree of a thousand uses." In the Philippines, coconut palms are "trees of abundance," and to Indonesians, "three-generations trees." These names reflect the fact that every part of the palm tree is useful to humans. Coconut meat is a nourishing food and coconut water provides drink. Palm branches can be woven into baskets, carpets, or roofs. The wood from palm trees is used to build furniture, canoes, or even entire homes. Coconuts have also been incorporated into traditional medicines to counteract poisons, treat menstrual issues, reduce pain, kill bacteria, ease inflammation, and treat diarrhea, among other things.

A cup of shredded fresh coconut delivers 280 calories, about 90 percent of which is saturated fat. A cup of coconut meat also provides these nutrients:

- Protein: 3 grams
- Carbs: 10 grams
- Sugar: 5 grams
- Fiber: 7 grams
- Manganese: 60 percent of the daily value (DV)
- Selenium: 15 percent of the DV
- Copper: 44 percent of the DV
- Phosphorus: 13 percent of the DV
- Potassium: 6 percent of the DV
- Iron: 11 percent of the DV
- Zinc: 10 percent of the DV

The Coconut Water Craze

Probably the biggest business boom in coconut sales in the last decade has been in coconut water, which reached the shelves of stores all over Latin America, Indonesia, India, and the Philippines long before becoming popular in the United States around 2004. The sales of coconut water hit $674 million as of January 2024, and today consumers rely on coconut water for everything from sports hydration to smoothies and mixed alcoholic drinks.

Coconut water is the clear liquid inside young, or "tender" coconuts that are around six months old, and it has long been considered a nourishing beverage against heat and dehydration in the tropics. A single green coconut typically yields ½ to 1 cup of water. Coconut water contains electrolytes—charged minerals that can keep you hydrated—like potassium, sodium, and manganese. This makes it a restorative drink in the tropics for hydrating people suffering from bouts of dysentery or cholera as well as for athletes in training. Having said that, we want to be careful about implying that electrolyte drinks are automatically healthy for us. It's true that coconut water contains these electrolytes in more natural ratios with, for example, more potassium than sodium compared to manufactured sports drinks, but the ratios in even natural coconut water can vary a lot. Check the labels of any coconut water you buy to make sure you're not getting a version too high in sodium.

Various long-term studies have shown that the magnesium found in coconut water may prevent blood glucose disorders and reduce the risk of developing diabetes, as in one 2021 study using rats with diabetes. That study demonstrated that giving the animals coconut water significantly reduced the retinal damage associated with diabetes and lowered their blood sugar. Scientists are also examining the potential of coconut water to lower blood pressure because of its high potassium content, since potassium has been shown in various studies to lower blood pressure in humans.

Coconut oil for heart health

With such a high saturated fat content, should we be eating coconuts at all? The answer is yes. Coconut meat and coconut oil were once widely shunned by Western nutritionists because they believed the high level of saturated fatty acids in coconuts would raise the level of our blood cholesterol, clog our arteries, and raise the risk of cardiovascular disease. However, there was one odd fact that researchers couldn't explain: Why did Indigenous people in the tropics, who have always consumed great amounts of coconut meat and oil as part of their traditional diets, experience only a minimal incidence of cardiovascular disease? For example, despite the large consumption of coconut oil, the people of Sri Lanka can expect a higher life expectancy than those in countries where people consume comparatively little coconut oil.

Dietary fats are essential to good nutrition because they help our bodies store energy, absorb and transport fat-soluble vitamins, supply essential fatty acids, and help build up cell membranes, among other functions. As we've already discussed, what matters more than *how much* fat you eat is *what kind* of fat you're eating. For decades, nutritionists drummed it into the public health sphere that increased consumption of saturated fat increases the risk of cardiovascular disease, with the standard dietary advice being to cut down on saturated fat intake to bring down the risk of heart disease and stroke. But to truly assess the value of consuming any particular food for our long-term health, it's crucial to look at the food as a whole. This is abundantly true when it comes to considering the saturated fat content in any food, since recent scientific studies demonstrate that some foods high in saturated fat may help protect our health.

As Dr. Cordain explained in his last book, *The Paleo Answer*, and as we mentioned previously in this book, consuming saturated fat increases total cholesterol (TC), and years ago, this was the measure being used to predict cardiovascular disease. However, researchers later discovered that increasing saturated fat increased HDL cholesterol to the point that the TC/HDL ratio (a much better predictor of cardiovascular disease) *decreased* as a result of increased saturated fat intake. In other words, saturated fat (in the amounts that our ancestors would have eaten, which was no more than 15 percent of their caloric intake) is healthy.

This certainly seems to be the case with coconuts. Various studies have shown that because consuming coconut oil has the potential to increase HDL, the "good cholesterol" in your blood, consuming coconut oil may help protect you against elevated LDL (the bad cholesterol), which in turn helps us fight obesity, type 2 diabetes, hypertension, chronic inflammation, and cardiovascular disease.

Why should this be true? Fatty acids are generally classified according to the number of carbons chained together in the fatty acid's backbone. They're also classified by how "saturated" those carbons are with hydrogen ions. Most saturated fats—the ones that tend to get a bad rap—are long-chain fatty acids (LCFAs) with 13 to 21 carbons strung together. Coconut oil is rich in medium-chain fatty acids (MCFAs), which have only 6 to 12 carbons in their chains. In coconut oil, lauric acid constitutes up to half of the MCFA, and researchers now theorize that lauric acid conveys special health benefits. That's because when compared to other saturated fats, lauric acid contributes less to fat storage, leading to less inflammation, which in turn cuts down on the risk of clogged arteries, high blood pressure, and cardiovascular disease.

Without digging too deeply into the chemistry here, LCFAs combine with proteins and produce lipoproteins, which can go straight into your bloodstream without having to pass through the liver. When lipoproteins circulate in your blood, their fatty components may accumulate in your tissues or coagulate on artery walls, leading to a higher risk of high blood pressure, heart disease, and other chronic diseases of aging. The reason MCFAs are healthier than LCFAs is because MCFAs are more easily absorbed by your liver and can be more readily used as energy than LCFAs. As they're metabolized by your liver, MCFAs produce ketone bodies like acetoacetic acid and acetone. These can then be efficiently channeled straight back into your organs and muscles as energy instead of being turned into fat deposits.

Perhaps even more importantly, ketones can be an important alternative source of energy in the brain, since the brain will preferentially use available ketones even if glucose is also present. That's because ketones can freely cross the blood-brain barrier, while glucose requires a more complex chemical process (involving insulin) to be made available to the brain. As you'll read below, this may provide important protection against Alzheimer's disease.

Coconut oil can help protect the aging brain

Most of the research on coconut oil to date has been devoted to its potential positive effects on cardiovascular health since it boosts the HDL in your blood. These high-density lipoproteins can reduce the risk of clogged arteries and heart disease by transporting phospholipids and cholesterols out of artery walls before fat deposits form. This is important because heart disease has been the leading cause of death in the United States since 1950, according to the National Center for Health Statistics.

Now, new studies are emerging that show coconut oil might also prove beneficial in preventing or treating neurodegenerative diseases like Parkinson's and Alzheimer's. The most diagnosed form of dementia, Alzheimer's is a progressive neurogenerative disease affecting more than 40 million people around the world, typically striking those over age 70. Parkinson's affects fewer people but is the second-most diagnosed neurodegenerative disease.

The risk factors associated with developing these diseases are strikingly similar to the risk factors linked to heart disease and diabetes, including lifestyle factors that aggravate chronic inflammation and oxidative stress, like obesity and high blood pressure. As we've already discussed, those factors can be greatly reduced through diet, so scientists are currently conducting studies to see if there are specific nutrients that might specifically be associated with a lower risk of Alzheimer's and Parkinson's. (We'll focus on Alzheimer's here, but we mention Parkinson's because the mechanisms of how coconut oil might protect the brain over time initially appear to be similar.)

One area of research is zeroing in on how coconut oil consumption can play a role both in reducing the risk factors of developing neurodegenerative diseases and in improving the cognition of those diagnosed with them. The theory here is that in addition to providing nutrients that might have antioxidant properties that protect your brain cells, the extra ketone body formation that results from the high levels of MCFAs in coconut oil offers an alternative energy source for the brain. This may provide health benefits for those with Alzheimer's, since one hallmark of this disease is the development of extracellular amyloid plaques, which impair the brain's ability to use glucose properly. Alzheimer's is also characterized by insulin insensitivity in the brain, which has led some in the medical world to refer to it as type 3 diabetes. Researchers theorize that the brain atrophies over time as glucose provides less and less available energy. In a healthy brain, about 100 trillion synapses make it possible for your brain to transmit signals rapidly, but postmortem examinations of patients with Alzheimer's show a significant depletion in synapse density. Synapse loss correlates with the cognitive decline experienced by people with Alzheimer's.

With few FDA-approved drugs for treating Alzheimer's, and none yet for preventing it, many dietary interventions are currently under scrutiny. While the evidence is still in the early phases, a multifactorial approach to Alzheimer's that includes diet, exercise, and reducing stress has shown promising signs of improving and potentially even reversing the condition. Scientists have also shown that a higher intake of fruits, vegetables, nuts, and other foods high in antioxidants and vitamins, along with cutting back on high-fat dairy foods and sweets, is associated with a lower risk of developing Alzheimer's or other cognitive deficits. This isn't surprising, since those foods are associated with increasing chronic inflammation, and in the past decade a third core pathology—in addition to plaque formation and neuronal tangles—has emerged for Alzheimer's: a sustained or chronic inflammatory response in the brain.

In addition to ketone bodies, consuming coconut oil means your body is receiving the benefit of phenolic compounds that you already know can combat oxidative stress, and this is another factor associated with developing Alzheimer's. Taking all of this into consideration, we can say that coconuts, and specifically coconut oil, have many properties that make coconuts powerful allies in combating the cognitive decline associated with Alzheimer's disease. In one small pilot study with 44 people, for instance, people who received the same diet were broken into two groups, one of which consumed additional coconut oil. Those who added more coconut oil to their diets exhibited significant improvement to their memories—especially women with mild or moderate cases of Alzheimer's. And, in another Sri Lankan study comparing the effects of enriching the diets of people with Alzheimer's with canola oil or coconut oil, researchers found that coconut oil improved performance on the MMSE (Mini-Mental State Examination) typically used in clinical settings to evaluate cognitive impairment without increasing their lipid profiles.

While of course many of these studies on the health benefits of coconuts are ongoing, early findings offer every indication that adding moderate amounts of coconut to your diet may be another nutritional strategy for healthy aging. See chapter 9 for ideas on how to use more coconut oil in your diet.

Add Avocados to Boost Vitality and Longevity

If you search for "avocados" on social media, you'll earn millions of hits. North Americans consume avocados in everything from smoothies to salads and even slice them into sandwiches. According to the World Population Review, people in the United States consumed an average of 8.43 pounds of avocados per person in 2020—and that's a good thing.

Avocados are high in potassium and contain over 20 vitamins and nutrients, including folate, vitamin A, beta-carotene, and the antioxidant lutein. They're also rich in the monounsaturated fat oleic acid, which can help improve lipid profiles, reducing the risk of stroke and cardiovascular disease. Among those with type 2 diabetes, researchers have conducted various studies demonstrating that avocado intake may help improve glucose/insulin homeostasis. In another 2022 comprehensive meta-analysis and systematic review of available studies, scientists also linked eating avocados to healthier lipid profiles.

Perhaps even more notable is the research supporting the association among older adults between avocado consumption and long-term brain health. For one 2021 study, researchers surveyed 2,886 adults age 60 and over and divided them into avocado or non-avocado consumers. When they evaluated the cognitive function of these older participants, they discovered that avocado consumers had significantly better cognitive scores on all tests.

Bananas: A Sweet Treat to Thwart Disease

One of the healthiest, least expensive fruits to add to your diet, bananas are packed with important vitamins, potassium, antioxidants, and other nutrients. A single medium banana gives you:

- Vitamin C: 12 percent of the DV
- Potassium: 10 percent of the DV
- Magnesium: 8 percent of the DV

Because they're sweet and relatively low in calories, many people trying to lose weight find that bananas make a good substitute for more sugary foods if they have a sweet tooth. Various studies have shown that bananas can help improve gut, heart, and kidney health. New evidence is emerging that green bananas may offer even more therapeutic health benefits than yellow ones. This is potentially due to the green fruit having a higher resistant starch content, lower glycemic index, and higher flavonoid and antioxidant content. Scientists are currently studying the impact of green banana consumption on diseases of aging such as ulcers, high blood pressure, and diabetes.

For instance, testicular dysfunction can be one unfortunate result of type 2 diabetes, and studies have demonstrated that green bananas helped correct testicular dysfunction in diabetic rats. Just beware: Because bananas are higher in carbohydrates than many other fruits, if you do have type 2 diabetes, it might be best to keep your banana consumption to a minimum, pair bananas with foods high in protein and fat, and consider eating green bananas since they have a lower glycemic index.

Cherries and Berries: Antioxidant Powerhouses

Few plant sources are richer in age-defying antioxidants than cherries and berries. The Montmorency tart cherry is the most popular sour cherry in the United States, and it is extensively used to make cherry pies as well as jams and preserves. Tart cherries are a nutritionally dense food rich in anthocyanins, quercetin, hydroxycinnamates, potassium, vitamin C, carotenoids, and melatonin. These nutrients help protect against inflammation and a wide variety of chronic diseases, including cancer, cardiovascular diseases, diabetes, and Alzheimer's. They also have a high level of antioxidants and a low glycemic response.

Berries, such as blueberries, blackberries, strawberries, and raspberries, are some of our favorite Paleo foods because they're rich in anthocyanins, which give these berries and many other plants their delightfully rich colors (see page 64). Also, they are high in healthy unsaturated fatty acids, which can help protect both heart health and brain function as we age. We'll go into more detail about the benefits of omega-3 unsaturated fats in part III of this book.

The importance of sleep to our health cannot be overstated, and one study showed that berry consumption was associated with a 10 to 17 percent decreased risk of short sleep. This was particularly true for strawberries and blueberries, but sleep difficulties were also reduced with blackberry consumption.

In addition, a recent review has shown that black raspberries and strawberries exhibit anticancer effects against esophageal cancer, one of the most fatal malignancies. The protective mechanisms were attributed to the high anthocyanin content of the berries.

When it comes to brain health, increased consumption of berries leads to higher levels of dietary flavonoids (in particular, flavones, flavanones, and anthocyanins), which have been associated with a decrease in subjective cognitive decline. In addition to berries, other flavonoid-rich foods (oranges, grapefruits, citrus juices, apples, pears, celery, peppers, and bananas) were shown to lower the odds of cognitive decline as well.

As you will learn in chapter 5, a key factor in supporting longevity is to keep *Candida albicans* at bay. One breed of strawberry, the Clery strawberry, has been shown to have anti-candida activity. These particular strawberries have also been shown to inhibit enzymes involved in the onset of diabetes, neurodegenerative diseases, and other chronic diseases. This activity likely extends to all strawberries; however, further research will be needed to confirm this.

Another dietary antioxidant, *fisetin*, found in strawberries, apples, onions, and other plant sources, has attracted interest in preventing cancer via multiple pathways. These mechanisms include a reduction in reactive oxygen species, cell cycle alteration, initiation of apoptosis, and activation of the autophagy signaling pathway. In our introduction to plant foods, we discussed the activation of sirtuins and their ability to delay cellular senescence (see page 39). Fisetin has also been shown to activate sirtuins.

Finally, in addition to the high polyphenol content of berries, blueberries, raspberries, and strawberries, they are some of the highest plant food sources of biotin (vitamin B7), which we discuss in detail on page 178.

The Coffee Cherry: More than a Wake-Up Call

Like the coconut, the coffee cherry and its seeds are technically a drupe fruit. And no, it's not a cherry that you eat with your morning coffee. Coffee cherries are the fruits that grow on the coffee plant. (The seed inside the coffee cherry is what we call a coffee bean.) The coffee cherry is considered a superfood because it's rich in vitamin B2 and magnesium, and because coffee cherries are filled with antioxidants and powerful polyphenols like chlorogenic acid and anthocyanin.

Among other benefits, the procyanidin and polyphenol content of coffee fruit can protect your brain from dementia and Alzheimer's disease because it raises your levels of brain-derived neurotrophic factor, a protein that protects your brain cells from damage and improves brain function. Another powerhouse antioxidant, chlorogenic acid, is found not only in coffee cherries but in coffee extracts as well. Studies have linked it to potentially decreasing blood pressure, which means coffee may lower your risk of heart disease and stroke. Chlorogenic acid has also been associated with reduced inflammation, mitochondrial health, and general longevity. Finally, some exciting early animal studies show that coffee fruit may have anticancer effects, especially when it comes to liver and endometrial cancer.

One of Nature's Top Longevity Promoters: Pomegranates

Pomegranates are one of the oldest known edible fruits and easily one of nature's best longevity foods. The primary edible portion of pomegranate fruit is called the *aril*, which consists of the plant's seed and the surrounding fruit. Most consumers consider the peel and the rest of the fruit inedible, though pomegranate juice can be extracted from the entire fruit. Fresh pomegranates are a great source of nutrients, as a 100-gram portion of this food (only 83 calories) provides:

- Vitamin C: 17 percent of the DV
- Folate: 10 percent of the DV

- Vitamin K: 21 percent of the DV
- Copper: 8 percent of the DV

While pomegranate juice is less nutritionally dense in vitamins and minerals than its aril, both are rich sources of the phytochemicals primarily responsible for pomegranate's many longevity benefits.

The authors of a 2024 paper summarize the many benefits of this delicious fruit in their title: "Pomegranates: A Nutritional and Medicinal Powerhouse." Here, the researchers synthesized evidence-based studies to examine the proven health benefits of pomegranates and found associations between consuming pomegranates and lower risks of developing high blood pressure, heart disease, inflammation, infections, and cancer because they're so rich in antioxidants. In addition, a wide variety of studies with people who have type 2 diabetes demonstrate that pomegranates can improve lipid profiles, reduce levels of fasting blood sugar, lower inflammation, and more.

CHAPTER SIX

The Mighty Mushroom

K aren was diagnosed with cervical cancer when she was 15 years old. At 47, she had surgery to remove one of her kidneys after being told she had kidney cancer. More recently, she has undergone surgery and treatment for breast cancer.

"I figure it's my body's way of saying, 'We're just going to try out all the cancers and see if you're going to die from any of them,'" she says with a laugh. "Then I don't die."

Karen feels lucky: Her cancers were caught early enough to cure. Now in her early 60s, she's still leading an active life and working full-time. She attributes this to her Paleo lifestyle.

The first person to describe Paleo nutrition to Karen was a yoga teacher who worked at the University of Colorado and knew of Dr. Cordain's research.

"My teacher thought it was absolutely the thing that made the most sense," she says. "This surprised me. Up until then, I thought going Paleo meant eating turkey legs or some other meat and not much else. Certainly not a typical yogi diet. But the Paleo Diet includes a lot of veggies, a proper amount of protein, and a little fruit."

Unlike many who ease their way into a Paleo lifestyle, Karen did it overnight, emptying her shelves of cans and boxes of processed food and restocking her kitchen with vegetables and natural grass-fed meat. She also learned how to make Paleo appetizers and desserts fit for a party, like her signature chocolate mousse (the secret ingredient is avocados) and a Paleo version of Reese's Peanut Butter Cups.

"I can modify any recipe to make it Paleo," she says. "It's all about finding the right ingredients."

For Karen, the most immediate consequence of going on a Paleo Diet surprised her: She lost 18 pounds, though she hadn't considered herself overweight and that was never her goal. She'd had a cholesterol problem for 20 years and took medication for it, but eating Paleo also improved her blood lipid profile to the point where she was able to stop the cholesterol medication.

In addition, Karen started sleeping better and had more energy overall. "Once I started eating Paleo, I experienced this overall feeling of well-being that I'd never had before," she says.

Among Karen's favorite foods these days are mushrooms, especially cremini and button mushrooms. "I make mushroom soup and add mushrooms to lots of different dishes for extra texture and flavor," she says.

As it turns out, adding more mushrooms for flavor means Karen is also getting additional nutritional benefits that contribute to her vitality. Mushrooms, long overlooked in American cuisine, aren't just delicious. They also have the power to help prevent many diseases of aging and may be one of our most accessible longevity foods.

We've Been Foraging Mushrooms for Millennia

In 1903, when archaeologists excavated El Mirón Cave in northern Spain, they discovered not only cave paintings done during the Upper Paleolithic era, but also the skeleton of a woman who died during that time, about 18,700 years ago. Because her bones were coated with red ochre, they fondly called her the "Red Lady."

The Red Lady has been a treasure trove of information about our ancestors. One of the most recent discoveries revealed that humans included mushrooms in their diets during the time the Red Lady was alive. In a 2015 study conducted by a research group associated with the Max Planck Institute for Evolutionary Anthropology in Leipzig, Germany, an examination of dental calculus found on the Red Lady's teeth showed that she had eaten mushrooms, giving us the earliest known evidence that our human ancestors consumed mushrooms as food.

Of course, there is also evidence from more recent historical records that people have long relied on mushrooms for nutrition. In ancient Greece, warriors consumed mushrooms to give them extra strength in battles, and the Chinese have prized the medicinal value of mushrooms for centuries. In Europe, people have long valued wild mushrooms as delicacies, especially porcinis, chanterelles, and oyster mushrooms. Mexican Aztecs revered the huitlacoche fungus for its flavor, and in Asia, cooks have long used mushrooms to add *umami* (a savory flavor) to a wide variety of dishes.

Until fairly recently, many Americans have given mushrooms a dietary shrug. Now, at last, the mushroom is getting the spotlight it deserves: None other than *The New York Times* named mushrooms "the ingredient of the year" in 2022.

Here in the United States, we each currently consume about 3 pounds of mushrooms a year, according to the US Department of Agriculture, and we should probably eat more. The available evidence points to a strong association between eating mushrooms and good health as we age, with studies linking mushroom consumption to a lower risk of diabetes, hypertension, heart disease, and cognitive decline.

What's in a Mushroom?

Mushrooms contain protein and fiber but are wonderfully low in calories. One cup of cremini mushrooms has a scant 15 calories, for instance, but gives you 1 gram of fiber and 2 grams of protein. You can add mushrooms for flavor to practically anything you're cooking or use them as a tasty side dish as often as you like.

Even better, mushrooms contain compounds like sterols and polysaccharides that help protect your health, along with many essential nutrients. These include vitamin B6 to help your body make red blood cells; potassium to help balance your sodium-to-potassium ratio; selenium, which helps your body make antioxidants to combat oxidative stress; and niacin, riboflavin, and pantothenic acid, all of which boost cellular energy production.

Some of the specific longevity-boosting nutrients in mushrooms include:

- Carbohydrates: Scientists have been studying the carbohydrates derived from mushrooms for their anti-inflammatory and antitumor activities, especially the monosaccharides that activate our body's cytokines, such as *interferons* and *interleukins*. These small proteins are crucial in supporting the activity of our immune cells. Glucans—one of the carbohydrates found in mushrooms— are especially potent when it comes to protecting us against carcinogens, pathogens, and toxins in the environment.
- Bioactive proteins: While mushrooms certainly don't pack as much protein as some other plant sources, they have higher levels of bioactive proteins such as lectins. If you are familiar with the Paleo Diet, you'll know to avoid cereal and legume lectins; however, mushroom lectins are different. They can bind to cell surface carbohydrates and act as antitumor warriors.
- Lipids: Mushrooms are low in fat, yet they're still a great source of essential fatty acids like linoleic acid. They are also a good source of oleic acid, a monounsaturated fatty acid. Additionally, mushrooms contain the bioactive compound ergosterol, which has demonstrated antimicrobial, antioxidant, anticancer, antidiabetic, and antineurodegenerative effects, which can help reduce the risk of many age-related diseases.

Is It Better to Eat Mushrooms Raw or Cooked?

While many people love the extra crunch raw mushrooms can add to a salad, we recommend cooking mushrooms before eating them. That's because the cell walls of mushrooms contain a fibrous polymer called *chitin*, and humans lack the chitinase enzyme to digest it. That means you won't get the same beneficial nutrients if you eat raw mushrooms as you would if you cooked them first. In addition, certain edible mushroom species might pose health concerns if eaten raw.

The Age-Defying Health Benefits of Mushrooms

From lowering your cholesterol to promoting a healthy gut, from keeping you cognitively sharp to fighting cancer, mushrooms have the power to help you live a longer, healthier life. Here are some of the potential health benefits of mushrooms in your diet.

Mushrooms improve lipid profiles

Using animal studies, scientists have shown that eating more mushrooms has the potential to improve our lipid profiles. That's because mushrooms contain compounds that block cholesterol from being absorbed and inhibit cholesterol production.

Mushrooms decrease cancer risk

When one group of researchers reviewed 17 scientific studies on cancer conducted between 1966 and 2020, the results were persuasive: Eating just two medium-size mushrooms (about 2 tablespoons) a day can lower your risk of cancer by 45 percent.

Mushrooms support a healthier immune system

Many of the macronutrients contained in mushrooms play a role in supporting our immune systems. For instance, mushrooms contain vitamin B6, which helps the body form red blood cells, and selenium, which supports the body's ability to fight against cell damage by making more antioxidant enzymes. Researchers have shown in animal studies that β-glucans in mushrooms even have the power to "train" immune cells.

Mushrooms protect brain health

Could eating more mushrooms keep you cognitively sharper as you age? The research seems to support this. A pair of wide-ranging 2024 scientific reports have concluded that adults who eat more mushrooms experience less risk of cognitive decline associated with aging than adults who don't.

Mushrooms keep telomeres healthy

You learned about the link between shortened telomeres and aging in chapter 2. As you'll discover in the next section, one of the most potentially powerful longevity benefits of eating more mushrooms is that they can help protect your body's telomeres from damage.

Two Potent Mushroom Longevity Nutrients

Two of the most powerful nutrients in mushrooms are currently in the scientific spotlight: the natural antioxidants *ergothioneine*—which our own bodies can't synthesize, and which acts as a potent protector of our telomeres—and *glutathione*. Both amino acids are natural warriors against the oxidative stress our cells suffer over time.

Mushrooms offer the highest dietary source of the amino acid ergothioneine. Ergothioneine is a powerful antioxidant in its own right. But this isn't the only way it helps longevity. It also plays a key role in preventing the potentially damaging shortening of telomeres we described in chapter 2 as an important hallmark of aging. It's such a powerful antioxidant that ergothioneine is known as the longevity vitamin in some research circles, especially when it comes to fighting the cognitive decline and mobility problems associated with growing older.

Among other things, ergothioneine also helps our bodies clear out senescent cells. As we discussed in chapter 2, senescent cells are those that have reached maturity and stopped multiplying but don't die off when they should, potentially causing damage to otherwise healthy cells.

A second powerful anti-aging component of mushrooms is glutathione. Emerging research demonstrates that glutathione promotes better cardiovascular and metabolic health as we get older by protecting living cells against toxic molecules. In one particularly exciting animal study, researchers compared young mice to older mice. Not surprisingly, they found the older mice had significant age-associated cognitive decline and brain defects, but giving the older mice glutathione supplements both improved cognition and reversed the brain defects.

Finally, glutathione may play a large role in protecting us against the cardiovascular diseases often suffered by those with type 2 diabetes. This is important because the leading cause of death among those with type 2 diabetes is heart disease—and many people with type 2 diabetes experience a glutathione deficiency. Scientists are now studying the benefits of glutathione supplements in combating diabetes-related cardiovascular disease.

Which Mushrooms Are Healthiest?

All edible mushrooms are nutrient-rich foods, but here are three of the most potent longevity mushrooms you'll likely encounter in your grocery store:

- Lion's mane mushroom: Best for promoting brain and immune system health and protecting against tumors. May also help protect against Parkinson's and Alzheimer's diseases.
- Maitake mushroom: Helps regulate blood sugar, blood pressure, and cholesterol levels, as well as boosting immunity.
- White mushroom: About 90 percent of the mushrooms consumed in the United States are white mushrooms (also called button, cremini, or portobello mushrooms, depending on their age). They contain significant quantities of the "anti-aging vitamin" ergothioneine and the powerful antioxidant glutathione, as well as the B vitamins, biotin, riboflavin, niacin, and folate. They also provide a host of important minerals. Mushrooms are a nutritional powerhouse that help support overall health.

When It Comes to Adding Flavor, Try These Mushrooms

Mushrooms are a cinch to add to your diet. Throw mushrooms into sauces, prepare a tasty side dish of mushrooms sautéed in olive oil, stir-fry them with other vegetables, add them to your eggs, or mix mushrooms into cooked lean beef or free-range chicken dishes and you'll be on your way to a healthier, longer life.

As you can see in the box above, we're in luck: The common white button mushroom is the one is the one you'll most easily find in your local grocery store, and it has some of the greatest health benefits of any edible mushroom. Still, many other delicious varieties are worth a try if you see them making their way onto the store shelves, including:

- Black trumpet: This dark-colored, cone-shaped mushroom has a rich, smoky flavor.

- Chanterelle: Shaped like a trumpet, the chanterelle has a lovely golden color and a rich, fruity smell.
- Enoki: Crunchy and long-stemmed, these mushrooms have small white caps and a mild flavor.
- King oyster: This thick-stemmed mushroom is also known as the French horn or king trumpet, and has a meaty texture.
- Lion's mane mushroom: This mushroom tastes a bit like shellfish and has a shaggy look.
- Maitake: Sometimes called hen of the woods, this mushroom is a particularly good substitute for meat because of its gamy flavor.
- Morel: Because of their short growing season and nutty flavor, morels have become highly popular and are often sold in dried form.
- Oyster: These mushrooms are well named for their fan shape and white color.
- Porcini: It's tough to find fresh porcini mushrooms in most American grocery stores, but the dried versions are delicious, with a woodsy flavor.

Are There Mushrooms We Should Avoid?

While they likely pose no threat to most people, raw or only slightly cooked shiitake mushrooms have been shown to cause a skin rash called "shiitake dermatitis" in some people. They also contain a biotin-binding avidin-like protein, meaning they can contribute to biotin deficiency. So, if you're going to consume shiitake mushrooms, you might consider having some strawberries for dessert because, as you read in chapter 5, they have a high concentration of biotin. We'll discuss avidin in more detail when we talk about eggs in chapter 12.

A little research on toxic mushrooms will lead you to realize that there are well over 100 poisonous fungus species. Mushroom poisoning occurs from the toxins that are secondary metabolites produced by the fungus and can lead to anything from slight gastrointestinal discomfort to death. Thankfully, unlike our Paleolithic ancestors you don't have to risk any trial-and-error analysis to determine which mushrooms are edible and should be part of your longevity plan.

Also known as magic mushrooms or shrooms, psilocybin mushrooms contain the psychedelic compound *psilocin*, as well as *psilocybin*, which, upon ingestion, converts to psilocin. While they historically have a cultural application as well as being used as a recreational drug, they have the potential for mushroom poisoning and even myocardial infarction. Consequently, they should not be part of your diet.

The Dark Side of Fungus: *Candida Albicans*

The popular TV show *The Last of Us* opens with two scientists being interviewed about global pandemics on a talk show in 1968. One of the scientists declares that viruses and bacteria don't scare him. What scares him is fungus. He talks about how deeply they can infect our bodies but correctly points out that most fungi can't survive in the human body because of our body temperature.

The rest of that fictional interview revolves around fungi controlling our minds, which was just an exposition to set up the future zombie apocalypse of the show. That was more fiction than science, of course, but what was interesting was that the show got the first part of that interview right.

In nature, *eukaryotic cells* (cells with a nucleus and organelles) are divided into eight major categories. Animal cells fit in the *Opisthokont* category, while plants fit in the *Archaeplastid* category. Bacteria and viruses aren't even eukaryotes, but fungi are opisthokont cells just like human cells. So, if a fungal cell could survive in the human body, it could cause some trouble—potentially worse trouble than any virus or bacteria.

This is important because there is one common fungus that can infect our bodies: *Candida albicans*. Every year, 90,000 people in the

United States are infected with *candidiasis*, more commonly called thrush. Immunocompromised patients are particularly susceptible. Oral and vulvovaginal candidiasis (VVC) are the most common infections, but candidemia can become systemic if severe enough or if the person is infected long enough. It has been associated with various inflammatory conditions, including periodontitis, inflammatory bowel disease, and skin and respiratory disorders.

More importantly, *Candida albicans* has been linked to poor aging. It can repress the insulin signaling pathway; increase age spots; and increase superoxide dismutase (SOD-3), a powerful enzyme that can protect cells from oxidative stress.

Candida albicans is commonly found in our gut microflora. The trick is to prevent it from infecting other parts of our bodies. We can do this by keeping our guts healthy and averting an overgrowth of candida. A recent review of candida provided several suggestions, including eating *diallyl disulfides* (DADS), which is a garlic extract; keeping our immune systems strong; consuming herbal extracts with antifungal properties; using regular pre- and probiotics for gut health; keeping blood glucose levels down; and avoiding smoking. Taking *Trachyspermom ammi* and *tryptophan* can also help. Finally, be careful of broad-spectrum antibiotics, which can allow candida to flourish.

CHAPTER SEVEN

Add Age-Defying Herbs and Spices to Your Plate

Few people embrace the health benefits of herbs and spices more than Crystal, who freely admits she had a "garbage diet for the first twenty-two years of my life, subsisting on meat, bread, sugar, and dairy." She had been dealing with migraine headaches and digestive issues for years but figured that was "my lot in life."

Then, in her early 20s, Crystal developed Hashimoto's disease, an autoimmune disorder that affects the thyroid gland. A few years later she moved to Portland, Oregon. "It was during all of the crazy pandemic lockdowns and riots," she says, "plus all of Oregon was on fire. It seemed very apocalyptic." That, combined with working full-time, plus 30 hours weekly of trade school, a bad diet, and lack of sleep put her under constant stress. "I'm sure that all of those factors combined into a perfect storm that made my immune system inflamed at all times."

During the pandemic, Crystal was diagnosed with ocular rosacea, a type of inflammation that causes itchy, burning eyes. She was in so much pain that sometimes all she could do was lie in the dark and keep her eyes closed. "Doctors said to use eye drops and warm compresses, but nothing helped. I started to feel that if I had to live the rest of my life like this, I'd become suicidal."

At last, Crystal went to an integrative eye specialist who asked about her diet, then scanned her for carotenoid levels and told her they were too low. "You're going to have to start eating more fruits and vegetables," the specialist advised.

Not long after that, Crystal read about the Paleo Diet. "I ate more grains than anybody in the world, and I decided I needed to find out why the Paleo Diet recommended getting rid of the grains in your diet," she says. The deeper she dug into the Paleo Diet research, the more convinced she became that the science behind it made sense. "I figured I had nothing to lose, so in 2021 I cold-turkeyed it and got rid of sugar, bread, dairy, and processed foods." She started making veggie and fruit smoothies and bought only salmon and grass-fed meats.

For the first two weeks, "I felt sick," Crystal admits, "but I've read that a lot of people have that experience because your immune system is detoxifying." She stuck with her new regime, however, and gradually began to normalize. About three months into her Paleo lifestyle, she was walking through the grocery store and stopped halfway through her shopping, shocked by how good she felt.

"Oh my God, I felt amazing," she says. "It stunned me. All my life, I'd had stomach pains and thought that it was a normal thing to be sick to my stomach. Everybody in my family gets migraines, so I thought that was normal, too. But now my stomach issues have gone away completely, and I have only a couple of migraines a year." Her ocular rosacea is much improved as well, and the ovarian cysts that had plagued her for years have disappeared.

Crystal has also started adding herbs and spices to her daily regime through smoothies, teas, and ingredients in her meals. "Turmeric and ginger both help with inflammation, and black cumin seeds help with Hashimoto's," she reports, "and I've found that holy basil helps lower my stress and improves my acne." Crystal adds that maqui berry helps greatly with her dry eyes, which isn't surprising since it's "highest in antioxidant activity out of any other fruit," she says. "The Paleo Diet has totally changed my way of thinking. Clearly, your body can often heal itself as long as you're getting the nutrients you need."

You probably already use herbs and spices to flavor your foods—a pinch of basil here, a quarter teaspoon of thyme there, maybe a cup of herbal tea after dinner—as if herbs and spices are complements to the "real" food. In reality, herbs and spices are as important as any food we consume. They are plant foods, and plants provide powerful nutritional benefits. The right plant foods are packed with longevity nutrients such as flavonoids, many antioxidants, phytochemicals, and polyphenols as well as vitamins and minerals. But when you add herbs and spices to your daily diet, you're upping your intake of health-boosting bioactive compounds.

Why Herbs and Spices?

Certain herbs and spices have far and away the highest concentrations of polyphenols (peppermint and oregano) and antioxidants (cinnamon and spearmint). Just as importantly, there are probably as many, if not more, undiscovered longevity nutrients in herbs and spices as the ones we've identified. Our ancestors understood the value of herbs and spices; they used them for centuries not only to color, flavor, and preserve food, but for their medicinal properties as well.

A great example of this is the Kawymeno tribe in South America, one of the last remaining Indigenous hunter-gatherer societies left on Earth. Since they live in a tropical region, their diet is rich in fruit and hunted animal food. While most have probably never heard the term "phytochemical," they seem to have an innate ability to "smell" when the phytochemical content in the indigenous fruit is strong. Their fruits are available year-round, but they prefer to eat each type of fruit only when they can sense the phytochemical content is at its peak. Researchers studying the tribe have theorized that this has given them a natural ability to maximize the medicinal value of the foods around them.

We've lost our ability to sense the nutrients in fruit, but rest assured that herbs and spices come pre-packed with many of the most important longevity nutrients.

What's the Difference Between Herbs and Spices?

While many people use the words "herbs" and "spices" interchangeably, an herb is the green, leafy part of a plant, like basil or parsley, while spices are derived from a plant's root, seed, fruit, flower, or stem (or even tree bark). We most often consume herbs as fresh greens, while spices are almost always dried. Any way you add them to your diet, though, it's increasingly evident that "spices and herbs are the treasure house of useful bioactive compounds," as researchers reported in a 2022 paper reviewing the health benefits of phenolics derived from dietary spices.

As they point out, many phenolic compounds in herbs and spices, as in other plant-derived foods, offer us so many health benefits that they should be considered natural therapeutic agents. Even better, because we ingest them as foods, the valuable phenolic compounds in herbs and spices reach our intestines in an intact form, followed by enzymatic digestion and fermentation in the colon—all of which means they're more readily absorbed by body tissues and can go straight to work in fighting infections and diseases.

Today's nutrition science is still in its infancy (or maybe its toddler years) when it comes to fully understanding the impact that individual herbs and spices have on health and longevity, but there is no doubt in our minds that they should be included as part of a nutritious Paleo lifestyle to support long-term health.

Many researchers are now looking at the value of phytochemicals found in plant food as natural medicinals. The most current research demonstrates that the high concentrations of phytonutrients and other bioactive compounds in herbs and spices can strengthen immune defenses, leading to decreased health risks and quicker recovery times from disease. They can also reduce the effects of pro-inflammatory cytokines that are associated with pain and ramp up the risk of chronic, life-threatening conditions like heart disease, hypertension, type 2 diabetes, painful joints, Alzheimer's, cancer, and even the worst effects of COVID-19, which are characterized by what scientists call a "cytokine storm."

We'll drill down on research regarding specific top longevity herbs and spices later in this chapter, but for now, we'll just say that many of them are rich in polyphenols. We discussed the value of polyphenols in our introduction to chapter 2, so you already know they act as antioxidants fighting the oxidative stress that serves as one of the top causes of cellular aging over time. Because diabetes and oxidative stress are inextricably connected, causing your insulin and glucose levels to go haywire, researchers are now exploring the value of phenols and polyphenols from spices to actively interrupt glucose metabolism signaling and regulate the absorption of glucose, which can lead to a more balanced sugar level.

And, when it comes to battling cancer, researchers are looking at the ability of certain polyphenols to interrupt the cell proliferation that serves as cancer's hallmark. Adding particular spices and herbs to your diet may contribute to lowering your risk for those conditions.

Your immunity, too, might be much improved by adding herbs and spices to your diet, since maintaining your immune system's healthy functions calls for a rich supply of nutrients. In one 2020 research study devoted to examining the impact of nutrient deficiencies on people's health during the COVID-19 pandemic, for example, researchers discovered that adding herbs and spices to a balanced, diverse diet supported better immune responses. These researchers noted the powerful disease-fighting herbs in the *Lamiaceae* family in particular, like basil and spearmint, as well as spices like clove, ginger, and turmeric for their antiviral and antibacterial properties.

Polyphenolics and Antioxidants in Herbs and Spices

	Total Polyphenols mg/100 g		Antioxidants mg/100 g
Peppermint	11,960	Cinnamon	9,070
Mexican oregano	2,319	Spearmint	6,575
Celery seed	2,094	Basil	4,317
Sage	1,207	Marjoram	3,846
Rosemary	1,018	Sage	2,920
Spearmint	956	Caraway	2,913
Basil	322	Rosemary	2,519
Caraway	33	Peppermint	980
Cinnamon	27		
Marjoram	23		

Add Spice and Herbs to Your Life

Herbs and spices have long been used in traditional Asian medicines for their therapeutic effects, and today's scientists are exploring the most effective ways to add herbs and spices to our daily menu, boosting the nutritional value of every meal and beverage so we can strengthen our immune systems and combat chronic diseases of aging. For instance, green tea, which is rich in polyphenols, is now routinely added to smoothies and desserts, while pro skateboarder Tony Hawk is currently pushing the use of turmeric supplements to fight inflammation and joint pain on TV. Remember, however, that while a supplement may give you one nutrient that you need, you'll probably be missing out on the hundreds of longevity nutrients you're not aware of by skipping out on eating the entire herb.

We could devote an entire book to detailing the benefits of various herbs and spices, but in this chapter we'll focus on our top contenders when it comes to preventing or lessening the most common diseases of aging.

Basil

Basil has a rich culinary history in many countries around the world. In recent years science has confirmed its health benefits, particularly as a potent source of polyphenols and flavonoids. Researchers have confirmed the beneficial antibacterial properties of basil, for example, which is of special interest because the medical community is concerned about the rise of antibiotic resistance. Basil has also been shown to help prevent blood clotting, and other studies have suggested that basil might be beneficial in protecting against Alzheimer's and other neurodegenerative disorders. Animal studies demonstrate that the compounds in basil can lower blood pressure and lipid levels—even if the compounds are inhaled rather than consumed.

Berberine

Berberine is a *yellow alkaloid* (an organic compound containing at least one nitrogen atom) found in plants like tree turmeric, goldenseal, *Phellodendron*, and European barberry. It's somewhat bitter tasting but commonly used as an extract in clinical practice because of its proven health benefits. In examining 11 meta-analyses from 235 different papers published between 2013 and 2022, researchers reported that berberine has a positive impact on reducing blood glucose levels and lipid levels, lowering inflammation markers, and more. When it comes to fighting harmful bacteria, berberine has demonstrable effects against various bacteria, protozoa, and fungal infections, and can help modulate a healthy gut microbiome. Berberine also has proven neuroprotective effects against cognitive disorders associated with aging.

Black pepper

One of the oldest and most popular spices, black pepper is derived from the seeds of a tropical evergreen plant originally from the Malabar Coast of India and is now grown in many different countries. The most

active—and useful—compound in black pepper is *piperine*, a plant alkaloid that has been shown in various research studies to protect against
cancer. In particular, researchers have shown that piperine can effectively
inhibit the growth of breast cancer and pancreatic cancer stem cells. Piperine also has anticonvulsant effects and might be useful in treating pain
and epilepsy.

Cayenne pepper

If you like spicy food, you're probably already familiar with cayenne
pepper. Originally from Central and South America, cayenne peppers
are now grown in tropical climates worldwide. The spice—usually consumed as a dried powder—comes from the long, thin, bright red chili
pepper and is part of the nightshade (*solanaceae*) family. It's also related
to sweet bell peppers, jalapeños, poblanos, and serranos. Cayenne pepper has been used for centuries for medicinal purposes in Eastern and
Ayurvedic traditions, typically for digestion and circulation issues. Both
fresh and dried cayenne peppers are packed with beneficial antioxidants
and nutrients. Cayenne peppers are also rich in capsaicin—the chemical
that gives these peppers a distinctive burning sensation on the tongue—
which provides some remarkable health benefits.

Most notably, capsaicin can block pain messages from your nerves.
When you apply it topically, capsaicin blocks substance P, a chemical
messenger that tells your brain, "This hurts." For this reason, capsaicin
is often used in creams or patches to treat neuralgia in older people with
rheumatoid arthritis, osteoarthritis, or other joint pain. It can also reduce
itching and inflammation for people with psoriasis, and it can stimulate
the stomach to produce more digestive fluids, which aids digestion and
helps maintain a healthy gut biome. Animal studies have shown that
consuming capsaicin helps prevent the risk of developing metabolic disease, too. And, although the research is in its early stages, scientists are
exploring capsaicin's potential to slow the growth of cancer cells or even
kill them.

Perhaps even more pertinent to this book are studies showing an association between spicy food intake and longevity. Put simply, people who regularly eat chili peppers appear to live longer and stay healthier than those who don't. For instance, a study in the United States with 16,179 adults and a 23-year follow-up showed that those consuming hot chili peppers experienced a 12 percent reduction in total mortality rate. Of course, this is only an association and leaves a lot of questions: Do spices change our physiological conditions, and that's what reduces our mortality rate? Do people who love spicy food share something about their lifestyles or physiology that might lead them to live longer? Or are there components in hot chili peppers that are actually responsible for helping people celebrate more birthdays? All of these questions demand further study before they can be answered.

Cloves

It's always easy to tell when a beverage or food is spiced with cloves because of the distinctive fragrance and flavor. Derived from the dried flowers of the clove tree, cloves can be used whole or ground and are a favorite spice for curries, baked goods, teas, and Chinese food. As for health benefits, there are many. For instance, cloves are rich in manganese, a mineral that acts as an antioxidant and can help boost the body's ability to make hormones and heal broken bones. Cloves are also rich in vitamin K, potassium—good for keeping our salt levels in check, as we learned earlier—and eugenol, another powerful antioxidant that has been linked to reduced inflammation, potentially lowering your risk of arthritis and heart disease.

Ginger

Closely related to turmeric and cardamom, ginger belongs to the *Zingiberaceae* family and is harvested from a flowering plant originally grown in Southeast Asia. We commonly use the spice derived from the underground part of the stem and may consume it in fresh, dried, or powdered forms or as an oil. The plant's most important bioactive compound is gingerol; traditional medicine practitioners have relied on ginger for centuries to treat patients with colds and flu, help lessen nausea, or ease digestive problems.

Today's researchers are exploring and validating ginger's therapeutic benefits. In one systematic review of 109 randomized controlled trials using ginger for clinical applications, researchers found significant evidence that ginger supported lower inflammation, decreased the risk of metabolic syndrome, and improved digestive function. And, in an umbrella review of orally consumed ginger and human health, scientists reported that ginger can have beneficial analgesic effects in people with osteoarthritis and helps patients maintain a healthier glycemic blood level. In this same report, the researchers also noted that ginger was associated with improving metabolic conditions and supporting weight loss while lessening gastrointestinal issues, among other things—issues that most commonly affect people in the second half of life.

Ginseng

Probably few herbs are as popular in the United States today as ginseng. The American ginseng plant has umbrella-shaped, yellowish-green flowers and isn't ready for use until it's about six years old. Consumable products are typically made from the ginseng root, which is light tan and looks a bit like those screaming baby Mandrake roots in the *Harry Potter* movies, and from the root hairs. The ginsenosides in both Asian and American ginseng give this herb its medicinal properties.

In traditional Chinese medicine, ginseng has been used for thousands of years for a multitude of medical purposes, including improving memory, boosting the immune system, and reducing the risk of cancer. Today's scientists are conducting studies on ginseng to confirm how it can be used to help improve the immune system, fight inflammatory diseases, support healthy liver and kidney functions, lower blood sugar in people with type 2 diabetes, and inhibit tumor growth in cancer patients. In one 2022 paper, researchers looked at the association of ginseng consumption with mortality using a large women's health study in Shanghai, China. They found that long-term ginseng use was associated with a decreased mortality risk, especially from cardiovascular disease. Their results suggest that regular ginseng consumption may support longevity. And, in another paper reviewing ginseng and health outcomes, Chinese researchers culled 19 meta-analyses from 1,233 scientific papers and concluded that ginseng intake is beneficial in lowering inflammatory markers, treating respiratory diseases, improving sexual function, and boosting energy.

Mint

Scientists are excited about the potential benefits of peppermint and menthol in treating migraine headaches. In one study using an animal model, inhaling or applying peppermint essential oil greatly reduced migraine symptoms. And, in a study in which people were given either a nasal application of peppermint oil or lidocaine (a synthetic medication) to treat headache pain, the two proved to be similarly effective in relieving headache symptoms.

When it comes to promoting health in our older years, mint is rich in antioxidants and a good source of vitamin A, which plays a critical role in long-term eye health. There is even evidence that smelling peppermint oil may produce improvements in alertness and memory.

Nutmeg and mace

Check out the spice rack of any friend's kitchen and you'll probably spot a jar of nutmeg, a spice with a nutty flavor that's used in both sweet and savory dishes as well as in teas and cocktails. This spice—which is made from the seeds of *Myristica fragrans*, a tropical evergreen tree native to Indonesia—also happens to convey powerful health and longevity benefits. Nutmeg is rich in antioxidants like cyanidins, essential oils like terpenes and phenylpropanoids, and phenolic compounds. It even offers antibacterial effects that can fight potentially harmful bacteria like *Streptococcus mutans*, a big contributor to tooth decay, and inhibits the growth of the harmful bacteria *E. coli*.

Nutmeg is now widely grown in Asia, South Africa, and the United States. The seed is a brown kernel inside an outer red aril, called the mace, and both are used as spices. In one recent overarching review of nutmeg's biological and pharmacological activities, researchers from India confirmed that clinical and experimental investigations support nutmeg's anticancer, antimicrobial, antioxidant, and antimalarial benefits, among others.

Thyme

A versatile herb with a variety of uses in the kitchen, thyme also smells good—so good that the ancient Greeks used thyme as incense. As for medicinal qualities that might help you stay healthy and vital into your 80s and 90s and beyond, studies have shown that thyme may boost immunity, lower blood pressure, prevent bacterial infections, and increase your body's ability to stop certain cancers from spreading.

In one wide-ranging review of the nutritional health benefits of wild thyme, researchers noted that studies have demonstrated thyme's therapeutic effects in a variety of arenas important to healthy aging. For instance, pre-clinical studies corroborate thyme's potential to lower inflammation, especially in irritable and inflammatory bowel disease, as well as in managing metabolic syndrome and cardiovascular health issues. And, in a study using orange thyme, researchers cataloged the herb's high antioxidant capacity and concluded it may potentially be beneficial in fighting inflammation in the body and offering neuroprotective benefits.

Turmeric and curcumin

One spice to regularly command today's health food spotlight is turmeric, a yellow spice that has been used for centuries in India as a medicinal herb and for food flavoring. Many believe turmeric might be the most powerful longevity spice available because it's rich in compounds called *curcuminoids*, phenolic compounds with validated therapeutic anticancer, anti-inflammatory, antioxidant, and neuroprotective effects. Turmeric is about 5 percent curcuminoids, the most important of which is curcumin (see below). A 3-gram dessert spoon of turmeric typically contains 30 to 90 mg of this powerful antioxidant, which can help regulate several essential factors in the metabolic pathway of lipids and lipoproteins.

Curcumin has been used for centuries in traditional Chinese and Indian Ayurvedic medicines to treat everything from liver disorders and respiratory problems to allergies and rheumatism. It's such a powerful anti-inflammatory that contemporary scientists have focused specifically on trying to understand the mechanisms and potential therapeutic impact of curcumin, typically in studies using dosages too high to consume simply by spicing your food. People seeking the benefits of turmeric and curcumin usually take supplements. When advising people to take curcumin supplements, experts suggest taking them with black pepper because curcumin doesn't absorb very well in your bloodstream, and the piperine in black pepper greatly enhances that absorption. In fact, if you check out the labels on curcumin supplements, the odds are good that the supplements will also contain piperine.

Animal studies have shown that in addition to acting as an antioxidant that reduces inflammation, curcumin can boost brain-derived neurotrophic factor, which is important in memory and learning. In addition, studies have shown that taking curcumin can reduce the amyloid plaques caused by Alzheimer's.

Researchers are also examining the link between curcumin consumption and a lower risk of heart disease, investigating the theory that this antioxidant helps improve the function of the endothelium, the lining of your blood vessels that helps regulate blood clotting, hypertension, and other disorders. In one of the most extensive reviews examining studies conducted on the effects of curcumin on metabolic syndrome, scientists published a paper in *Nutrient* magazine concluding that curcumin supplementation has a positive impact on people with metabolic disorders like polycystic ovary syndrome, metabolic syndrome, glycemic disorders, cardiovascular disease, and nonalcoholic fatty liver disease.

As a longevity-booster, scientists point to curcumin's potential to lower the level of proteins associated with the aging process. In addition, curcumin has been shown to activate sirtuins, those key "longevity proteins."

Just one warning to our endurance athletes: You need some oxidative stress from exercise to produce fitness gains. Curcumin is such a powerful antioxidant that it has been shown to reduce adaptations in athletes. If you're an endurance athlete taking curcumin, try to take it as far away from your exercise sessions as possible.

————————

After reading about the health benefits of these herbs and spices, you may be thinking, "I have all of them on my spice rack and I'm not feeling any benefits." That might be because as we started this chapter, you were just lightly sprinkling them into your food and not getting enough to truly see the benefits. Our suggestion is to find ways to increase the use of these herbs and spices in your diet. Remember that although our culture classifies herbs and spices differently than plant foods like vegetables and fruits, they're essentially the same things.

CHAPTER EIGHT

Salt

E va's happy place these days is on a surfboard. A competitive athlete all her life, she was a member of the US ski team for 12 years, earning six national championships in alpine skiing and a world championship bronze medal. She was awarded a medal of honor by the US Ski and Snowboard Hall of Fame.

"A sport like mine takes a toll," Eva says, noting her multiple knee surgeries, but she went on to earn a Masters National Championship title in Olympic weightlifting. She stopped weightlifting because of her knees and because she was at risk for more joint damage after years of intensive CrossFit training. She then had to recover from a traumatic brain injury and shattered leg when the small plane she was piloting crashed as the result of unexpected wind shear.

As Eva prepares to celebrate her 60th birthday, she credits the Paleo Diet for her ability to enjoy an active life despite her injuries. "Eating healthy foods, as well as getting good sleep and proper movement, are the biggest things you can do to heal your body," she says.

Eva had an inside track in learning about the Paleo Diet. Her father, an Olympic fencer, met Dr. Cordain at the University of Nevada

107

when her father was a doctoral student and taught Dr. Cordain's under-graduate class. The two became lifelong friends, and when Eva first decided to eliminate gluten and most dairy from her diet twenty years ago, Dr. Cordain helped support her decision by explaining the science demonstrating how a typical Western diet with too many processed foods contributes to chronic inflammation and can lead to joint pain and disease.

"Eating Paleo was a way for me to reverse the clock," says Eva, who reports that a Paleo lifestyle helped her joints stop hurting and her thinking become more focused. "It was a different world because I didn't have the same persistent aches and pains." She eats mostly good-quality protein and vegetables, "though I do allow myself an occasional bowl of ice cream or pasta for a treat. I want to maintain strength and mobility as I age. With the Paleo Diet, I have a better chance of achieving that."

The most commonly used spice in the United States is black pepper. Naturally, when people pass the pepper, they also pass the salt—a lot of salt. Many people consider salt to be a spice, but it's actually a mineral. Salt is essential to maintain homeostasis in our bodies, but physiologically speaking, there's always an optimal amount of most nutrients to ensure our health. Too much or too little of something isn't good for us. Sodium is a classic case of this. Without consuming salt, we die, but eating too much is associated with a host of diseases. The optimal amount of salt fits in a very tight range, which happens to be well below what people eat on a typical Western diet.

According to the US Food and Drug Administration's latest tally, Americans consume an average of more than 3,300 mg of sodium per day—well above the federal recommendation of less than 2,300 mg of sodium daily for teens and adults. This is also far more salt than our hunter-gatherer ancestors consumed. If we assume that the content of the minerals in the wild animals our ancestors hunted was roughly the same as in present-day cows and sheep, their daily intake of sodium would have been less than 1,000 mg per day. In other words, we're consuming at least three times more sodium than our hunter-gatherer ancestors did. Meanwhile, someone on a standard Western diet consumes far less potassium than those ancestors did because of our relatively low intake of fruit and vegetables in proportion to the rest of our diet, and as we explained before, what may be even more important than the absolute amount of salt we eat is the sodium-to-potassium ratio, which affects a host of things in our bodies, including blood pressure.

Our high consumption of salt began 5,000 to 12,000 years ago, when people began farming and discovered that salt had antimicrobial properties, which made it great for preserving food, particularly fresh meat. We don't know exactly when this practice began, but there is evidence that the Egyptians were using salt to preserve meat as early as 2000 BCE. About 1,000 years ago, salt intake in the Western world had risen to about 5,000 mg per day, and salt consumption continued rising until the introduction of refrigeration.

Of course, most of the salt you consume isn't even coming out of that shaker on your table but through processed foods. You might not even think those foods taste salty. For instance, pickles and soy sauce taste salty, but other foods that contain a lot of sodium, like pastries or cereals, taste sweet. So, it may surprise you to learn that bread is one of the biggest sources of salt in the Western diet. Many of the foods you might typically eat several times a day, like bread, can increase your sodium intake even if the individual servings aren't especially high, so it pays to read the labels of any food you consume from a package or jar. Also, keep in mind that those "gluten-free breads" may have taken the wheat out, but they're just as high in salt.

In an effort to lower the average American's high salt intake, the FDA recently asked food companies to voluntarily reduce the sodium content of their products. Since a large portion of added sodium in the average American diet comes from processed food, the idea is that this shift will help bring the average American diet down to the recommended daily allowance (RDA) of 2,300 mg of salt per day. We applaud the FDA's efforts to help Americans cut back on sodium, since a low-salt diet is a key part of the Paleo Diet. We also recognize that this is a tough challenge. Humans crave salt and will favor foods that are high in sodium. Let's dive into why that is.

Why Do We Crave Salt and Sugar?

The two foods humans crave above all else are salt and sugar and, on average, we crave them about equally. There's an evolutionary explanation for this. We do need small amounts of salt and some glucose to survive. Our bodies require sodium for almost all physiological functions, and despite some ketogenic diet misconceptions, our brains need glucose to function. They can't survive solely on ketones. If you don't eat glucose, your liver will convert ketones to glucose for the brain.

It's important to remember that we evolved during a time when we couldn't walk to the corner store and buy a salty bag of chips or a pack of candy. Our ancestors were always struggling to get enough calories and the nutrients they needed. Our bodies evolved around this scarcity, so we developed cravings for the nutrients that were critical for survival but hard to find. Conversely, if a nutrient was in abundant supply, we didn't evolve to develop a strong craving because we'd overconsume it.

So our strong craving for salt and simple sugars makes sense if they were rare in Paleolithic times. That was the magic formula—necessary but rare—for the evolution of strong cravings. It's also the only way we can explain why we crave something so bad for us in large portions. Overconsumption back then was never an issue, since salt and sugar were so rare that our ancestors necessarily kept their intake low—that is, until modern times. Driven by consumer demands, the food science industry has developed foods to appeal to these cravings, which is why you see sugar and salt as primary ingredients in most processed food products.

Talk to food industry scientists and they'll tell you that if you create a product with lots of salt, sugar, fat, and a good artificial flavor, you'll have a profitable, hyperpalatable product.

Scientists have long agreed about the dangers of overconsuming sugar—particularly processed sugar—because sugar acts as one of the main drivers of our current epidemics of obesity, metabolic disease, and diabetes. More recent research supports the idea that salt also contributes greatly to chronic diseases, including cardiovascular disease, autoimmune disease, and certain cancers. Some health advocates will say we have to learn to fight our sugar cravings, yet in the same breath, they'll insist that a high-sodium diet is healthy and our craving for salt is the proof. Below, we give you our reasons for refuting the idea that a high-salt diet is healthy.

Why do some people say a high-sodium diet is healthy?

While most influencers in Paleolithic eating were quick to recognize the dangers of consuming too much sugar, even shifting to a ketogenic lifestyle to completely eliminate it, many of these same influencers have taken a very different direction with salt, promoting a trend toward higher salt consumption. This trend grew out of some highly publicized research, specifically two studies published in 2014 showing that while people on a very high-sodium diet had much higher rates of heart disease, surprisingly, so did people on a low-sodium diet. This created a U- or J-shaped relationship, which meant that according to the studies, the healthiest people—the ones at the bottom of the "J" curve—were eating around 3,000 to 6,000 mg of sodium per day. Even on the low end, this was well above the government's recommendation of 2,300 mg of sodium daily. This has led some to believe that eating even twice the RDA of sodium would improve their health.

The problem is that these studies had two fundamental flaws that caused them to misrepresent the data. First, the researchers didn't use the gold standard of 24-hour urinary sodium measurement. Second, and more critical to understand, is that the researchers didn't control for people who already had heart disease at the start of the study. That's a serious flaw because when someone is diagnosed with heart disease, one of the first things their doctor generally recommends is cutting salt from their diets. So it wasn't a very low-sodium diet causing high rates of heart disease—it was heart disease causing people to eat a very low-sodium diet.

A research team identified this second flaw, and in 2016, they analyzed data from a larger study tracking 3,126 subjects over 20 years. This time, the researchers controlled for subjects who had been diagnosed with heart disease before the study. When they did that, the J-shaped relationship disappeared and became a straight line—the lower the sodium in the subjects' diets, the lower the risk of heart disease. In fact, the risk of all causes of death were lower. Unfortunately, there are still people in the Paleo community who are citing the original two 2014 studies and claiming that a high-sodium diet is healthier.

Supported by science, we promote a lower-sodium diet here at the Paleo Diet, and we believe the current RDA of 2,300 mg per day is at the high end of what we should consume. Fortunately, if you're eating mostly natural Paleo foods, it's nearly impossible to eat too much sodium. We've run dietary analyses of virtually every combination of Paleo foods within the plant/animal subsistence range from Dr. Cordain's research and have never been able to see sodium levels exceed the levels we're recommending. A typical modern Paleo Diet with no added salt usually falls in the 1,600 to 2,200 mg range, and even lower if you eat more fruits than vegetables.

Four Reasons the Paleo Diet Is a Lower-Sodium Diet

We have written extensively about sodium and its health implications over the past few years. Since there is so much information to comb through, here are four of our key takeaways to help you understand why we support a lower-sodium diet.

Too much sodium increases inflammation

Too much sodium can lead to many chronic diseases. The science behind how excess salt contributes to inflammation is complex, but as a quick explanation, salt collects in our cells, which causes an increase in two highly inflammatory immune cells called CD14+ macrophages and Th17 cells. Imbalances in these two cell types have been linked to almost all autoimmune diseases, heart disease, and some cancers.

Too much sodium increases the chance of heart disease

There's a straight-line relationship between sodium consumption and heart disease when you consume sodium in amounts greater than contained in natural foods. In other words, the more salt you consume, the higher your risk of heart disease. This is due in part to the inflammation mentioned above. Plus, as Dr. Cordain has written elsewhere, too much sodium can contribute to key steps in the formation of atherosclerotic plaque in our arteries that can in turn lead to heart attack and stroke.

Too much sodium can contribute to cancer

An increased risk of cancer is another potential consequence of accumulating excess sodium within our cells. It does so by damaging our DNA, increasing oxidative stress, and fundamentally impairing metabolism within the cells. Increasing the ratio of potassium to sodium in our diets can prevent many of these negative effects. That brings us to our fourth and most important point.

Increasing potassium while reducing sodium can reverse negative health effects

As we discussed in chapter 1, the ideal sodium-to-potassium ratio in our bodies should be 1:5 and even as much as 1:10. But the typical Western diet flips the ratio, with people consuming twice as much sodium as potassium or worse. Our bodies use potassium to pump sodium out of cells, which helps reverse many of the inflammatory effects detailed above. When the sodium-to-potassium ratio in our diet resets to its natural level, research shows that it can have a protective effect against cancer, reduce blood pressure, and even prevent bone loss. Our best sources of potassium are vegetables and fruit. A recent study found that a healthier sodium-to-potassium ratio was associated with fruits, vegetables, and fresh meat, while a poor ratio was associated with bread, processed meats, and butter. Keep in mind that it is nearly impossible to eat enough healthy fruits and vegetables while on a high-sodium diet and still reach a healthy ratio of 1:5 or better.

CHAPTER NINE

The Near-Magical
Properties of Olive Oil

Steve first learned about the Paleo Diet when his wife showed him an article about it. He had exercised all his life and thought of himself as healthy, he says, but "over the years, I became increasingly aware of how the food we eat can impact our health." In addition, he had developed an interest in evolution. "The Paleo Diet made so much sense to me, I went into it 100 percent."

Before choosing a Paleo lifestyle, Steve, who immigrated to Canada from Greece at age 12, had been eating "mostly Mediterranean," with an emphasis on potatoes, rice, and macaroni. On the Paleo Diet, he began losing weight "rather quickly," dropping from 180 pounds to 150.

"I became concerned about that because I lift weights and didn't want to compromise my lifting capacity," says Steve, who's 5 feet 7 inches tall. "To my complete surprise, I need not have worried; I still lifted the same weight a few months later at 135 pounds. I was shocked."

Now 69 years old, Steve says he's about 90 percent Paleo and typically eats 4 ounces of meat, chicken, or fish at each meal with about 10 ounces of vegetables. Snacks are predominantly fruit, nuts, and seeds. The main benefits of his new lifestyle haven't been weight loss, he adds, but his improved lipid profile. "My triglycerides practically disappeared, my HDL started going up, and my LDL went down," he says.

As a lab technician who was employed by a hospital for 14 years, Steve is surprised that nobody he worked with seemed motivated to change their own eating habits, "even though quite a few people I knew talked about diet and weight loss." His advice to anyone who wants to try Paleo is simple: "The Paleo Diet isn't written in stone. Pick some ideas you can make changes with and apply them to your lifestyle. Take it step by step and you'll see a lasting difference for the better in how you look and feel."

Our Paleo Ancestors Never Consumed Olive Oil, So Why Should We?

The Mediterranean diet features olive oil and the foods our friend Steve grew up eating. As we discussed in chapter 1, we disagree with many aspects of this diet, like the inclusion of grains, legumes, and dairy. However, we agree wholeheartedly with the diet's efforts to include less processed, nutrient-dense Mediterranean favorites to your plate, like vegetables, fruits, meat, fish—and olive oil. Vegetable oils were obviously not a component of any hunter-gatherer diet, simply because the technology to produce them did not exist then, but some vegetable oils provide so many health benefits that we're happy to add them to our Paleo plates. Top among these is olive oil—especially extra-virgin olive oil (EVOO)—because it's rich in bioactive phenolic compounds and monounsaturated fatty acids (MUFAs) that help protect us against diseases as we age. (We'll cover the other oils we like later in this chapter.)

Fossils from wild olive trees (*Olea europaea*) around the Mediterranean date back some 20 million years, and there is evidence of humans eating olives and using olive trees for fuel 100,000 years ago along the coast of Morocco. Humans first domesticated the fruit thousands of years ago, with olive oil being produced as early as 2500 BCE for cooking, soap, cosmetics, lamp fuel, and medicine. In ancient Greece, olive trees were considered sacred symbols of wisdom, peace, and prosperity, and you can still visit the alleged descendant of the Sacred Olive Tree in Athens today. Olive oil was used to help light the Olympic flame, and olive trees and their fruits make appearances in both the Bible and the Quran.

Producing olive oil takes several stages, starting with harvesting and cleaning the olives, then washing them to eliminate leaves, dirt, and other impurities. The clean olives are crushed into a paste through a press or a centrifuge before filtering the oil and storing it in a cool, dark place. We emphasize EVOO as the healthiest choice over more refined olive oils because it's produced without heat or chemicals, thus preserving its nutrients.

EVOO is 98 to 99 percent fatty acids, with the highest proportion (between 55 and 83 percent) of those being MUFAs such as oleic acid. The remaining 1 to 2 percent of EVOO is made up of phytosterols, tocopherols, squalene, and phenolics—up to 100 different phenolic compounds. The most important of these are the antioxidants hydroxytyrosol, oleocanthal, and oleuropein, all of which help give olive oil its potential to increase lifespan.

Why Olives Aren't Paleo but Olive Oil Is

The fruit of the olive tree is a drupe (a stone fruit) in which a hard inner seed is surrounded by a fleshy outer portion. The olive has a low sugar content (less than 6 percent) compared with other drupes (apricots, peaches, plum, etc.), which may contain 12 percent or more sugar. Olives have a high oil content (12 to 30 percent) depending on the time of year and variety of olives harvested. The olive fruit generally can't be consumed directly from the tree because it contains a strong bitter component, *oleuropein*, which can be removed or lessened in concentrations by a series of processing techniques.

All olives are typically treated in diluted lye solutions (sodium hydroxide or potassium hydroxide) to eliminate the oleuropein and transform the sugars into organic acids that aid in subsequent fermentation. Olives are then washed and placed in brine—a concentrated solution of water and salt—before canning; the brine stimulates the microbial activity for fermentation and also reduces the bitterness of the oleuropein.

In other words, to make fresh olives edible requires massive additions of salt at nearly every stage of processing. A 1,000 kcal serving of green olives would supply you with 10,730 mg of salt, and the same serving of jumbo black olives would give you 9,074 mg. The recommended daily intake of salt is 2,300 mg for adult men and women; accordingly, even modest consumption of olives gives you far too much.

Now contrast the salt concentrations in a 1,000 kcal serving of olive oil, which is 2.26 mg—or 0.02 percent of the amount found in a 1,000 kcal serving of green olives. In chapter 8, we described how too much salt in your diet can promote cardiovascular disease, cancer, autoimmunity, chronic inflammation, immune system dysfunction, and ill health. The bottom line is that processed olives are high in sodium and should be eaten very sparingly on the Paleo Diet. If you want to enjoy olives, rinse them well before serving and pair them with foods high in potassium to maintain a sodium-to-potassium ratio as close to 1:5 as possible.

How Extra-Virgin Olive Oil Can Add Years to Your Life

As we said earlier, research shows that consuming EVOO helps our bodies maintain oxidative balance, reduce inflammation, and prevent a host of age-related diseases. Scientists attribute these positive effects in part to the higher MUFA content of olive oil, particularly oleic acid, which can help support the body's immune response.

EVOO is also rich in polyphenols like carotenes, hydroxytyrosol, oleocanthal, oleuropein, and tyrosol. These powerful antioxidants are linked to treating and preventing inflammation and a slew of noncommunicable diseases, so it's no wonder that EVOO consumption is linked to lower rates of cardiovascular disease and all-cause mortality. In fact, one large cohort study in Italy involving 22,892 men and women with an average age of 52 showed that a high intake of olive oil is associated not only with a lower risk of death from cancer and cardiovascular disease, but with a lower risk of mortality from all causes. Those researchers, who published their paper in 2024, showed that people who consumed the most olive oil (over 30 g daily) had a 20 percent lower risk of all-cause mortality and a 25 percent lower risk of death from cardiovascular diseases when compared to participants with the lowest intake of olive oil (no more than 15 g daily).

Here are some of EVOO's many well-documented health and longevity benefits:

EVOO reduces inflammation

EVOO has a concentration of 284 to 711 mg/kg oleocanthal, which acts as a powerful anti-inflammatory that has been shown to slow or prevent the spread of joint-degenerative and neurodegenerative diseases. Many scientists see the potential of oleocanthal as a naturally occurring nonsteroidal anti-inflammatory drug (NSAID) that can replace manufactured NSAIDs like ibuprofen to reduce inflammation and treat or prevent degenerative joint diseases. Other researchers have linked EVOO consumption to reduced oxidative stress on our cells; for instance, one study demonstrated that 25 middle-aged participants consuming 10 to 20 g of EVOO daily significantly decreased their production of oxidative markers after eating.

EVOO helps strengthen the heart

Various randomized trials and epidemiological studies have demonstrated that adding EVOO to your diet reduces the risk of heart disease and improves cardiovascular outcomes. Researchers theorize this is because consuming EVOO is associated with reducing negative clinical biomarkers like high blood pressure and unhealthy blood lipid levels.

Compared to a low-fat diet or refined olive oil, EVOO can help lower the risk of stroke by boosting endothelial function and lowering the aggregation of platelets. Both factors are related to blood clots. In one study, 3,042 Greek men and women eating a Mediterranean diet with EVOO lowered their cholesterol levels and systolic blood pressure. It was also shown that EVOO has a lipid-lowering effect by increasing HDL capacity and promoting cholesterol efflux, as well as by lowering LDL levels.

EVOO moderates blood glucose levels and insulin sensitivity

Oleic acid, the primary fatty acid in EVOO, can help maintain healthy glucose levels in the blood. And, in a 2024 meta-analysis of randomized clinical trials, researchers examined 33 trials involving 2,020 participants and concluded that adding EVOO to the diet can have a positive effect on maintaining healthy blood insulin levels. This is important because insulin helps move glucose from the blood into cells that metabolize sugar into energy.

EVOO protects against cancer

The fatty acids in olive oil can help tame the body's production of prostaglandins, possibly inhibiting cancerous tumors from developing and slowing their growth. Likewise, certain polyphenols in olive oil, like hydroxytyrosol and oleuropein, support the body's synthesis of cytokines, white blood cells, and other factors that support the immune system. Laboratory studies have also shown that oleuropein inhibits the growth of cancer cells and can cause those cells to die.

EVOO boosts brain health

Parkinson's, Alzheimer's, and other neurological diseases associated with aging share a certain pathology that involves inflammation, oxidative stress on cells, and abnormal protein aggregation, among other things. The polyphenols in EVOO help protect brain health; for instance, studies have shown that EVOO polyphenols can modify a cellular mechanism at fault for Parkinson's disease. In addition, olive oil is being studied as a tool to treat and even cure multiple sclerosis, a disease of the central nervous system that causes inflammation, blood-brain barrier breakdown, and demyelination. Rodent studies highlight how orally administering EVOO or its specific phenolic compounds can reduce the accumulation of plaque deposits in the brain, which can help improve memory and cognition.

EVOO keeps your gut healthy

Many recent studies have demonstrated that EVOO consumption has a positive effect on gut health by reducing the population of pathogenic bacteria, supporting the growth of healthy bacteria, and increasing the body's production of short-chain fatty acids that help reduce inflammation. EVOO can also support the health of the mucus lining of the intestines by promoting the production of immunoglobulin A, an important antibody.

Olive Oil for Better Skin

The outer layer of our skin consists of 30 to 40 layers of dead skin cells that act as a protective barrier for the body. Embedded within these layers are lipids. Very little that comes into contact with the skin can penetrate it, other than some fatty acids. One of these fatty acids is oleic acid, which is found in high concentrations in olive oil. Olive oil is also high in polyphenolic compounds, and when olive oil is put on the skin, oleic acid can penetrate the barrier and pull these compounds in with it. These compounds have strong antioxidant properties and can attenuate the wrinkling process.

EVOO activates the body's own natural defenses

While it is important to consume antioxidants to reduce reactive oxygen species (ROS) in the body, it has been shown that activating the body's natural antioxidant defense mechanisms is the best way to keep ROS low and help longevity. One of the most powerful natural mechanisms in our bodies is the transcription factor Nrf2, which we introduced in chapter 3 as one of the most important proteins in regulating our health.

Which Plant-Based Oils Are Healthiest?

It wasn't until the beginning of the 20th century, with the advent of mechanical extraction processes, that vegetable oils contributed significantly to the Western diet. Today, vegetable oils used in cooking, salad dressings, margarine, shortening, and processed foods supply 17.6 percent of the total daily energy intake in the US diet.

The enormous infusion of vegetable oils into the Western diet started in the early 1900s and represents the greatest single factor responsible for elevating the ratio of dietary omega-6 to omega-3 to its current and unhealthful value of 20:1 or more—a ratio that can promote inflammation and chronic disease. Fortunately, some plant-based oils promote healthy aging by supporting the balance of good fats in your diet. These include flaxseed, walnut, olive, macadamia, coconut, and avocado oils.

When you're choosing which oil to use, one of the biggest health factors to consider is the smoke point, which is determined by the fatty acid composition. When oils get so hot that they start smoking, this means that they've reached their stability point and begin to decompose, releasing free radicals along with toxic fumes. Oils are often refined to raise their smoke point through heating, neutralization, filtering, and processing with chemicals and bleaching agents. These modifications are why these oils can damage your health—even though they may come from healthy sources in their pure state. While this section is about the best plant-based oils to use for health and convenience, we always support using pure animal fats, such as lard, tallow, duck fat, and chicken fat. These fats can withstand very high temperatures without oxidizing and provide a healthy and natural fatty acid composition.

Olive oil is our top choice among plant-based oils, but if you don't have it on hand, here are the other healthy plant-based oils we include on the Paleo Diet. Please note that flaxseed and walnut oils should never be used for cooking because they contain high concentrations of poly-unsaturated fats. This makes them fragile and susceptible to degradation when heated. The most stable oil to use for cooking is coconut oil because of its high concentration of saturated fats. Here's how you can best use each cooking oil:

Flaxseed oil

While flaxseed oil has healthy omega-3 fatty acids, which you already know can help battle chronic inflammation and the risk of heart disease, use it only in salads or in recipes that are served cold or at room temperature because its low smoke point means it can break down at high temperatures.

Walnut oil

Walnut oil possesses many antioxidants, including ellagic acid, which research suggests prevents the buildup of plaque in the arteries and supports bone health. It's a great source of omega-3 fatty acids. Although the refined version is often labeled safe for high-heat cooking, like flaxseed oil it is best not to heat it to high temperatures. Not only will the omega-3s be damaged, but the oil will also develop a bitter taste. The unrefined version has a smoke point of 320°F, but there are better options even for low-heat cooking, so save your walnut oil to drizzle on salads.

Macadamia nut oil

Macadamia nut oil is higher in monounsaturated fats than olive oil and provides a low level of omega-6 fats. It is also high in phytochemicals like squalene, tocotrienols, and tocopherols that protect against oxidation. Macadamia nut oil has been shown to improve the biomarkers of oxidative stress and inflammation and to reduce the risk factors for coronary artery disease. With a smoke point of around 400°F, macadamia oil can be used for almost any dish, whether you're grilling, sautéing, or stir-frying.

Coconut oil

Coconut oil is more than 90 percent saturated fat. Specifically, it's high in medium-chain triglycerides (MCTs). MCTs do not require bile acids for digestion, which makes them easy to digest and available immediately as an energy source. Coconut oil is also rich in lauric acid, a fatty acid found in human breast milk that has antifungal, antibacterial, and antiviral properties. Unrefined coconut oil, which has not been bleached or filtered to remove impurities or natural flavors, has a smoke point of between 350° and 380°F. You can use coconut oil as a replacement in any recipe that calls for butter, such as coating a whole chicken before roasting. We use it regularly to sauté vegetables, like kale or onions, as well as to grease the pan before cooking eggs.

Avocado oil

Cold-pressing avocados retains their high concentrations of vitamin E and chlorophyll, which gives the oil a green tint. Research shows that consuming avocado oil enhances carotenoid absorption from vegetables and can decrease your risk of coronary artery disease. Similar to olive oil, avocado oil has a higher omega 6:3 ratio (13.1:1) than flaxseed, walnut, and macadamia nut oils. Unrefined avocado oil has an exceptionally high smoke point of 482°F and can be used in any high-heat cooking. Use this instead of canola or other vegetable oils.

CHAPTER TEN

Chocolate for Healthier
Hearts and Minds

When Inés had her fourth child after age 40, "all of my friends thought I was crazy," she says. Yet, medical tests demonstrated that she was as healthy as a 25-year-old woman. Inés credits the Paleo Diet for being able to keep up with her work as a physicist and happily running around after her children. "If you take care of your body, your body will take care of you," she says.

Inés didn't always enjoy such abundant energy. Her health problems began as a university student in 2001 after she broke her leg and could no longer exercise. That sedentary lifestyle, plus her fast-food diet and even faster-paced university schedule, led to obesity in her 20s. Meanwhile, her husband's weight also skyrocketed, and he developed nonalcoholic fatty liver disease.

Her doctor put Inés on a "typical 1,200-calorie diet," but eating less caused her blood pressure to plummet and she felt faint. "My doctor told me I couldn't diet anymore," she says. "I felt trapped in my body and had no energy to play with my kids."

Then, in 2013, her husband discovered the ECCO (Evolution, Complexity, and Cognition) multidisciplinary research group and began reading about the Paleolithic model of evolutionary well-being. This led him to Dr. Cordain's books. "Everything clicked for him," Inés says, "but I was reluctant to try that lifestyle."

Her hesitance stemmed from their Spanish cultural background, she explains. They'd always eaten a Mediterranean diet with bread at every meal and plenty of grains and legumes, but she finally agreed to try Paleo for a month. "The more we read about Paleo, the more we understood we were starving our bodies because the foods we were eating weren't very nutritious," she says.

One month of eating Paleo turned into six, and Inés found herself at a healthy weight for the first time in 20 years. More importantly, "I felt so energized," she says. "I slept well, woke up happy and relaxed, and could run around with my kids. The difference was completely mind-blowing." Their doctor couldn't believe the difference at their next physicals and wanted to know what Inés and her husband had done to reach such healthy levels on their blood panels.

These days, instead of a typical Spanish breakfast of coffee with toast and cereal, Inés is more likely to make eggs. Dinner is apt to be salmon or chicken with vegetables and the occasional sweet potato. "One thing I love about the Paleo Diet is that you're never craving food," she says. "You feel full from giving your body the proper combination of nutrients."

As Inés discovered, it's easy to beat back cravings and feel satisfied on the Paleo Diet because you're filling up on the nutrient-dense foods your body needs. Even better, many foods we include on the Paleo Diet are deliciously surprising—like dark chocolate. We never included chocolate on our previous lists of Paleo foods, but the latest science is solid when it comes to showing how chocolate's unique bioactive compounds help promote longevity—especially when it comes to supporting long-term heart and brain health. Today's researchers are exploring the association between consuming chocolate and a decreased risk of many chronic diseases associated with aging, including cancer, cardiovascular disease, cognitive issues, diabetes, gut health, metabolic disorders, and osteoporosis.

Not Just Any Chocolate

Just keep in mind that we're talking about dark chocolate—very dark chocolate—to get the most health benefits. The inexpensive milk chocolate you find in the candy aisle of most grocery stores has more sugar, milk, and other ingredients in it than actual cacao. A quick explanation here: We're going to use both the terms "cacao" and "cocoa" throughout this chapter. While the terms are often used interchangeably, cacao refers to the seeds from which cocoa and chocolate are made. Cocoa is just the powder form of roasted cacao seeds. As you'll learn in this chapter, it's the cacao that gives chocolate its magical longevity properties.

The first people to recognize the benefits of consuming chocolate were the Olmecs of Central America some 3,900 years ago. The Mayans cultivated the cacao tree to create a chocolate drink made by mixing cacao with hot water and sweetening it with spices, and the Aztecs relied on chocolate for ceremonies and medicinal purposes.

Cacao first appeared in Europe in 1528, when the Spanish conquistador Hernán Cortés brought samples of it to King Charles of Spain. Thus began the spread of chocolate to Europe and elsewhere. The Swedish scientist Carl Linnaeus named the plant *Theobromo cacao*, from the Latin name *theobroma* ("Food of the Gods"). Manuscripts published between the 16th and 18th centuries reveal that Europeans relied on chocolate for over 100 medicinal uses, including stimulating the nervous system and improving digestion and elimination. Furthermore, chocolate was considered such a powerful aphrodisiac that theologians believed monks wouldn't be able to stay abstinent if they ingested it, and many in Europe believed cultural morals were slipping when chocolate houses opened in Europe. None of these scandalous rumors kept chocolate from becoming popular. The 2024 revenue for chocolate confectionery in the United States hit $23.21 billion and is expected to continue growing.

Research on the longevity benefits of chocolate is still new, but we have plenty of anecdotal evidence from centenarians and supercentenarians supporting the notion that life is better, and longer, with chocolate. For instance, in a 2010 review of the planet's longest-living humans (115+ years), researchers noted that "three of the longest-lived women were all great consumers of chocolate," including Jeanne Calment, the longest-living human (she lived to 122), who claimed to eat a kilogram of chocolate every week.

In 2005, William Baldwin, senior contributor for *Forbes*, had the opportunity to interview Albert H. Gordon, who took over in 1931 as chairman for the Wall Street firm Kidder, Peabody & Co. Gordon celebrated his 104th birthday that year, and interviewer Baldwin asked him about the secrets to his health and longevity. Some of Gordon's regimen is standard fare: He didn't smoke, drink much alcohol, or salt his food. He also exercised regularly. Regarding chocolate, Baldwin wrote of Gordon, "He consumes prodigious quantities of dark Côte d'Or chocolate, high in cocoa solids, low in sugar."

According to a 2018 article in *The Chicago Tribune*, Eunice Modlin, who had just celebrated her 102nd birthday, attributed her long life to chocolate and naps. Later that same year, *The New York Times* wrote, "As one of the exceedingly rare members of her species to live beyond age 110, Goldie Michelson had divulged her secrets to longevity countless times before dying last year at 113 years, 335 days. "Morning walks and chocolate," the Worcester, Massachusetts, resident and onetime oldest living American told the steady stream of inquisitors who asked the secret to her longevity.

While these are only anecdotes, plenty of solid science supports the theory that chocolate has anti-aging benefits—especially if you reach for dark chocolate instead of the milk or white varieties.

Health Benefits of Chocolate Are Linked to Production

Turning the oblong fruit pods growing on the bark of the cacao tree into an edible food is a complex process. There can be as many as 50 seeds inside the cacao fruit's shell. Workers crack open the fruit to scoop out the seeds and let them drain for up to 10 days. This phase is a time when the seeds are undergoing natural fermentation, which, as we'll explain in a minute, is a critical part of what gives cacao its health benefits. During this controlled activity when microbes ferment the seeds, the bitter cacao beans begin producing the flavors we associate with chocolate.

The quality and flavor of chocolate are dependent both on the region the beans originate from and on the production process they undergo after harvest. Chocolate is typically classified as dark, milk, or white. Dark chocolate is made primarily from cocoa solids, cocoa butter, and a small amount of sugar; while milk chocolate has more sugar and also milk powder or condensed milk added to give it a milder taste. White chocolate has no cocoa solids at all, which means it's creamy and sweet on the tongue but devoid of most of the beneficial phenols. That's why we recommend eating only dark chocolate with a high cacao content, preferably at least 70 percent.

Put simply, a 100 g piece of 90 percent dark chocolate contains very little added sugar or sodium, but a whopping 715 mg of potassium and 228 mg of magnesium, which is nearly 60 percent of your daily requirement. It also has nearly all of your daily requirements for copper and manganese.

Cocoa beans are composed of 33 to 62 percent cocoa butter, which is primarily made up of triacylglycerols, an important energy source for your body, and contain palmitic, stearic, and oleic acids, as well as low amounts of linoleic acid. You've already learned about the longevity-boosting potential of oleic acids on page 76. Because of the cocoa butter, chocolate is mostly fat, but it's one of the richest food sources of longevity-boosting polyphenols, including several of our most important longevity vitamins.

What's in a Cacao Bean?

While we like to talk about cacao beans, technically it's the seed from a fruit and not a bean (although we'll keep using the word "bean" here). "Chocolate" is the food we typically consume after the cacao has been cleaned, roasted, shelled, ground up, and refined. Frequently manufacturers then add milk, sugar, and other ingredients.

Cacao, and the processed cocoa, contains about 300 natural components and a surprising mix of beneficial nutrients, including these:

- Fiber (26–40 percent)
- Micronutrients—minerals, such as calcium, copper, potassium, magnesium, sodium, phosphorus, and zinc, and vitamins A, B, E, and K
- Methylxanthines—theobromine and caffeine
- Phenolic compounds (13.5 percent)—Chocolate is actually among the top five foods for phenolic content.

One of Chocolate's Secret Longevity Agents: PQQ

We discussed the power of some polyphenols to act as free radical scavengers in chapter 1, describing how these antioxidants help ease inflammation and protect healthy cells in our bodies from the ravages of disease and damaging environmental toxins. Cacao beans are a rich dietary source of polyphenols like catechins, epicatechins, and procyanidins. Most importantly, cacao powder contains *pyrroloquinoline quinine (PQQ)*.

PQQ is the most important antiaging antioxidant you've never heard of, because this water-soluble quinine plays a critical role in maintaining essential physiological functions such as reproduction and growth, reducing inflammation, protecting the brain from neurodegenerative diseases targeting metabolism, ensuring mitochondrial health, and maintaining adequate blood flow. PQQ is so crucial to our health that scientists are now suggesting it acts more like an essential vitamin when it comes to disease prevention and longevity. In 2003, a paper published in the highly respected journal *Nature* stated that PQQ was indeed a new vitamin. This led to controversy in the science community, but in 2018 Dr. Bruce Ames agreed that PQQ was an important longevity vitamin. To that point, PQQ has even been linked to slowing down the aging process in various animal studies.

Laboratory studies conducted on everything from fungi to mice have shown that PQQ deficiency is associated with a wide range of abnormalities, and researchers have demonstrated that PQQ affects some of our most basic biological processes, like *mitochondriogenesis* (the growth and division of mitochondria to meet the energy needs of a cell), reproduction, and aging. PQQ is also associated with reducing ischemia, inflammation, and toxic lipid levels.

When it comes to keeping your brain healthy as you age, PQQ is a great ally. Laboratory research shows that PQQ has great promise in protecting us against the neurodegeneration associated with Parkinson's disease, traumatic brain injury, and stroke. But the positive effects of PQQ don't stop there: Recent studies with laboratory mice showed that PQQ prevented age-related osteoporosis in the animals. As we discussed in chapter 2, cellular senescence is the process by which cells age but don't die, and excess cellular senescence is a hallmark of poor aging. One of the things cellular senescence can drive is bone loss. Now, scientists have made the exciting discovery that PQQ supplementation can help slow the osteoporosis brought on by the estrogen deficiency that occurs as we age. PQQ does this in part by stimulating bone formation and inhibiting the resorption of bone cells.

In clinical studies with human participants, researchers have shown that eating chocolate with a high PQQ content (that is, dark chocolate) can help people better perform continuous, challenging cognitive tasks. And, in a 2024 study with older adults experiencing mild cognitive decline, PQQ supplementation was linked to enhanced brain metabolism and mental orientation.

Another Great Reason to Eat Chocolate: Methylxanthines

In addition to PQQ, cacao provides your body with *methylxanthines* like caffeine and *theobromine*. Historical evidence suggests that humans have long been consuming drinks not only for the calories, but for the feelings of well-being associated with those drinks. Many of those drinks, like coffee, tea, and cocoa, are rich in methylxanthines. For instance, when researchers examined ceramics from Cahokia, a large pre-Hispanic site in Illinois, they found residue from a black drink that contained theobromine, caffeine, and ursolic acid.

Why should drinks containing methylxanthines make us think and feel better? It's largely because they act on the central nervous system's adenosine receptors to boost mood and concentration. Theobromine has other benefits as well. For instance, methylxanthines are associated with improving blood lipid profiles, stimulating the heart muscle, and relaxing the smooth muscles in the lining that help transmit signals between cells. And, in studies examining the use of theobromine to suppress cough in both humans and guinea pigs, researchers concluded that it was effective without the usual adverse side effects of codeine or other cough suppressants—so much so that theobromine has completed trials in South Korea to be sold as a cough-suppressing, nonopioid, noncodeine drug.

Fermentation: What Chocolate, Cheese, Kombucha, Kimchi, Yogurt, and Some Seafood Delicacies Have in Common

When you unwrap that bar of silky dark chocolate, it probably seems like a stretch to imagine that this sweet treat has anything in common with kimchi, cheeses, sourdough bread, fish sauce, or kombucha, but these foods all go through a unique process to be edible: fermentation.

According to archaeological records, humans have relied on fermen-tation since around 8000 BCE to help produce and preserve food and to make certain foods more beneficial to health. However, based on DNA and on how the human gut microbiome might be a biological marker for fermented food use, some researchers are now making the argument that humans, like other primates, might have developed a taste for fermented foods even earlier than that.

Their theory goes like this: Because the common ancestor of humans and other primates relied heavily on fruits for nutrition, and because ripe fruits have a higher ethanol content than fruits that aren't yet ripe, early humans would have developed a sensory bias for the smell of eth-anol in fermented fruits. Other early humans may have sought out fer-mented foods because these foods were essentially predigested, which would have made it easier for foraging humans to get the nutrients they needed. Finally, early humans often had to eat the remains of kills from larger animals. As a result, they didn't always have the option of fresh meat and had to eat animal remains that had started to rot or ferment. And of course, they didn't have refrigeration, so they often didn't have the option to eat fresh food. For whatever reason, early humans devel-oped two specific gene variants associated with increased fermented food consumption about 10 million years ago, before humans diverged from African apes.

Today, the International Scientific Association for Probiotics and Prebiotics (ISPP) defines fermented foods as "food made through desired microbial growth and enzymatic conversions of food components." In essence, this means that healthy microbes are allowed to partially digest the food before we eat it. In this case, the cacao bean is broken down by microorganisms like bacteria. That taste you associate with chocolate is the result of hundreds of individual compounds generated through microbial activity. Yeasts in cacao digest the pulp around the beans and produce alcohol, which creates esters (fruity flavors) and fusel alcohols (flowery flavors). These compounds soak into the beans. As the pulp breaks down, oxygen allows bacteria to turn the alcohol into acetic acid, which also soaks into the beans. This acid helps enzymes break down proteins into peptides and separate antioxidant polyphenols.

Microbial fermentation can convert food into nutritionally richer products by adding microorganisms that help your body fight against gastrointestinal diseases and provide metabolites that support the gut biome. When administered in adequate amounts, these microorganisms confer healthy benefits and are called "probiotics," according to the ISPP. The microorganisms most often used in fermented foods include acetic acid bacteria, yeasts, and lactic acid bacteria.

Consuming probiotic fermented foods is associated with a number of health benefits, including preventing and treating atherosclerosis, cardiovascular disease, cognitive issues, and metabolic disorders. These foods are also associated with boosting the immune system and supporting a healthy gut biome. And, when researchers screened the American National Health and Nutrition Examination Survey to identify links between diseases and live microbe intake, they found that eating fermented foods may be beneficial in lowering systolic blood pressure, inflammation, and insulin and triglyceride levels. However, because so many popular fermented foods also contain a great deal of salt, like kimchi, or are dairy-based, like yogurt, we don't include most of them in the Paleo Diet.

There is another side to fermentation and how our ancestors ate that despite being part of our Paleolithic history, we can't recommend on a modern Paleo Diet. But it's important to point out that when meat and seafood start to go bad, they also undergo a bacterial fermentation process. As we said earlier in this chapter, it's been shown that our Paleolithic ancestors would have regularly eaten meat that was starting to go rancid. In Southeast Asia, a part of the world known for its longevity, burying fish to allow some fermentation before eating it is considered a delicacy. There are now 18 known fermented fish products from this region that are recognized for their probiotic diversity. Given the health risks of eating rancid meat, we can't recommend consuming it except as a delicacy prepared by skilled chefs, but eating safe fermented food is an important part of a healthy diet focused on longevity. In this next section, we explain one of the most important reasons why.

Chocolate's coolest longevity vitamin: Menaquinones (vitamin K2)

Scientists recognized the importance of vitamin K decades ago when they realized it plays a crucial role in helping blood clot and in supporting other physiological functions. Since then, they've recognized two different forms of this essential nutrient. One of these is vitamin K1 (phylloquinone), which is synthesized in algae, plants, and some bacteria. The other is vitamin K2 (menaquinone), which is divided further into MK-4 through MK-13 subtypes. All menaquinones are fat-soluble. Animals, including humans, have difficulties excreting fat-soluble vitamins, so we tend to store them in our fat tissue. While they've all been grouped under the name vitamin K2, that's a bit of a misnomer. It has been shown that each menaquinone is unique, with discrete physiological functions. In other words, we need to make sure we are getting adequate MK-4 through MK-13, though the longer-chain vitamin K2 (MK-7 through MK-13) appears to be most effective at combatting chronic disease.

While our bodies can convert vitamin K1 into MK-4, all other menaquinone variants can be produced only by bacterial fermentation. So, we can get them in only three ways. The most common is by eating fermented foods like dark chocolate. The second way is for the bacteria in our guts to produce some menaquinones like MK-7 by fermenting the food that we eat. Finally, we can get them by contamination in the food chain. For example, pork has one of the highest concentrations of menaquinones because pigs like to eat rancid food, which is high in long-chain menaquinones. The menaquinones they eat are stored in their fat. (We'll talk more about this in chapter 12.)

Clearly, eating fermented food would have been a key part of the diet since our genus *Homo*'s first appearance more than two million years ago, which means menaquinones from bacterial fermentation would have been an important part of our evolutionary template. Unfortunately, because fermented foods have become such a small part of our diet, the typical Western diet is low or deficient in total menaquinones.

Scientists have shown that menaquinones make up a major class of growth factors that keep our gut biomes healthy. That's key to long-term health because many age-related diseases like cancer, type 2 diabetes, and heart disease are linked to issues in the gut biome, as well as with overall nervous system health and mental health disorders. Vitamin K2 has also shown its effectiveness as an anti-inflammatory by exerting a protective effect against oxidative stress, osteoporosis, and heart disease.

In one study conducted with 564 postmenopausal women in the Netherlands, dietary menaquinone helped protect them against coronary calcification. Interestingly, dietary phylloquinone (vitamin K1) didn't have the same beneficial effect. In another Netherlands study with 4,807 men and women age 55 and older, scientists discovered the same protective effect: Menaquinone intake was associated with reduced aortic calcification and with a lower risk of all-cause mortality, whereas phylloquinone supplements didn't have the same health-boosting impact. Finally, in a study with 6,759 women designed to determine whether vitamin K2 was effective in treating osteoporosis after menopause, the researchers reported that treating the women with K2 improved bone mineral density and reduced the risk of fracture. On the flip side, several chronic age-related diseases, including chronic kidney disease, osteoarthritis, and cardiovascular disease, have been associated with vitamin K deficiency.

As you can see, menaquinones may very well be one of our most important longevity nutrients identified to date. The issue is how to add healthy sources of menaquinones to our diet if, as we've already mentioned, we can get menaquinones only from bacterial fermentation. Although we get some menaquinones from natural bacterial fermentation in our guts, that doesn't give us the full range of MK-4 to MK-13. While many fermented foods are high in menaquinones, they often have a negative impact on health. For example, cheese is high in vitamin K but is a non-Paleo food and is very high in salt. Likewise, kombucha tends to be extremely high in sugar.

Thankfully, two of the foods with the highest concentrations of menaquinones are Paleo-friendly: cacao and pork. We've already shown the large number of the world's oldest living people who included dark chocolate as an important part of their diets. Likewise, in four of the five identified Blue Zones (regions with a high percentage of centenarians), pork was an important part of the regions' diets.

It's hard to believe that dark chocolate and pork are part of the secret to longevity, but now we have the science to back it—including the high concentration of longevity nutrients like menaquinones. Just remember that as with all foods, quality is everything. Bacon is heavily processed and loaded with salt and nitrates, so sorry, it's still not good for you. Likewise, heavily sweetened milk chocolate is going to do more harm than good. Seek the healthier cuts of pork, the minimally sweetened 85 percent or higher dark chocolate, or, better yet, straight cacao powder in hot water, and you're on your way to better health.

Other Benefits of Dark Chocolate

In addition to PQQ and vitamin K, dark chocolate offers a host of age-defying antioxidants and other beneficial nutrients that confer a variety of other important longevity benefits:

Dark chocolate reduces your risk of dying from all causes

Because cacao is an excellent source of antioxidants and because, as we discussed on page 19, oxidative stress on cells is one of the primary forces behind inflammation and age-related chronic diseases, researchers have been exploring the possibility that cacao consumption—typically in the form of dark chocolate—can help extend our lives. One study, published in 2021, followed 91,891 people age 55 to 74 years old for 13.5 years. Using a questionnaire-based study, the researchers concluded that eating chocolate was associated with a reduced risk of dying from Alzheimer's, cardiovascular disease, or all causes.

Another study, this one published in 2023, included 84,709 postmenopausal women through the Women's Health Initiative. Here, researchers
concluded that chocolate consumption was linked to a reduced mortality
risk from all causes, cardiovascular disease, and dementia if the women
consumed a moderate amount of chocolate (1 to 3 servings) each week.

Dark chocolate keeps your blood flowing and your heart healthy

Dark chocolate is high in flavanol content. As we saw in chapter 2 and
elsewhere in this book, many studies show that consuming foods high
in flavonoids can help protect against cardiovascular disease. Not surprisingly, then, cacao is also directly associated with supporting heart
health. For instance, researchers noticed the heart-protective effects of
chocolate among the Kuna people who live on islands off Panama's coast.
They make a chocolate drink by grinding up the seeds and adding hot
water; they typically drink many cups a day of this special brew instead
of downing Stanley mugs of water as we do. Scientists have observed
that the Kuna people have much lower rates of heart disease than most
people—even compared to others in that part of the world—and theorize that the cacao flavonoids are responsible for that healthy outcome.

Other wide-ranging epidemiological studies have also demonstrated
that consuming cacao products can lower your risk of cardiovascular disease. One meta-analysis was conducted on the association of chocolate
with cardiometabolic disorders; this study, with 114,009 participants,
linked higher chocolate consumption with a reduction in the risk of cardiovascular disease by one-third. In addition, a study published in 2024
demonstrated that eating dark chocolate improved coronary artery vasodi-
lation and endothelial function, both factors in avoiding essential hypertension. Researchers in Japan also showed a link between eating chocolate
and lowering blood pressure, which reduces the risk of heart disease.

Many investigations worldwide have looked at the relationship
between endothelial function and cacao flavanols and have demonstrated
that flavanol-rich cacao products are associated with a healthier vascular

system. In fact, the health benefits of cacao are so numerous that in 2012, the European Food Safety Authority declared that people might benefit from consuming cacao flavanols daily.

Dark chocolate boosts the immune system

Because the antioxidants in cacao reduce inflammation and oxidative stress, researchers have been exploring the impact of cacao on the immune system. Laboratory studies both in vitro and with animals have demonstrated that a diet supplemented with cacao can help modify the synthesis of antibodies and reduce inflammation.

Dark chocolate improves memory and brain function

Research studies have highlighted different ways in which the consumption of dark chocolate can enhance brain function. As we noted above, cacao contains the compounds theobromine and caffeine, both of which act as stimulants on the brain. Scientists have demonstrated that the polyphenols in cacao can activate intracellular pathways that help enhance your body's ability to make the neurotrophic factors the human brain needs to grow new neurons. In addition, the flavonoids in cacao, especially the procyanidins, stimulate blood flow in the brain and support changes in the neurons that enhance memory and learning. Consuming cacao and its flavonoids can help protect against neurodegenerative diseases that result from oxidative stress, too, like Alzheimer's and Parkinson's, as well as reduce the cognitive decline associated with aging and inflammation.

Why should cacao consumption be linked to cognitive improvements? Researchers believe there are two possible mechanisms of action. One involves the flavonoids interacting with signaling pathways that support healthy brain cell functions; the other is related to the impact cacao consumption has on improving cerebral blood flow, which could improve memory processing.

Dark chocolate for bone and artery health

Osteocalcin is the most abundant protein in our bones and plays a crit-ical role in maintaining bone mineral density. Menaquinones have been shown to play an important role in maintaining both osteocalcin levels and its integrity so that it can continue to perform its key functions. As a result, menaquinones have been shown to help protect bone health.

Osteocalcin also appears to play an important role in preventing the body from depositing calcium in our soft tissues and endothelial cells. This is very important because our arteries are lined with endothelial cells, and it's well known that a key event in the development of ath-erosclerosis is the calcification of the arterial endothelium. There is pre-liminary evidence that a menaquinone deficiency, which impacts the functioning of osteocalcin, can increase the deposition of calcium in the arterial walls and increase the risk of atherosclerosis.

The other side of chocolate

In the spinach section of chapter 4, we mentioned that the only food with a higher concentration of the antinutrient oxalate is chocolate. Con-sequently, just as we advised in the spinach section, if oxalate is an issue for you, try heating the chocolate and then refrigerating it to harden it again. But if you find even that doesn't work for you, avoid chocolate. Just like those who have to avoid spinach, you'll still be able to obtain all of the nutrients chocolate offers from eating a balanced Paleo diet. For instance, if it's menaquinones you're after, don't forget that you can obtain a very healthy amount by eating your St. Louis–style pork ribs!

PART III

Add Animal Foods
to Promote Longevity

Mark's Paleo Story

I was born in Germany and moved to England when I was five. My dad was an art lecturer, and my mother went back to school when I was young and then worked as a neonatal nurse, so my dad jumped in to help out with the cooking. Our meals were made from scratch and were usually healthier than today's typical Western diet of processed foods, but they certainly weren't Paleo. For instance, my breakfast was often an oat-based hot porridge called Ready Brek served with milk.

In college, my diet went downhill because I rarely cooked meals from scratch. Dinner was often a takeout curry with rice or fish and chips. When I started graduate school at Colorado State University, which is where I first met Dr. Cordain, I was eating a little better, but not much. Fortunately, I was a competitive rugby player who burned a lot of calories and I had no major health issues.

Dr. Cordain became my advisor for my master's degree in 1988. At the time, he was deep into researching Paleolithic nutrition, but he hadn't yet made his findings public. The first time he spoke to me about it was when I was beginning work on my doctorate in 1990. I was researching the impact of diet, low-dose aspirin, vitamin E, and beta-carotene on atherosclerosis (arterial plaque formation), and when Dr. Cordain started sharing his discoveries about the Paleo Diet with me it all made perfect sense. *If you believe in evolution, how could foods we never naturally evolved eating, including grains and dairy, be harmonious with our physiology?*

As Dr. Cordain introduced me to the science supporting his ideas, I recognized immediately that the Westernized food pyramid was absolute nonsense. I stopped eating grains, legumes, and dairy. The Paleo Diet became my guide, but not my religion. (I still treat myself occasionally to non-Paleo meals and snacks.)

The most immediate and visible effect of the Paleo Diet was an improvement in my skin. As a kid, I had developed a butterfly rash around my nose, and the doctor gave me a cortisone cream that would literally rip away the skin to treat it. Psoriasis became an issue for me as an adult; when I went Paleo, however, my skin problems cleared up. Even now, I can tell if I've overindulged on non-Paleo foods because my skin breaks out.

Over the past 30 years, I've helped a lot of people begin a Paleo lifestyle and I've seen the benefits for them as well—even in my own family. My sister had breast cancer, and the Paleo Diet helped her skin, body composition, and tolerance to the side effects of cancer treatments. It may have even helped her stay cancer-free for 20 years. My mother had rheumatoid arthritis, but when we took away her dietary triggers, she was like a new woman.

One of the main tenets of the Paleo Diet is the *optimal foraging theory*, which basically means that our ancestors would hunt and gather the foods that would give them the most calories for the least amount of energy expended to get the food. They were omnivores, but the biggest caloric bang for the buck came from large animals. Here's where my coauthor Trevor and I disagree a little: While he believes plant foods should dominate a Paleo Diet, I'm inclined to add more animal foods. This is in keeping with Dr. Cordain's original paper on the wide-ranging diets of our hunter-gatherer ancestors. We have never told people how much plants or meat they should eat. Your own metabolism should dictate the best ratio for you. Ultimately, we must fine-tune our diets to suit our own bodies.

Having said that, I want to emphasize that even though you can get most of the nutrients you need from plants and plant protein, if you could eat only one thing to survive, I would have to say the most nutritious choice would be animal protein. Eating "nose to tail" provides you with virtually every nutrient you need to survive.

While I firmly believe that eating at least some animal foods is essential for optimal health, the Paleo Diet is often confused with an entirely meat-eating carnivore diet. It's a myth that eating Paleo is the same thing as following a carnivore diet. Let me explain why.

Mark's Take on the Carnivore Diet Versus the Paleo Diet

Given what I said above about eating animals nose-to-tail to get all of the nutrients you need to survive, you might be wondering why the Paleo Diet emphasizes the importance of fruits and vegetables. Or maybe at this point you're thinking, "Fine, I'll just go on the carnivore diet." But that's not at all what we're suggesting.

First, let's define a carnivore diet: In simple terms, people following this popular plan restrict their food consumption to meat, poultry, eggs, seafood, some dairy products, and water. This makes it a zero-carbohydrate, or ketogenic, diet because we generally get our carbohydrates almost entirely from plant foods.

While some people do well on this diet, humans evolved eating a mix of plants and animal foods, and we still don't know the long-term consequences of eating only animal foods. When Amber O'Hearn, founder of CarnivoryCon, an annual conference dedicated to the carnivorous lifestyle, reviewed the available data on whether a carnivore diet can provide all of the essential nutrients, she concluded, "Historical and clinical data suggest that all acute micronutrient needs can be met without plants, but long-term consequences are unknown. Calcium levels in particular may be compromised over time."

This is in line with research conducted by Dr. Cordain's late friend and colleague, Dr. Staffan Lindeberg, who studied the diet of the Inuit people. The Inuit ate almost entirely animal foods out of necessity and shared a concern for an increased risk of osteoporosis. Advocates of the carnivore diet argue that the regular consumption of bone broth and small fish bones would fix any calcium deficiencies, but we don't support a long-term carnivore diet. While I believe the carnivore diet may be extremely beneficial in the short term for people with certain health issues, if you buy into Dr. Bruce Ames's proposal that proteins and vitamins be classified according to survival versus longevity (see page 17), eating only meat means you'll miss out on the Paleo plant foods that contain many nutrients that simply aren't available in animal-sourced foods.

In the more than thirty years I have been helping people implement a Paleo Diet, I have never told anyone how much of any food they should consume. I simply provide a list of allowable foods and encourage people to listen to their bodies to determine the best ratio of animal to plant foods to support their own unique metabolisms. I'm confident this will work for you, too.

In this section of the book, we focus on the impact that eating animal proteins can have on supporting healthy longevity. Chapter 11 focuses on terrestrial animal proteins. Chapter 12 highlights the benefits of adding eggs to your Paleo lifestyle, and we devote chapter 13 to the amazing longevity benefits of fish and shellfish.

CHAPTER ELEVEN

Slow Aging with Beef, Chicken, Turkey, and Pork

O nce a nationally ranked gymnast, Rachel first noticed something
was very wrong when she was 16. She'd been suffering pain in her
toes for a couple of years, something she attributed to the hazards of her
athletic career, but then the pain turned crippling and spread to her fingers and jaw. She also experienced severe irritable bowel syndrome (IBS)
starting at an early age.

A specialist finally diagnosed Rachel's rheumatoid arthritis (RA)
as the cause of the sometimes excruciating pain in her joints, but her
parents were reluctant to let her start taking the medications available
to treat RA at that time, since she was still growing and there were
potential side effects. As she entered adulthood, Rachel noticed her IBS
continued to worsen; it was only later that she learned that most people
with autoimmune diseases like RA also have gut issues.

Just before she started college, Rachel saw a naturopathic doctor
who suggested that she try eliminating gluten from her diet to see if
that might help her digestive issues. Rachel readily agreed, since she

had already noticed that eating wheat and dairy products always left her "bloated and in pain."

Ditching gluten, dairy, and legumes helped settle her gut. In her 20s, she also went on Enbrel, a new medication for RA that she describes as a "game changer." Rachel finally felt healthy and energetic enough to continue her education, this time pursuing a master's degree in anthropology at San Francisco State University. While there, she did a research paper on RA post-agriculture and industrialization. That's when she discovered the Paleo Diet, and everything clicked into place.

Now 45, Rachel works in a hospital surgery unit and is happily married. She says that she and her husband are 70 to 80 percent Paleo, and the results have been nothing short of remarkable. Her husband, who struggled with weight most of his life, is now fit and trim, and Rachel's health has never been better.

"I've seen a notable decrease in inflammation from Paleo," she says, explaining that making this lifestyle choice has tamed the gastrointestinal symptoms that had plagued her since adolescence. "Paleo controls my gut inflammation and even helps with excess joint inflammation. I believe that Paleo is part of why I've been able to cut my Enbrel dose in half."

Interestingly, there has been another, unexpected effect of a Paleo lifestyle as well: Neither Rachel nor her husband has had an upper respiratory infection in seven years. This is remarkable, given that they live in an area of California subject to wildfires, and her husband is a former firefighter.

"He got valley fever in 2017 while fighting fires, which is a fungal infection from ingesting too much dirt while working next to the bulldozer," Rachel says, "and I lost sleep when he was admitted to the hospital. That's the last time we were sick."

Her theory: "Meat has a lot of important nutrients and vitamins that protect us and keep our immune systems healthy. When you're displacing the amount of meat your body needs with processed food and cereal grains, your immune system can't fight off infection." On the other hand, "when you mostly eat meat, vegetables, and fruit, your body thrives. Plus—getting enough sleep and living a stress-free life is huge, too."

As Rachel has discovered, eating a balanced, nutritious Paleo Diet of meat, vegetables, and fruit can help you defeat many health issues. Yet animal protein—particularly red meat—has gotten a bad rap in the past few decades. (When we write about red meat here, we include beef, pork, lamb, and game meat such as venison and elk.) Let's take a closer look at some of these nutritional misconceptions and why they exist.

How Red Meat Became the Darth Vader of the Nutrition World

Over the past few decades, as researchers looked at the associations between the consumption of red meat and disease, there have been studies suggesting that red meat is to blame for everything from heart attacks and stroke to diabetes and kidney disease. One of the most alarming studies was published in *The Journal of the American Medical Association* (JAMA) in 2005, where the authors argued that the prolonged high consumption of red and processed meat may increase the risk of cancer in the large intestine. Another study, published in 2019, linked the dietary intake of red meat and dietary iron with metabolic syndrome. And in 2024, a group of researchers published a paper claiming they'd found a significant link between higher intake of red meat and an increased risk of developing type 2 diabetes.

The truth is that all of these studies are *epidemiological* in nature, and that limits the conclusions we can draw from them. For example, an epidemiological study looks at the people who eat more red meat and then looks at the data to see if these people also have higher rates of cancer. In other words, they suggest a link or an association, but they can't claim that red meat causes cancer or heart disease. That's because the researchers in these studies didn't control for other variables, like the fact that people who eat a lot of red meat may have other lifestyle factors that increase their risk of cancer, such as lack of exercise or smoking. Unfortunately, by the time the information from these studies was made public, the media and many readers leapt to what we think are inappropriate conclusions.

A growing body of evidence supports the idea that inconsistent findings in nutritional epidemiology studies are the result of investigators making different analytic choices when they look at the same data. For instance, a group of researchers reviewed all published observational studies on the effect of unprocessed red meat on all-cause mortality in 2024. From these, they selected 15 publications to examine in detail and identified 70 unique analytic methods that were used by the original researchers. In other words, none of these scientists were using the same method to analyze their data, making their findings somewhat subjective.

Of the 48 methods the researchers deemed statistically significant, eight of them indicated that consuming red meat increased mortality, while 40 showed that eating unprocessed red meat *reduced* all-cause mortality. This is important because depending on which methods the researchers chose, that influenced their views on whether eating red meat is good for you or not.

Another problem with many of these studies is that data collection is often unreliable. If researchers collect information by asking participants to complete questionnaires asking things like "How often did you eat beef, pork, or lamb as a main dish, and how many ounces?" they have to rely on faulty human memory. (Do *you* remember what you ate last week?) Worse, the classification of red meat consumption in these instances might include foods such as grain-heavy lasagna, which is not simply red meat. But the good news here is that science is constantly evolving, and today's researchers are fine-tuning their methods for analyzing the true impact of eating animal foods on the human body.

Meat and colon cancer

When it comes to the association between red meat and colon cancer, people have been eating red meat for millions of years, but the rates of colon cancer have risen substantially since 1950, and particularly since the 1980s, when fat became the boogeyman and people started eating more refined carbohydrates. If eating red meat is causing an increase in colon cancer, we should expect to see an increase in red meat consumption, right? Not so. Red meat consumption has been declining since its peak in the mid-1970s. According to the US Department of Agriculture, Americans ate 4.2 percent less beef between 2023 and 2024. We can hardly lay the primary blame for colon cancer on red meat if cancer rates are going up while meat eating is going down. There must be other contributing factors that weren't revealed in the epidemiological studies.

Processed versus unprocessed meat

Another problem with these and many other studies on the impact of meat consumption is that some scientists group processed and unprocessed red meats together in one big red-meat bucket. There's a big difference between the two. Think about it this way: kale and jelly beans are both plant-based foods, but if you argued that kale is bad for you because jelly beans are bad for you, people would think you were being ridiculous. Yet some of those epidemiological studies showing a link between meat consumption and cancer are looking at people who eat fast-food hamburgers or processed meats almost daily.

Many canned, cured, and processed meats are prepared using ingredients that are toxic to our health. These include too much salt, corn syrup, high-fructose corn syrup, dextrose (glucose), sucrose (table sugar), and modified food starches made of wheat, corn, potatoes, soy, and so on. As if that weren't enough, these ultra-processed meats might also contain sodium lactate, potassium lactate, calcium sulfate, citric acid, propyl gallate, silicon dioxide, sodium nitrite, sodium nitrate, potassium nitrite, potassium nitrate (the nitrites and nitrates have been shown to have carcinogenic properties), sodium tripolyphosphate, hexametaphosphate, acid pyrophosphate, orthophosphates, erythorbate, oleoresins, monosodium glutamate (MSG), sodium diacetate, hydrolyzed proteins (wheat, soy, milk), sodium caseinate, and dried whey.

In addition, unless you can find a supplier who manufactures their processed meats from wild game or grass-fed animals, any processed meat you consume originates mainly from feedlot animals eating virtually nothing but grains (corn primarily) before they are slaughtered. This practice produces inferior meat with an unnatural fatty acid balance characterized by high omega-6 fatty acids, low omega-3 fatty acids, a lower protein content, a higher-than-normal unhealthy fat content, and many other important nutritional shortcomings. In 2002, Dr. Cordain was the lead author in a study analyzing the fatty acid profile of game meat compared to free-range and feedlot meats, and the differences in the fatty acid profiles were staggering. Grain-fed steer had over double the saturated fat content of free-range cattle and over triple that of elk, while game meat had up to five times more omega-3s.

Ultra-Processed Foods

In 2009, the NOVA scale was created to classify foods into four levels of processing, from unprocessed to ultra-processed. While we have spent decades arguing whether plant foods or animal foods are better for us, research looking at processed foods has been showing in pretty stark detail that ultra-processed foods—whether plant-based or animal-based—are associated with most chronic diseases, and unprocessed or minimally processed foods—whether plant-based or animal-based—are associated with better health and longevity. This is part of why we believe that the debate shouldn't be vegan verses carnivore, but about how processed the foods are.

The bottom line is that processed meat is typically a nutritionally inferior product to start with even before it's transformed into ham, bacon, lunch meats, bologna, hot dogs, salami, sausage, deli meat, canned Spam, or Vienna sausage. Fortunately, today's researchers are starting to make the distinction between processed and unprocessed meats, and when they do, most associations between unprocessed red meat and disease risk will likely go away.

The anti-protein faction

The anti-protein crowd believes protein rots in your gut—the technical term is *putrefaction*—and is the root of all diseases. Technically, putrefaction is defined as "the anaerobic breakdown of undigested protein in the colon by microbiota," but many researchers refer to the putrefaction process as protein fermentation. (See chapter 10 for more on fermentation.) Fermentation of both protein and fiber is actually a normal physiological function in the digestive tract.

Many compounds are produced during protein fermentation, including ammonia, phenols, and indoles, which anti-protein advocates believe are harmful to the body and associated with a higher risk of colon cancer. However, this argument doesn't hold up. The increase in some of these volatile compounds might be an issue if a person ate only meat and nothing else, but most people eat meat combined with other foods. Consuming protein with vegetables and fruits counteracts the possible detrimental effects of protein fermentation. For instance, if you eat animal protein with a source of fiber such as vegetables, the combination of compounds diminishes the protein's negative effects.

One 2024 study showed that consuming just 30 grams per day of leafy vegetables significantly reduced the risk of mortality. In another relatively recent review of the research connecting red meat to colon cancer, the authors pointed out that most studies "used levels of meat or meat components well in excess of those found in human diets." They also made the point that in most studies the subjects were eating a typical Western diet high in processed foods, unhealthy fats, too much salt, and added sugars. When *protective dietary compounds* such as fruits and vegetables were added to the diet and grains were reduced, red meat was actually protective against colon cancer. The Paleo Diet is effective because it combines natural protein sources with vegetables and nonsugary fruit and eliminates grains.

What's the Difference Between Plant Protein and Animal Protein?

People often ask whether plant-based proteins are just as good as animal proteins. The answer is no. The science clearly shows that meat, seafood, and eggs are far superior protein sources than plants for several reasons. The first and most important of these is that animal proteins are a complete source of all essential amino acids in the correct ratios. Conversely, since almost no plant foods have a complete profile of amino acids, you'd need to eat a specific variety of plant-based foods, and enormous amounts of them, to get your daily fill.

To understand what determines a protein's quality, we must consider two main factors: its amino acid profile and its bioavailability.

All proteins are made up of strings of amino acids such as histidine, isoluecine, lysine, and valine. When we eat a protein, our bodies break it down to absorb the resultant amino acids, which we then use to build the proteins our bodies need. Of the 20 common amino acids, 9 are considered essential because our bodies can't synthesize them. That means we need to get them from food. The quality of the protein we consume is partially determined by whether it contains all these essential amino acids and how closely it has them in the ratios we need. This is referred to as the amino acid profile of a protein.

Just as important as a protein's amino acid profile is its bioavailability, which refers to how easy it is to digest. A protein source may contain the essential amino acids, but if it's hard for our digestive systems to break it down and absorb its amino acids, that protein isn't a great source for us—it has a low bioavailability. A high-quality protein has a good profile of both essential amino acids and amino acids that are highly bioavailable for breakdown and absorption. When we consider plant versus animal foods using these two simple criteria, it's clear that animal foods are a better source of protein.

Do Your Protein Needs Change as You Age?

While we all need protein, some of us need a little more than others, including athletes and older adults. Evidence from the PROT-AGE Study Group shows that older adults need more dietary protein than younger adults to support good health, promote recovery from illness, and maintain function. This age-related increased need for protein is due to changes in the way our bodies metabolize protein over time.

When differentiating between plant and animal proteins, it's important to look at the essential amino acid profile, and particularly at the branched-chain amino acids (leucine, isoleucine, and valine). As an example, the adult RDA for leucine is 42 mg/kg of body weight, which is 2.94 grams for a 70-kilogram person. That RDA can be accomplished with the consumption of just 100 grams of beef skirt steak—that's only a 3.5-ounce steak. You would have to eat twice the amount of firm tofu or almost five times the amount of canned navy beans to obtain the RDA for leucine! And those quantities still don't consider whether tofu or canned beans supply the other essential amino acids—never mind the fact that soy and legumes may have a negative impact on your health. Similarly, you would have to eat over 2.5 times the amount of pumpkin seeds compared to beef skirt steak to obtain the same amount of lysine.

To put it into perspective, we can compare animal and plant protein sources using the DIAAS (digestible indispensable amino acid score) protein quality rating (see table 2 in appendix). This rating factors in both the amino acid profile of a protein and its bioavailability. Eggs rank the highest at 113. The lowest animal protein is chicken at 108, and the highest plant protein is chickpeas at 83. The scientific data is very clear that animal proteins, pound for pound, are significantly superior in quality to plant proteins.

Why Vegetarians Are Missing Out

If anyone had ever tried telling Nicole in her 20s that she'd be eating Paleo one day, she wouldn't have believed them. "I'm still surprised," she says. "Everyone I know is surprised that I adopted Paleo as a lifestyle."

Nicole, who is now 53 and works in public health, became a vegetarian in college largely because her grandfather owned a meatpacking plant. "We'd go to the plant and see raw meat hanging up, and we ate meat at every single meal," she remembers. "I hated meat because I thought it was gross."

She remained a vegetarian for 10 years, until she attended a barbecue one day and ate a bratwurst. Still, despite eating meat again, she remained overweight and had little energy. Her health deteriorated as the years passed. In 2019 she was diagnosed with a herniated disc "and I had a lot of inflammation. Something was always hurting," Nicole says. She also suffered from frequent headaches.

Then, in November 2023, Nicole caught COVID-19 for the first time and was "really, really sick." She spent three weeks in bed and suffered from long COVID after that. "I was so tired I couldn't stay awake past 2 p.m.," she says. "I became desperate. I didn't want to feel this way for the rest of my life, so I finally tried Paleo on the Tuesday after Thanksgiving."

She hasn't looked back. Nicole has lost 22 pounds and now weighs the same as she did in high school, "but the important thing is that I feel better than I ever have in my entire life," she says. "I don't have any pain in my body, and I no longer get headaches. The biggest miracle is that I've always had horrible seasonal allergies, but this season I didn't. For me, Paleo has been life altering."

Previously, Nicole had relied on canned or boxed processed foods when she cooked, but now she shops "the edges of the grocery store" for fresh produce and meats. On a typical day, she starts the morning with eggs and a salad or a cup of fruit. She might have nuts for a snack, then lunch is typically a salad with grilled chicken "and any vegetables I feel like throwing in there. Instead of living to eat, I now eat to live. It's kind of amazing to feel this good."

Did we have vegetarian ancestors?

Although the practice of vegetarianism dates back to at least 500 BCE with such ancient Greeks as Pythagoras and Plutarch eating no meat, that's a blink of an eye compared to our evolutionary timescale. In a comprehensive analysis of 229 hunter-gatherer diets, Dr. Cordain and his research group found no evidence that any foragers were purely vegetarians. Why? Because animal-sourced foods were optimal in terms of giving them more calories and nutrition for the energy expended to obtain the food, which makes sense in terms of the optimal foraging theory.

Our natural human preference for meat, marrow, organs, and other animal foods is supported by the discovery of fossils in Africa of butchered animals with stone-tool cut marks on their bones. On the flip side, there is no credible fossil, archaeological, anthropological, or biochemical evidence to suggest that preagricultural humans ever consumed all plant-based diets. Scientists are also able to determine the relative percentage of plant and animal food in extinct human (hominin) species by analyzing the element isotopes within their fossilized bones, which show the isotopic signature characteristic of meat-based diets dating back 2.5 million years.

The discovery of stone-tool cut marks on these fossilized bones supports the idea that our earliest ancestors were increasingly exploiting animal foods for nutrition. As their diets began to shift and include more proteins, the bodies of these early hominins began to change as they consumed more fatty acids and foods with higher energy density. Thanks to that improvement in dietary quality, more energy went from sustaining their guts to feeding their brains, which led to today's humans having enormous brains that use up to 25 percent of our total resting metabolic rate. (The brains of other primates use only 8 or 9 percent.)

For this to have happened, the earliest hominins—who were small and unsophisticated when it came to hunting—would have been opportunistic foragers, eating whatever animal foods they could scavenge from carcasses killed by other predators, disease, or accident. This would likely have been the parts left over by other, stronger predators like lions or scavengers like hyenas; those powerful animals would have eaten most of the flesh of the animals they killed, while leaving bones with intact marrow and skulls with intact brains. Scavenged marrow would have therefore been the most reliable source of fat, which was very high in omega-3 fatty acids—a necessary component to develop larger brains. The bottom line is that today's humans, like our Paleo ancestors, benefit from animal protein and fat when it comes to feeding our big brains and keeping our tissues and bones healthy.

Health Benefits of Animal Protein

Getting adequate protein is important for maintaining both muscle mass and bone health. These two things become increasingly important as we age and try to maintain our mobility. Researchers have demonstrated in a variety of studies that it's simply not possible for older adults to consume adequate protein on a vegan diet, and a vegan diet has been associated with increased risk of bone fracture in older adults.

More specifically, there are many health benefits of animal protein:

Animal protein promotes better performance and recovery

Protein contains the amino acids your body needs to build and maintain lean muscle mass. As you go throughout your day and complete your workouts, you're tearing your body down. We require adequate dietary protein to promote muscle growth, repair damaged cells and tissue, synthesize hormones, and assist in a variety of other metabolic activities.

High-quality protein contains the essential fatty acids and selenium we need to combat inflammation, carries the most readily available heme iron our bodies need to prevent anemia, carries zinc for immunity, and provides vitamin B12 for proper cell formation and energy level support.

Animal protein promotes improved bone and muscle health

The intestinal absorptive properties of the calcium in animal proteins facilitate the most rapid and sustained delivery of nutrition to your bones. For instance, a study published in 2023 using data from 1,570 adults over age 65 showed that total protein intake was associated with a higher total body and spine bone mineral density, as was animal protein intake. Plant protein intake, on the other hand, was linked to lower spine and total body bone mineral density.

Animal protein is also a powerful ally when it comes to keeping aging muscles strong and supple. In one recent study examining the emerging evidence on how dietary protein intake influences the muscles of older adults, the authors reported that diets that included sufficient dietary protein to maximize protein anabolism promoted muscle function and size in otherwise healthy older adults. For older adults diagnosed with acute illnesses or medical conditions, specialized protein supplements helped slow down the loss of muscle mass and function. The researchers also discovered that observational studies favored animal versus plant protein sources.

Animal protein promotes enhanced brain health

A less obvious and often ignored reward of a high-protein diet is the long-term health of our brains and improvements in both cognition and mental states. Multiple studies have shown dramatic improvements in the treatment of anxiety, depression, and dementia with dietary changes leading to a greater consumption of animal-based, high-quality proteins. Essentially, the healthy fats, vitamin B12, choline, and energy that these proteins provide contribute to enhanced emotional regulation and cognitive achievement.

Animal protein promotes improved kidney function

In the first meta-analysis to compare the intake of plant, animal, and total protein intake with the risk of developing chronic kidney disease (CKD) in 2024, researchers reported that the data from six studies with 148,051 participants showed a lower risk of CKD associated with higher levels of protein, especially from fish and seafood sources.

Animal protein promotes overall longevity

In 2022, researchers examined the association between life expectancy and meat consumption using ecological data published by the United Nations from 175 different countries and territories. Even taking into account established risk factors to life expectancy like education levels, obesity, urbanization, and others, these scientists found that meat intake was positively correlated with life expectancy, while carbohydrate crops were apt to decrease longevity.

Essentially, this means that while it's possible to get the nutrients we need, including our full range of amino acids, from an omnivore diet, a vegetarian or vegan diet can lead to deficiencies in several key nutrients that contribute greatly to our health and longevity. One of the most common deficiencies among vegetarians is vitamin B12 because it's difficult to consume it in sufficient amounts from nonanimal sources. Vitamin B12 is essential to the folate cycle, which we touched on in chapter 4 and will delve into more thoroughly later in chapter 12. When the folate cycle doesn't function properly—such as when a person is B12 deficient—the body has a reduced ability to methylate DNA, a key aging factor, and overproduces homocysteine, which correlates more strongly with heart disease than cholesterol does.

As an example, many Indians are vegans for religious reasons and don't supplement with vitamin B12, and researchers have generally pointed to the prevalent high levels of homocysteine among many Indian vegans to explain India's high rate of heart disease.

Animal protein promotes a full complement of essential vitamins and nutrients

Vitamin B6, or pyridoxine, is also important to the folate cycle, and many plant forms of B6 are not bioavailable. This means our bodies have a hard time using the form of B6 found in plants, which may explain why even vegans who eat high amounts of B6 are often still diagnosed as being deficient.

Another important longevity nutrient is omega-3 fatty acids. We'll cover their health benefits in more detail in chapter 13, but for now it's important to understand that we can get two extremely important forms of these fatty acids, EPA and DHA, from animal foods and seafood. However, other than seaweed and algae, we can't get them directly from plant foods because the form of omega-3 fatty acids found in most plant foods is the essential fatty acid ALA (alpha-linolenic acid), and our ability to convert ALA to EPA/DHA is extremely limited. As a result, many vegans and vegetarians can be deficient in important omega-3 fatty acids.

That goes for taurine, too

Taurine, which we highlight in chapter 13, is an amino acid that we can get only from animal foods. It is one of our most important longevity nutrients, and we've known for a while that vegans who do not supplement with taurine are usually deficient.

Taurine deficiency can contribute to many adverse health effects, including vision problems and neurodegeneration. Both taurine and vitamin B12 are important for maintaining our vision. So, while so far only case studies have been done on poor vision health in vegans, the signs point to vegans being at risk of age-related macular degeneration. If seafood isn't your thing, another great animal protein rich in taurine is bone marrow.

What About Plant-Based Meat Substitutes?

Plant-based meat substitutes may taste like meat (most do not), but they're usually made with unhealthy, highly processed seed oils, grains, soy, and lectin-filled legumes. What's worse, the protein quality doesn't come close to that of high-quality, animal-based sources. In one study looking at young men in New Zealand, the participants ate standardized meals containing either a plant-based meat substitute, lamb, pasture-raised beef, or grain-finished beef. When the researchers tested the participants' blood after eating, they discovered that the plant-based substitute resulted in lower levels of amino acids in their subjects' blood plasma than beef or lamb. Regarding amino acid consumption, there were no differences between pasture-raised or grain-finished beef (cattle that start their lives feeding in pastures but are given grain at the end of their lives).

Is Poultry a Healthier Protein Choice than Red Meat?

While many imagine that people who follow the Paleo Diet must be tossing beef steaks onto the grill every night, the truth is that we advocate for including seafood (see chapter 13), pork, and poultry in your animal protein choices.

The total amount of poultry consumed in the United States has tripled over the past six decades, with chicken being the most commonly consumed. Each American eats about 100.6 pounds of chicken and 14.7 pounds of turkey annually, but only 59.4 pounds of beef and 51.4 pounds of pork. Poultry consumption continues to rise as beef consumption falls. As with studies on red meat, research on the health benefits of eating poultry is marred by scientists failing to separate people who consume unprocessed poultry meat from those who eat highly processed poultry foods. Even so, observational studies have shown that eating lean, unprocessed animal proteins, including chicken, can help people lose weight. Studies show that consuming this kind of protein has either no impact or a beneficial impact on the risk of cardiovascular disease, kidney disease, and other chronic diseases associated with aging.

Here's why we like naturally raised chicken or turkey on our Paleo plates:

- It's affordable and easily accessible.
- Chicken provides up to 31 grams of protein in a 3.5-ounce serving.
- Like naturally raised red meat, unprocessed chicken and other poultry meats provide many essential nutrients beneficial to health and longevity, including the nine essential amino acids and other key nutrients like the minerals magnesium, potassium, selenium, and iron; and B vitamins such as thiamin (B1), riboflavin (B2), niacin (B3), choline (B4), and cobalabin (B12).

As with all meat, we advise buying fresh, naturally raised, unprocessed cuts of poultry to avoid consuming high levels of salt and preservatives.

What About Organ Meats?

Most of the meat sold in grocery stores is muscle meat, which isn't the most nutrient-dense part of the animal. To get the full benefits of eating animal foods, we should eat nose-to-tail, including animal organs.

Organ meats like liver—otherwise known as offal—used to be common on American plates. People around the world also eat tongue, heart, kidneys, brain, sweetbreads (made from the thymus gland and pancreas), tripe (the lining of the animal's stomach, usually a cow's), and testicles (Rocky Mountain oysters). Organ meats are nutritious, packed with vitamins including folate and B12, and a great source of protein and iron.

Organ meat is also very high in coenzyme Q (CoQ10), a powerful antioxidant that many people buy as expensive supplements. The levels of CoQ10 in organ meats are 10 to 50 times higher than what we consume in other meats or plants. As we discussed in chapter 2, the leakage of reactive oxygen species (ROS) by mitochondrial membranes is an important factor in the pathophysiology of aging. Over time, our mitochondria produce a lot more ROS; how much they produce is partly determined by the amount of available CoQ10. CoQ10 has been shown to reduce mortality by 50 percent in cardiovascular disease, help glycemic control, improve renal function, and reduce inflammation. So even if you remember hating the liver your mother tried to force you to choke down, remember it's far and away the most nutrient-dense part of the animal. Our suggestion is to make a flavorful Paleo sauce and put it on the liver; keep eating liver to do your body good.

Animal Protein and Environmental Concerns

Given our ongoing struggle to combat global climate change, the impact of food production on carbon emissions is a topic of utmost importance. Even if some causes of climate change are beyond our control, we all need to contribute to the solution instead of the problem.

Many claim that plant-based diets are not only best for our health but also better for our environment. We've covered the first point in this chapter, but what about the second? Is it true that we should remove animal foods from our diet for the sake of the environment?

Agriculture does contribute to global greenhouse gas emissions, and cows are frequently singled out as major contributors responsible for anywhere from 3.7 percent to 14.5 percent of these emissions. That said, there is a wide variation in the carbon footprints among different production systems. We must take steps to further improve sustainable agricultural practices such as regenerative agriculture, a new approach to farming that aims to fight climate change. Regenerative agriculture (and specifically regenerative grazing) is a means to sequester carbon by improving soil health. This leads to healthy grassland systems with more methanotrophs (prokaryotes that metabolize methane) and lower methane emissions. Ultimately, regenerative grazing can produce a negative carbon footprint. In other words, "It's not the cow, it's the how."

How to support regenerative agriculture

Regardless of dietary preferences, supporting regenerative agriculture is crucial for rebuilding our land and soil so that we achieve a livable future that is abundant, healthy, and resilient. Here's how:

- Buy local: Purchase food from local farmers who use regenerative practices.
- Check labels: Look for certifications like Regenerative Organic Certified, Regenified, or Ecological Outcome Verification (EOV) to ensure your food comes from verified regenerative systems.
- Grow your own food: Even small efforts, like container gardening, contribute to food sustainability.

To learn more, consider watching documentaries like *Kiss the Ground* and *Common Ground*, which explore the transformative potential of regenerative agriculture. Better yet, take *Kiss the Ground*'s Regenerative Agriculture Essentials, a 90-minute on-demand course for anyone interested. For all this and more, visit KissTheGround.com.

"By addressing the root causes of soil and ecosystem degradation—such as harmful agricultural and livestock practices—humanity can tackle the climate, health, and water crisis more effectively," says thought leader Finian Makepeace, cofounder of the advocacy organization Kiss the Ground, which promotes improving soil health to combat climate change. "Regenerative approaches offer a path toward healthier landscapes, more resilient ecosystems, and a truly healthy food system."

Why Pork Is So Good for You

According to the website Worldometers.info, Hong Kong had the highest life expectancy in the world, followed closely by Japan. The people of Okinawa Island are famous even in Japan for their longevity; however, male longevity in Okinawa has declined dramatically in recent decades. This decline has been attributed to the Westernization of their diet. The biggest change in their diet may surprise you: It's the decrease in the amount of pork consumed. Pigs were traditionally the most important domesticated food animals on the island and an important part of their culture. The recent decline in pork consumption among Okinawans corresponds with their drop in longevity. And, when Dr. Cordain examined the records of supercentenarians in each of the US states, he discovered a direct correlation between longevity and each state's pork production.

Does this mean you should eat bacon and sausage? No. As we pointed out earlier, the levels of salt and other additives in those low-quality processed meats are too high to be healthy.

The healthiest cut of pork is one you probably haven't given much thought to: St. Louis–style pork ribs, which represent a specific cut of pork ribs recognized by the USDA. Because of their anatomical location slightly above pork bellies (the pork cut used for bacon), this cut represents the highest fat (combined muscle, bone, and fat) in the entire pig. While the official USDA position to prevent cardiovascular disease is to eat less saturated fat, we believe there is a nutritional factor present in unadulterated, fatty pork meat like St. Louis–style pork ribs that may not only prevent cardiovascular disease but may also prevent osteoporosis and be therapeutic for a wide variety of diseases that afflict the Western world. The secret lies in vitamin K2 or menaquinones, which we covered in depth in chapter 10.

Pork and chocolate have some of the highest concentrations of menaquinones of any foods. Chocolate has them because it is created through the fermentation of cacao beans. Pork is so high because pigs tend to eat a lot of rotted and rancid foods that are high in vitamin K.

Menaquinones are a fat-soluble vitamin, so they can't simply be excreted in urine. Instead, they're stored in the fatty part of the pig.

Fatty pork cuts such as St. Louis–style ribs represent one of the best dietary choices for maximizing your intake of K2 without increasing your salt intake or compromising that important sodium-to-potassium ratio in your diet.

Whether you choose to add unprocessed red meat, poultry, or St. Louis–style ribs or some other healthful cut of pork to your menu, remember that today's humans, like our Paleo ancestors, benefit from eating animal proteins and fats to keep our tissues, bones, and brains healthy—especially as we age.

CHAPTER TWELVE

Eggs for Energy, Better
Vision, and Brain Health

B y the time Lynda had bariatric surgery at age 64, she weighed 340
pounds despite trying to diet for decades. "I was like a yo-yo,"
she says. "I could lose the pounds but couldn't keep them off because I
couldn't find a way of eating that satisfied me." Her weight affected her
mobility because of pain in her hip. She started seeing a chiropractor,
"but nothing he did seemed to help me walk better."

The surgery did help Lynda tip the scale in the right direction, partly
because she was too nauseated to eat for about three months afterward.
She could tolerate only liquids during that time, mostly tomato juice and
chicken broth, eventually graduating to soft foods like scrambled eggs
after six months. She dropped to 221 pounds but gained 43 pounds back
a year later.

When her doctor diagnosed Lynda with type 2 diabetes in May
2024, "that's what changed my thinking," she says. Her aunt had recently
died; she was obese like Lynda and also had type 2 diabetes and heart
problems. "I knew I didn't want to end up like that," Lynda says.

Lynda saw an herbalist and asked if there was anything natural she could take to lower her blood sugar instead of the medication her doctor prescribed. The herbalist suggested some natural remedies, but strongly advised Lynda to go on the Paleo Diet. Coincidentally, Lynda's granddaughter had also discovered the Paleo Diet and was encouraging her to try it.

With her granddaughter's help, Lynda filled notebook pages "with what I could and couldn't eat on Paleo." She spent the next two weeks cleaning out her cabinets and refrigerator, and as she shopped for food, she began reading labels for the first time in her life. She also joined a Paleo support group on Facebook.

Soon after starting Paleo, Lynda was walking better and had more energy. This surprised her. "I hadn't realized before then that the Paleo Diet helps with getting rid of inflammation," she says. The weight started coming off as well, and at her next checkup, her blood tests showed that her glucose levels, blood pressure, and lipid panel were much improved.

Lynda's weight has now dropped to 183 pounds. "This is the lowest I've weighed in 54 years," she says. Best of all, she recently went to Busch Gardens with extended family and was able to "walk all day long. I've never walked that much in my entire life. Paleo has been a lifesaver for me. I can live this way and be perfectly content," she says, noting that where other diets left her hungry, on Paleo she feels satisfied. "Recently I had a pineapple, mango, and kale smoothie, and it was absolutely wonderful," she says. "Fruit has never tasted sweeter."

———

As we wrote in chapter 1, our hunter-gatherer ancestors were optimal foragers who searched for foods that gave them the most calories for the least amount of energy expended. Because they didn't farm the land or raise their own animals, hunter-gatherers typically preferred eating large animals if they were available, for that reason. However, they were also opportunists who ate whatever other foods were in season and were easy to gather, like roots, fruit, honey, and nuts.

From archaeological digs around the world, we can be certain that our earliest human ancestors also enjoyed eggs as a source of nutrient-rich food whenever they could find them. Records show that people in India were domesticating jungle fowl as early as 3200 BCE and that the Egyptians and Chinese were raising egg-laying birds around 1400 BCE. Although the first domesticated fowl probably didn't reach North America until the second voyage of Columbus in 1492, it's a safe bet that Native Americans were eating eggs gathered from turtles, turkeys, ducks, and other wild fowl long before that. For people like Lynda, eggs provide a source of protein that can help satisfy hunger and maintain weight loss, as well as being a terrific source of essential longevity nutrients.

Possibly the Best Reason to Eat Eggs: Choline

There are many good reasons to include eggs in your diet. For starters, eggs are one of the cheapest, most easily accessible high-quality proteins. However, there's an even better reason: The *choline* in eggs can positively impact our cognitive health as we age. In one 2023 study, researchers followed 617 men and 898 women living in Rancho Bernardo, California, all of whom were age 60 or older. For over 16 years, the men in this study who consumed more eggs did significantly better on both short- and long-term memory tests. Most importantly, these associations were independent of other health factors like cholesterol level, histories of heart disease or hypertension, cigarette smoking, and educational level. There were no similar positive associations between egg consumption and cognitive function in women, but the scientists theorized this might be because the men ate more eggs overall than the women.

Additional reports are now emerging worldwide linking egg consumption to cognitive health in our later years. While we don't fully understand the reason for this, scientists speculate that it might have to do with the choline in egg yolks. Choline is an organic, water-soluble compound that scientists are just beginning to study as a nutrient that is essential in many different bodily processes, including fat transport and metabolism, DNA synthesis and integrity, and helping maintain the nervous system and regulate mood and memory. Researchers are now starting to refer to it as vitamin B4, but dietary guidelines are still not established.

Your liver can make a small amount of choline, but we rely on consuming foods containing choline to meet our requirements. Currently, the average choline intake in adults is far below adequate intake levels. Recommended daily values for choline have been established at 550 mg for men and 450 mg for women, but only about 8 percent of adults meet these guidelines. (Young women have less need for dietary sources of choline because estrogen drives choline production.)

Despite being recognized only recently as an essential nutrient, there is already plenty of evidence that choline is truly a longevity powerhouse. If you remember the key factors affecting longevity that we described in chapter 2, choline has an impact on nearly all of them.

For instance, choline deficiency has been associated with DNA strand breaks and can alter genes that are critical to DNA repair. Deficiency can also cause radical oxygen species to leak from the mitochondria, increasing oxidative stress. A choline deficiency even impairs folate metabolism and can lead to increased homocysteine levels. Multiple studies have also linked choline intake to improved brain function, including better memory and processing. For example, one 2024 Chinese study followed 1,887 older adults for an average of 12 years and found that those who were given choline supplements were less apt to develop cognitive decline as they aged.

It is important to emphasize again that choline has only just recently been identified as an essential nutrient, and the impact of what appears to be widespread deficiency still isn't fully known. What we do know is that egg yolks are rich in choline (there's none in egg whites), with one large egg providing 113 mg of this essential nutrient and up to 25 percent of your daily requirement. More importantly, a study exploring the best ways to meet our daily requirements found that short of supplementing with choline—which can have the negative side effect of raising the risk of cardiovascular disease—it is almost impossible for adults to meet the recommendations without eating eggs.

Eggs Boost Healthy Brain Function and Vision

In addition to choline, eggs are also a great source of the antioxidants lutein and zeaxanthin, which are carotenoids that support cognitive functions as we age. These molecules are characterized by a yellow-orange color and are found in significant amounts in certain vegetables, fish, and eggs. In one study of 220 centenarians and 70 octogenarians from the Georgia Centenarian Study, higher serum and brain concentrations of these carotenoids were linked to better performance on memory, language, and executive function tests.

As antioxidants, lutein and zeaxanthin help protect your cells from being damaged by oxidative stress. This is especially important for aging eyes, since lutein and zeaxanthin, along with meso-zeaxanthin, make up the macular pigments forming the yellow spot of your iris, which is important to good vision. One of the main reasons we suffer from macular degeneration and cataracts as we age is because of the oxidative stress inflicted on the photoreceptors in rod and cone cells in our eyes by UV radiation and the blue light of our TVs and computer screens. (As you can imagine, the amount of blue light we expose our eyes to has gone up drastically with online shopping, gaming, and streaming services.) Lutein and zeaxanthin protect against the photo bleaching of our retinal pigments, age-linked macular degeneration, and cataracts, supporting eye health as we age.

The Truth About Cholesterol and Eggs

If eggs contain so many healthy nutrients, why do so many people worry about eating them? The answer lies in dated research generating pervasive fears about dietary cholesterol that have never really gone away. According to the American Heart Association, about half of all Americans are living with cardiovascular disease (CVD), which includes stroke, hypertension, congestive heart failure, and coronary heart disease. Currently, CVD is the leading cause of death for both women and men nationwide.

High levels of blood cholesterol, specifically LDL, are linked to a higher risk of CVD, so it's not surprising that in 1961 the American Heart Association and a host of other global health organizations recommended limiting dietary cholesterol. Since America's dietary sources of high-cholesterol foods are mostly red meat, dairy products, and eggs, eggs were struck off the list of healthy foods. The science on cholesterol has changed a lot, but that hasn't changed the fact that these foods got a bad rap for a long time.

Eat the whole egg

In particular, egg yolks were axed from so-called "heart-healthy" diets because that's the part of the egg that contains the cholesterol—as much as 200 g of it in a large egg. Many restaurants in the United States began showcasing egg-white omelets, and people found a myriad of ways to eliminate egg yolks from recipes. Egg whites are made up of 90 percent water and 10 percent protein, so eating only egg whites was popular among calorie-counters and those concerned about upping their risk of heart disease and other conditions associated with higher cholesterol.

But there's a problem here: While egg whites are low-calorie and cholesterol-free, they offer no nutrients beyond that small amount of protein. The most powerful longevity nutrients your body craves are in the egg yolk, as you can see from the table below:

	Egg White	Whole Egg
Calories	18	71
Protein	4 g	6 g
Fat	0 g	5 g
Cholesterol	0 g	186 mg

	Egg White	Whole Egg
Vitamin A	0% of the DV*	27% of the DV
Vitamin B12	0% of the DV	19% of the DV
Vitamin B2	11% of the DV	18% of the DV
Vitamin B5	1% of the DV	15% of the DV
Vitamin D	0% of the DV	19% of the DV
Choline	0% of the DV	27% of the DV
Selenium	8% of the DV	27% of the DV

*DV = Daily Value

As nutrition science has progressed in recent decades, it's now clear that unless you're allergic to eggs or have an autoimmune condition, they're a great Paleo food, and you're better off eating the whole egg than just the whites. If you've been told to avoid egg consumption, try eating only the yolk, since the whites contain the problematic proteins.

The science behind eggs and a lower risk of heart disease

Today, researchers consistently report that the high cholesterol in eggs doesn't translate to a higher risk of heart disease or other conditions associated with high blood cholesterol.

For instance, one 2021 paper bluntly titled "Eating Eggs Is Not Associated with Cardiovascular Disease" published in the journal *American Family Physician* highlighted a meta-analysis of 23 studies on the effects of egg consumption among 1.4 million participants, with an average follow-up of about 12 years. The authors of the metaanalysis concluded that eating an egg a day didn't raise the risk of cardiovascular disease; in fact, they found the opposite was true: Eating an egg a day *decreased* the risk of developing coronary disease by 11 percent.

While the researchers conducting this study couldn't rule out all dietary variables—for instance, the participants who ate an egg a day might simply have had healthier lifestyles overall—other researchers have demonstrated similar results worldwide. In one major study of 177,000 people in 50 different countries published in 2020 in *The American Journal of Clinical Nutrition*, researchers examined the associations between eating eggs, blood lipid levels, heart disease, and mortality. These scientists grouped participants into categories of how many eggs they ate weekly, ranging from less than one to more than seven. Their conclusion was the same as above: They found no correlation between "moderate egg intake" (one a day) and higher blood lipid levels, heart disease, or death. That research also supported the idea that an egg a day seems to keep people healthier than not eating any eggs at all.

Why should this be true? How can we eat a high-cholesterol food like eggs without raising our risk of higher blood cholesterol and CDV?

As one 2021 research paper by Japanese scientists pointed out, to truly understand the effects of egg consumption on blood cholesterol levels and disease, we must take into account the other foods people are eating with their eggs daily. This is important because most of the research showing that eggs hurt our health are epidemiological studies. In other words, the studies just show a correlation between egg consumption and disease, but don't mention anything else people might have on their plates. Bear in mind that most Americans tend to pair eggs with non-Paleo foods. Instead of having some salmon and an avocado with our omelet, we're more apt to heave piles of highly processed bacon or sausage onto our plates, along with home fries and toast.

What's even more important to understand is that most of the science of the 1980s and '90s that scared us about consuming cholesterol has since been updated or thrown out. The original research on cholesterol came out of the Framingham Heart Study in Massachusetts. When researchers created a formula showing which factors most closely correlated with heart disease, cholesterol was number one by a large margin. However, those calculations were revisited around 2010, and it was found that there were significant errors.

And it's not about cholesterol, anyway

Another important thing to understand is that the issue is not cholesterol. Cholesterol exists on the membranes of every cell in our bodies. Without cholesterol, we'd die. When we talk about LDL or HDL, we're talking about the transporters that carry cholesterol to our cells. The transporters are created in our livers and depend on the types of fats we eat—not whether we consume cholesterol or not. Eating a diet high in omega-3 fatty acids and low in omega-6 fatty acids leads to a healthier blood lipid profile. In fact, a very high correlation between the omega-6/omega-3 fatty acid profile in our diets has been associated with our cholesterol profile, with a ratio that's high in omega-3s and low in omega-6s leading to more HDL formation and less LDL formation.

Eggs contain only 1.5 grams of saturated fat and 1.8 grams of omega-6 fatty acids. Pay a little more for pasture-raised or omega-3-enriched eggs, and you can get close to that ideal 1:1 ratio of omega-6 to omega-3 fatty acids. But pay attention to what you're cooking those eggs in. For instance, a mere tablespoon of sunflower oil has 8.9 g of omega-6 fatty acids and kills the ratio.

Homecysteine

When it comes to heart disease, what's more important than the cholesterol in your diet is something many of us have never even heard of: homocysteine. Homocysteine, which is produced in our bodies during the folate cycle, is highly correlated with heart disease. When the folate cycle is functioning properly, homocysteine levels are kept very low. It's only when the cycle breaks down that homocysteine levels increase.

This is important because the folate cycle relies on three key nutrients: vitamin B12, vitamin B6, and folate. We can get folate from both animal and plant sources. Vitamin B6 is also found in plant and animal food, but the plant sources of B6 have a pyridine ring attached to them, which prevents our bodies from using it. In other words, if your only

source of B6 is plants, you're likely going to be deficient in the forms of
B6 your body can use.

Your best sources of B12 are seafood and liver, but if you don't like
either of those, next best on the list is eggs. Two eggs offer about half
of the daily value for vitamin B12. A single egg has about 10 percent of
the daily value for vitamin B6 and 6 percent for folate. One other thing
to know about the folate cycle, besides its important role in heart health,
is that the cycle plays a key role in DNA repair, and as we discussed in
chapter 1, keeping your DNA healthy is essential for successful aging.

Biotin Versus Avidin

One of the vitamins you might not recognize is vitamin H, but you probably know it by its other name: biotin. Like all B complex vitamins,
biotin helps your body metabolize fats and turn food into fuel, convert-
ing carbohydrates into glucose to produce energy. Biotin also supports
liver health and helps your nervous system function efficiently. A biotin
deficiency can cause you to experience hair loss, scaly skin, and depression. Biotin deficiency may also adversely affect your immune system,
increasing inflammation and inducing some immunological disorders.
Mice studies have also shown that biotin deficiency can cause an abnormal amino acid profile, and as you probably gleaned from our earlier
discussion of amino acids (see page 154), it's essential to maintain them
in the right ratios.

Biotin is water soluble, which means your body can't store it. However, bacteria in your intestine can make biotin, and good dietary sources
include liver, salmon, sweet potato, and eggs—especially the yolks. A
single egg yolk can provide a whopping 33 percent of your daily value
for biotin.

Raw egg whites, on the other hand, contain avidin, an antimicrobial protein that binds very strongly with biotin and creates a powerful
chemical bond called an avidin-biotin complex that your body can't
absorb. Some studies show that adults and teenagers who chronically

consume raw egg whites can suffer a biotin deficiency as a result. Multiple studies have been conducted to explore biotin deficiency. To induce deficiency in the subjects, the researchers didn't ask subjects to reduce biotin in their diets. Instead, they simply had the subjects eat an egg white–based beverage.

Generally, you would have to eat a lot of egg whites to impact your biotin absorption. Most people believe that cooking eggs denatures the avidin protein in egg whites, thereby reducing its ability to bind biotin, but research shows that the only way to completely inactivate avidin is by boiling the egg for at least 25 minutes. Accordingly, there is some evidence that marginal biotin deficiency—particularly during pregnancy, which increases the risk of birth defects—may be more common than we had originally thought.

So, if you're worried about the avidin in eggs binding with the biotin and having a negative impact on your overall health, you can consume foods high in biotin to counteract that. Our strongest suggestion, which will certainly turn heads at the health food restaurant, is to eat the nutrient-dense egg yolk and forgo the whites.

Which Eggs Should You Buy?

Most large grocery stores offer a large variety of eggs to choose from now. That's a good thing—but it's also confusing at times. For instance, what's the difference between "pasture-raised" and "free range?"

Here are some useful terms to help you navigate that tricky egg aisle:

- Cage-free: This is a term regulated by the USDA, and it means eggs that are laid by hens "able to roam vertically and horizontally in indoor houses"—in other words, not necessarily outside.
- Free-range: This is another USDA term, and it means cage-free, but the hens must have "continuous access to the outdoors during their laying cycle." Sounds great, but the outdoor area might be small and crowded.

- Omega-3 eggs: We have discussed the importance of omega-3 fatty acids throughout the book. Egg producers have also heard this message and have used it as a sales pitch by adding omega-3 fatty acids to chicken feed. Buying eggs supplemented with omega-3 fatty acids might be prudent if you can only get non-pasture-raised eggs, but your best bet is still to choose pasture-raised eggs, since they already have a better omega-6 to omega-3 fatty acid profile. They also provide a higher nutrient density.
- Pasture-raised: This is not a USDA term, which means it can vary by farm. Cartons labeled as "pasture-raised" that also include a Certified Humane seal mean the chickens get to roam freely in a pasture during the day and are provided tents for shade, water coolers, and even trees. They can forage, run around, and chat with other chickens. Every Certified Humane farm is audited by an inspector with a master's or doctoral degree in animal science.
- Organic: Eggs labeled with the USDA's National Organic Program label are defined as those eating organic feed without conventional pesticides or fertilizers. They must be uncaged hens with access to the outdoors and at least one square foot of outdoor space for each 2.25 pounds of poultry.
- 100% natural: "Natural" is not a regulated term, so it doesn't necessarily mean anything. It's often confused with "organic," but all this means is that nothing was added to the eggs.
- Hormone-free: This is a meaningless label, since it's illegal in the United States for chickens raised for meat consumption or egg laying to be given hormones.
- No added antibiotics: Farmers often give antibiotics to the animals they raise as food to prevent and treat disease. This label doesn't indicate anything about how the chickens are raised or what they ate.

Once you read through these definitions, you'll understand why we recommend eating organic eggs laid by pasture-raised hens whenever possible.

CHAPTER THIRTEEN

Why Seafood Is a Top
Paleo Superfood

In 2021, people participating in Paleo Diet focus groups told a consistent story about their eating habits: Most reported eating okay as children but lapsing into eating junk food diets through their teen years and college. They then extended those bad habits into adulthood partly because they were habits, partly because they never learned to cook, and partly because they simply didn't know which foods were healthy because of decades of food industry marketing. Generally, they didn't notice any negative health impacts until they graduated from college and started desk-based careers. That's when it all caught up to them, and they experienced weight gain and other negative health impacts from their eating habits.

Unlike those participants, Brigid says her diet was poor as a young child. "My parents let me eat as many sweets and drink as much soda as I wanted, so of course I did." Luckily, she'd always been a hiker, swimmer, and skier, so she was never overweight.

Brigid's diet improved when she married a hunter and moved to rural Oregon. Living on a farm with dairy goats, chickens, and a big garden, they grew a lot of their own food and ate game meat her husband killed. The nearest restaurant was so far away that "you cooked, or you didn't eat," she says, reflecting that she was "eating mostly Paleo" but didn't realize it.

Then Brigid had two children, returned to work full-time as a teacher, and suffered a curveball when she was diagnosed with thyroid cancer in her early 40s. After surgeries and radiation, she was constantly fatigued. "My body was falling apart, and I realized I needed to make some changes."

She was close to 50 by then. Her first attempt at improving her diet was trying keto, "but I just felt crappy on it." Next Brigid went to WeightWatchers, "but I was starved the whole time. Plus, I wasn't trying to lose weight. It was more about trying to be healthier."

Finally, Brigid landed on the Paleo Diet. "Right away I got rid of milk products. Then I started packing my own lunches, so I'd have a healthier midday meal. I took a lot of sugar out of my diet, too, like not having cereal for breakfast. The thing I liked about Paleo was that I could eat as much as I wanted of the foods that were allowed. I didn't have to be food-obsessed or count calories."

It has been 12 years now since Brigid first tried Paleo nutrition. Since then, she's been Paleo "on and off," so she has firsthand evidence that eating Paleo "makes a huge difference in how I feel," she says, "and it's always reflected in my blood tests."

When her last tests showed that she was inching toward kidney failure because of a medication she'd been taking after thyroid surgery, Dr. Cordain suggested that Brigid add more taurine to her diet. Now 67, she's currently following the Paleo Diet about 85 percent of the time. She adds taurine to her nutritional intake through supplements and plenty of seafood, like the skinless sardines she mixes with vegetables to eat on homemade flourless tortillas, or the smoked salmon her husband makes.

Today, Brigid credits eating Paleo for helping her qualify for an experimental drug to treat her kidney disease. Her recent blood tests led her doctor to comment on how well she has regulated her calcium levels—an important thing for kidney function.

"Taurine regulates your calcium at a cellular level as well as lowering your blood pressure. It's good for your brain, too," she says. "Best of all, I feel like a new person since going back on Paleo and adding more taurine to my diet."

The old saying that "fish is brain food" isn't just some advertising tagline dreamed up by the seafood industry. It's grounded in truth. There's no such thing as one perfect food for humans, but seafood comes close, providing your body with lean protein; vitamins A, E, and C; omega-3 fatty acids; iodine; and the mineral selenium, among other things.

Seafood's Powerhouse Nutrients

The powerhouse nutrients in seafood go a long way toward helping you win the longevity battle by lowering inflammation and decreasing the risk of age-related diseases like diabetes, cognitive decline, heart disease, and hypertension. Researchers recently published a paper showing several studies examining the positive impacts seafood can have on our overall health. In one of these studies, scientists demonstrated that among 3,500 men in South Korea who ate a diet high in fish consumption, these individuals saw a 57 percent reduction in their risk of developing metabolic syndrome. Another report featured in this paper was a five-year study in the United States with people who ate fish an average of five times a week; this study showed similar results.

That paper also highlighted a recent British study that followed 392,287 women middle-aged or older over a 10-year period, and revealed that the women who regularly ate oily fish—like salmon, trout, or sardines—had a lower risk of type 2 diabetes.

When it comes to keeping our cognitive faculties sharp, seafood also proves to be a stunning ally. This is especially important because we're a big-brained species. As we discussed in chapter 11, one of the most significant evolutionary changes of the last million years has been the development of the modern human brain. While some argue about whether our ancient ancestors got their omega-3s from fish or bone marrow, it's clear that their high consumption of omega-3s promoted their brain development.

As we get older, so do our brains, of course. Some of the age-related changes in our brain structure can lead to mild cognitive impairment (MCI), which manifests in memory problems. MCI can be an early sign of Alzheimer's, too, though not everyone who develops MCI will develop Alzheimer's. Now scientists are regularly demonstrating that a diet rich in fatty fish can have a positive impact on sharper cognitive function and brain health, as well as improved vision.

Why should eating more fish protect you against cognitive decline as you age? It's partly because fish contains a high level of omega-3 fatty acids, which are associated with boosting brain health by helping your brain maintain its structural integrity and overall volume. Several recent studies have even suggested that people who include fish regularly in their meals have fewer markers of Alzheimer's disease than those who do not.

Oily fish are a particularly good source of the omega-3 fatty acids DHA and EPA. Seafood is also rich in selenium, a mineral that researchers have demonstrated can help battle the cell damage we experience over time due to oxidative stress. Other studies have focused on the connection between eating seafood and a lower incidence of the chronic inflammation that so often leads to age-related diseases like diabetes, cancer, and cardiovascular disease.

It's certainly possible to get omega-3s from plant sources such as flaxseed and soybeans. But it's important to point out that the plant form of omega-3s, alpha-linolenic acid (ALA), must be converted to EPA and then to DHA. Our bodies can convert only about 1 percent of ALA, so seafood is a much better source of omega-3s than plants for humans.

What Is Oily (or Fatty) Fish Exactly?

Nutritionists and the media regularly tout the benefits of oily or fatty fish. What they're talking about is fish that contain high levels of oil in their body tissues. This oil contains two important fatty acids we've already mentioned here, EPA and DHA, both of which have proven wide-ranging health benefits.

The newest nutrition research illuminates two more key reasons why you should embrace the benefits of seafood. The first is taurine, an amino acid found in scallops, mussels, clams, and oysters. The other is astaxanthin, a red-orange pigment that's usually abundant in animals that feed on algae that contain it, like salmon, red trout, Arctic char, and crustaceans (shrimp, crab, lobster, and crayfish).

The Turbo Power of Taurine

Taurine—a sulfur-containing amino acid—is the most abundant amino acid in the human body, making up 0.1 percent of the total human body weight. In an average man, that amounts to about 70 grams of taurine, far more than any other amino acid.

While amino acids have other roles, their most important function is building proteins. Given this, you might logically assume that as abundant as taurine is, it must be essential for making proteins.

Surprisingly, it's not. Taurine isn't used to build proteins at all, but its list of functions in your body is impressive. For instance, taurine is important for regulating electrolytes and minerals across cell membranes, which helps support your cells as they metabolize energy. It is also contained in your bile salt, which helps you process cholesterol and digest food. However, taurine's most important function in mammals is to act as a powerful antioxidant.

Studies showing the benefits of taurine to humans have been rapidly accumulating since 1985, when Japan first approved taurine for treating heart patients. Researchers have since demonstrated that this amino acid is a reliable warrior in our body's fight against any of the age-related diseases associated with damage to the mitochondria in our cells, from cancer and cardiovascular diseases to hypertension and neurological disorders.

As such a powerful and abundant antioxidant, it's not surprising that taurine is associated with longevity. The longest-living organisms on earth include the bowhead whale, which can live up to 200 years. The Greenland shark is estimated to live up to 400 years, making it the longest-lived vertebrate on earth, and the ocean quahog clam lives up to 500 years, making it the longest-lived animal of all. What do these three animals have in common? They consume very high quantities of taurine. Clams get it from filtering algae—the ultimate source of taurine—while the bowhead whale and Greenland shark consume krill, scallops, clams, and mollusks, which are all good sources of taurine.

In animal studies, researchers recently reported in the journal *Science* that reversing age-related decline by supplementing taurine in studies with mice and monkeys led to an increased lifespan of up to 12 percent. More importantly, taurine supplements promoted an increased "health span" in these animals, meaning they weren't just living longer, but were healthier as they aged.

Another animal study—this one with mice—showed that taurine may help prevent the moisture loss, damage, and wrinkles we experience over time as our skin is exposed to the sun. In one study with hairless mice exposed to doses of UVB radiation for varying amounts of time, mice that received taurine supplements suffered less moisture loss in their skin—and therefore had fewer wrinkles than the mice that didn't.

Human studies with taurine have proved just as promising. For example, taurine can help people manage diabetes. Scientists have also shown that taurine has neuroprotective properties; it may help improve cognitive function and reduce the risk of neurological disorders such as

Alzheimer's disease. Additionally, research shows it may improve liver function in people with liver disease.

If that's not enough reason to celebrate taurine, this longevity ally can also help us combat the retinal disorders that may develop over time due to accumulated oxidative stress. That's partly because taurine plays a key role in the function of vitamin A in the visual pathways, which in turn can prevent retinol-induced damage in the eyes.

Cats are obligate carnivores and must get taurine from animal sources; there's a form of blindness found in cats fed a plant-based diet due to taurine deficiency. Unlike cats, humans can synthesize taurine in our livers. But as we age, our ability to produce taurine tails off, which makes it very important for us to get enough taurine in our diets in our older years. One major reason that eating adequate seafood is important is that there aren't any plant sources of this amino acid. Vegans can become taurine deficient. When this happens, there is research showing that they can suffer from neutropenia; this occurs when there are very low levels of important immune cells called neutrophils, and taurine is the primary fuel of neutrophils.

Taurine is considered safe and has no toxic effects for adults with doses as high as 7 grams per day.

The Amazing Longevity Power of Astaxanthin

As we discussed in chapter 2, living longer means that our bodies experience more oxidative stress due to decades of injuries, illnesses, UV radiation, and environmental toxins. Meanwhile, our antioxidant and cell repair processes become less effective as time goes by, leaving us more vulnerable to age-related diseases.

In recent decades, carotenoids—the yellow, orange, and red pigments synthesized by plants that serve as the precursors of vitamin A—have generated excitement in the research community because they act as powerful antioxidants, protecting our cells from oxidative stress. Carotenoids can help repair cell mitochondria and line up as a powerful defense against the most common diseases of aging, like cancer, heart disease, diabetes, and hypertension.

One carotenoid stands head and shoulders above the rest: *astaxanthin*. While many carotenoids are found in plants, as we covered in chapter 4, our best sources of astaxanthin come from seafood, particularly Antarctic krill, algae, and northern shrimp. Astaxanthin is considered safe by the US Food and Drug Administration with no known toxic effects, and you can consume up to 8 mg per day.

The Best Ways to Incorporate Fish into Your Diet

As a lifelong athlete and a chiropractor for over 40 years, David, 68, has always been interested in nutrition. He discovered the Paleo way of eating through a biochemist friend who was "big on the hunter-gatherer thing," he says, "and it all made sense to me."

David is quick to point out that he never diets. "As a chiropractor, my whole thing isn't about treating symptoms. It's about stimulating optimal function in my body and in the people I treat. I watch what I eat not out of vanity, but because I want to maintain my own optimal function and keep doing the fun stuff in my life."

For him, the "fun stuff" isn't sitting on the couch eating chips, he explains, but "being active with friends and family. That means skiing, hiking, golfing, or biking around the countryside."

Even so, "You can't outrun your fork," he says. "It doesn't matter how much you exercise if you're not going to give yourself a chance from the get-go to be healthy with the right nutrition." Or, to put it more simply, "Junk in, junk out," he says with a laugh.

David has maintained a healthy weight through the years and his blood pressure is a youthful 110/60. Today, he generally avoids the middle aisles of the grocery store and any processed foods, preferring to make salads or healthy shakes, and cooks his own vegetables and grass-finished meats at home.

"Anything that you can keep for years in your cupboard? Nothing good is in those boxes and cans," he warns. In fact, working in healthcare for so long has made him think that processed carbohydrates, along with things like high-fructose corn syrup and most vegetable oils, "should be listed as pre-diabetes foods."

The one place where his diet falls short is seafood, he admits. "Believe me, I'm well aware of the benefits of fish, but I still don't eat nearly enough of it."

David isn't alone. The most recent Dietary Guidelines for Americans 2020–2025 recommends that Americans should eat seafood at least twice a week. Sadly, fewer than one in five Americans reach that goal. About a third of us eat seafood only once a week, and nearly half eat seafood only occasionally or never.

With the Paleo Diet, we encourage you to include higher amounts of fish in your diet—at least four servings of 3.5 ounces every week. We'll address mercury below (see "Try a Little Seaweed for Variety"), but something to know is that mercury becomes more concentrated in fish higher up on the food chain. You can get the health benefits of oily fish from smaller bottom-dwelling seafood without having to ingest the mercury hit you'd get from larger fish.

As for what kind of seafood is best to buy, we recommend choosing from the following list:

Eel	Pilchards
Herring	Rockfish
Kippers	Salmon
Mackerel	Sardines
Mussels	Scallops
Ocean quahog	Trout
Oysters	Tuna
Pacific halibut	Whitebait

Try a Little Seaweed for Variety

As we discussed in our plant foods section, seaweed and algae are rich sources of protein, iodine, and omega-3 fatty acids. These are one of the few plant foods that contains EPA and DHA, so add a little crunch to your diet with nori, the seaweed used in sushi, or by snacking on crispy dried seaweed. Your smoothies can be made extra nutritious by adding chlorella and spirulina, too.

Tips on Buying the Freshest, Healthiest Fish

If you haven't had a lot of experience in shopping for seafood, you might be wary about adding more fish to your diet. It's important to always choose fish that's wild caught or farmed in environmentally sustainable ways. That's easy to do if you follow these simple guidelines:

Ask questions

Ask other locals and fish-loving friends for recommendations on where to buy good seafood. Then, begin to build your own relationships with fish sellers. Approaching the counter might feel a little awkward at first, but once you're used to doing this, it will be worth the effort. Your fishmonger should be able to tell you where your fish came from and the best choices for the freshest seafood that day. They might even have a few good cooking tips or suggestions.

Give it a sniff

If you are buying at a reputable location, you can always request to smell the fish before purchasing. Fresh fish will smell clean, not fishy. If your market doesn't let you smell the fish, you shouldn't be shopping there.

Look it over carefully

Freshness is really in the details. When whole fish are past their peak selling point, there are telltale signs, like sunken eyes or dullness. Make sure the fish's eyes are full and the body is bright and shiny. Gills should be red or have a pinkish hue—never purple or brown!

Consider your location

If you live on a coast, you'll want the freshest fish coming straight from the docks and not already frozen, as indicated by the word "refreshed." However, if you are far from the coast, perhaps pre-frozen fish is your best choice, as you don't want "fresh" fish that's been sitting on a truck way too long.

Check the source

When buying fish from a particular seller, ask about their sourcing and sustainability efforts. Are they selling wild-caught fish they've bought from fishers who use safe-practice fishing? Are the fish harvested from toxin-free waters? And, if the fish is farm-raised (as in today's aquaculture), are their fish free from added hormones and antibiotics? Remember: You're not just what you eat, but what you eat eats, so asking these questions can help you stay even healthier as you age.

If you want to be doubly sure that you're eating healthy seafood, check out the Monterey Bay Aquarium Seafood Watch at Seafood Watch.org for the most updated seafood recommendations.

What About Fish Oil Supplements?

When you hear about the benefits of a particular nutrient, like taurine, it might be tempting to think, "If I just buy it in supplement form, I'll get more of it, it'll cost me less, and I don't have to deal with all of the troubling cooking and preparation. It's a win-win-win situation."

Unfortunately, that's not how nutrition works. As we discussed in chapter 1, there's a very important concept in nutrition. In a nutshell, so to speak, it's this: A low dose of a nutritionally stressful stimulant activates the body to increase resistance to that stress through different mechanisms, including gene repair and cellular death. However, too much of certain foods can have a negative effect instead of helping our bodies build up an increased resistance to stress. For example, we need sodium in our diet to survive, but too much sodium can lead to conditions like heart disease and cancer.

This is always the challenge and danger with supplements. A particular nutrient may be highly beneficial for our health, but if you take it in pill form, you're likely to get a larger dose than what exists in nature. That means you're no longer consuming it in natural ratios with other key nutrients, and that superfood nutrient may be damaging your health.

However, one of the most recommended supplements is omega-3 fish oils, and there is plenty of research showing its benefits. So, should you take those? While some research supports the benefits of fish oil supplements, the results from long-term studies are hazier. Previously, we discussed the important ratio between sodium and potassium in our diet. Likewise, another key ratio for long-term health is that of omega-3-to-omega-6 fatty acids, which is optimally around 1:1. The typical Western diet has a ratio of around 15:1. This is concerning because when we consume too much omega-6 fatty acid relative to omega-3s, we can overproduce a molecule called cyclooxygenase-2, which may cause pain. In fact, some over-the-counter pain medications such as ibuprofen and naproxen are simply cyclooxygenase-2 inhibitors, so it's not surprising that some studies show that consuming more omega-3s and fewer omega-6s can reduce pain as much as those common medications.

We will always recommend getting your nutrients from natural foods, where you'll consume them in the right ratios and in balance.

The best way to achieve the optimal 1:1 ratio of omega-6s to omega-3s is through a healthy diet. Plus, as we've discussed, seafood offers many more benefits than just omega-3s, like providing you with astaxanthin, iodine, and taurine.

All that being said, when it comes to omega-3s, astaxanthin, and taurine, we can still justify some supplementation, if only because it's sometimes difficult to find good natural sources of these three nutrients. Just keep in mind that if you do supplement, more is not necessarily better. When it comes to omega-3s we wouldn't recommend more than a few thousand milligrams per day. Generally speaking, it is unusual to move the omega-6-to-omega-3 ratio to below one, but it's possible. If you have concerns about your over-consumption of omega-3s, this is something your healthcare provider can measure. Then you will know if you need to adjust your supplementation.

Is Seafood Healthy Even Though It Can Be High in Salt?

Scallops, mussels, and certain other types of seafood are very high in taurine. Some seafood is also very high in sodium, and as you know from chapter 7, the Paleo Diet recommends not consuming added salt, which lowers the sodium content of the diet compared to the typical Western diet. So how can we justify eating these foods?

The answer goes back to what we explained in chapter 1: There are key nutrient ratios in our diets and one of them is the sodium-to-potassium ratio. We should be eating more potassium than sodium—in a ratio of 5:1 or higher. Fortunately, most seafood that is high in sodium is also very high in potassium. For example, 1 cup of oysters has 210 mg of sodium, but 386 mg of potassium. No, you won't hit a 5:1 ratio eating just oysters, but if you combine them with plenty of vegetables and other seafood like salmon, which is low in sodium, hitting a 5:1 potassium-to-sodium ratio shouldn't be a problem.

What About Mercury?

Even though seafood is highly nutritious, delicious, and easy to prepare, and provides us with a source of healthy minerals, vitamins, protein, and fats, many people are afraid to eat it because they've heard that seafood is high in mercury, which can be toxic to our health. But if you eat smart, you don't need to worry, and the nutritional benefits of seafood far outweigh the risks.

Mercury levels in seafood depend on the age and size of the fish and where it was raised or caught. Tuna is the worst offender, especially if it's eaten raw, followed by swordfish. Seafood that's low in mercury includes cod, haddock, herring, salmon, sardines, and shellfish.

PART IV
Your Paleo Journey

CHAPTER FOURTEEN

Our 85/15 Guide to Natural, Healthy Eating

Tracy began studying health and nutrition in 2009 to help her husband manage his high blood sugar, cholesterol, and triglyceride
levels. Still searching for the healthiest possible lifestyle in 2015, they
adopted a keto-carnivore diet, but that turned out to be problematic.

"Because I didn't have enough stomach acid, I ended up with *H. pylori*
(a serious stomach infection). That led to all kinds of other problems. I had
pain in my joints, feet, and lower back; vertigo; and digestive issues."

Tracy saw specialist after specialist. When none of them had answers,
she took matters into her own hands and began cutting wheat, wine, and
sugar out of her diet. "I was going to try a Whole30 elimination diet, but
then decided to look at the Paleo Diet website. I read through a lot of the
information and printed out grocery lists and other resources. I finally
gave up all dairy except half-and-half in my coffee, and have been eating
more vegetables, animal protein, and fruit based on the grocery lists."

After a couple of weeks, Tracy noticed that her vertigo had gone away.
Next to disappear were the migraines. "I couldn't believe it, so I tested

this by eating wheat again, and that shifting feeling I associate with vertigo returned. That's when I realized I had a histamine intolerance."

Now 55, Tracy finds it's relatively easy to stay on the Paleo Diet. If she does venture off the diet and eat something like pasta with cheese and butter, "it's so rich I can barely eat it." She's more apt to crave her go-to vegetables, like a big green salad with asparagus, zucchini, or any other fresh vegetables in season.

"The Western diet has far too much processed food," says Tracy, who completed a nutrition certification program in 2021 and a health coach certification program in 2022, with the goal of one day working as a health and wellness coach. By eating Paleo, "I'm on a good, basic anti-inflammatory diet," she says, adding that she has the firsthand evidence she needs to prove this: "If I do decide to go off Paleo and eat bread, my feet hurt the next day."

Her husband's doctor wanted to prescribe metformin to control his blood sugar, Tracy adds, but thanks to the Paleo Diet, he's been able to lower his blood sugar without medication. "I wanted to tell that doctor sorry, but we're not going to help you fund those pharmaceutical companies," she says with a laugh. "We'll just keep doing what we're doing, focusing on fresh foods that have been around for many years."

———

For more than 20 years, Dr. Cordain has shared simple guidelines for how to practice a Paleo lifestyle, and as Tracy discovered, those guidelines have always focused on fresh, natural foods that we were meant to eat. In the past two decades, our team has learned even more about the practice of Paleolithic nutrition, but one thing remains true: We have confirmed that, for most people, it's unnecessary and unrealistic to eat 100 percent Paleo foods 100 percent of the time.

While our hunter-gatherer ancestors didn't have doughnuts, soft drinks, and other processed foods at hand, they did occasionally eat unhealthy foods like grass seeds, and they couldn't clean and sanitize their food the way we do today. Our bodies have evolved to handle a certain amount of less-than-optimal foods if it's kept to a small percentage of what we eat. In fact, as we discussed in chapter 1, many nutrition scientists and immunologists feel it's beneficial to challenge the body's digestive and immune systems with minor irritants to help keep systems regulated, primed, and functioning at their best.

Secondly, trying to stay 100 percent Paleo in today's fast-paced world is just too challenging for most people, and it's likely to cause frustration and failure. That's not how we want you to feel about food, eating, and health. Our hope is that you'll find the Paleo Diet to be a positive force of inspiration, not a source of disappointment. We would much rather see you sustain a mostly Paleo way of eating for a lifetime of health. After all, the Paleo Diet is not intended to be a short-term diet. We've designed it as a lifestyle that unlocks years of better health through smarter eating.

The Original 85/15 Rule

The best way to sustain the Paleo Diet for a lifetime is through flexibility. Dr. Cordain's first book, *The Paleo Diet*, introduced the 85/15 rule, which encouraged followers to eat Paleo 85 percent of the time and less restrictive foods 15 percent of the time. We still believe that's the best way to go.

For many of you starting out, even 85/15 may feel too hard, but that's fine. Any improvement is just that—an improvement. If someone is eating only 25 percent Paleo and they can double that to 50 percent without too much difficulty, they will still reap benefits. While some people enjoy the challenge of jumping into the deep end and going right to 85/15, and others might decide for health reasons that strictly adhering to a Paleo lifestyle is better for them, most people experience the greatest success in the long run by starting slowly and gradually making a habit of Paleo choices on their plates. Even a small shift in the way you eat will make a big difference—and feeling better can help motivate you to keep moving forward.

Trevor learned this as a cycling coach. He worked with athletes who had just bought their first bikes and athletes who raced the Tour de France. When his new athletes rode 20 miles for the first time, he celebrated with them. He didn't say, "So what, the Tour guy did 100 yesterday." Developing as an athlete is a journey where you celebrate your successes along the way. Moving toward a healthier diet is the same.

One way to think about the 85/15 rule is to focus on how you eat non-Paleo for that 15 percent of the time. Ideally, you want to think of it as the 85/10/5 rule, where the non-Paleo category is split into a goal of 10 percent minimally processed food, such as legumes and dairy, and 5 percent highly processed foods like packaged snacks and desserts. Categorizing your non-Paleo foods into "minimally processed" and "ultra-processed" can help remind you that not all non-Paleo foods are highly processed foods, and that there are tiers of healthy foods instead of just "good" or "bad" foods. In fact, it might help to mentally color code foods according to traffic light colors: green for Paleo, yellow for unprocessed non-Paleo foods, and red for processed foods.

If you're eating a typical American diet, you're likely consuming 25 percent Paleo-friendly foods; 25 percent minimally processed, non-Paleo foods like grains, legumes, and dairy; and a whopping 50 percent processed or even highly ultra-processed food. Here's an achievable stepping-stone approach: Start by simply replacing 25 percent of your processed foods with optimal Paleo foods.

Why go this route instead of changing your diet cold turkey? Because if you make the shift to eating Paleo 50 percent of the time, your palate will change and you'll start wanting to eat those healthier foods. Plus, you're sure to see breakthroughs in your health and weight that will motivate you to keep moving up in compliance.

Many people may end up short of the final goal and cap out at around 75 percent optimal foods, 15 percent minimally processed foods, and 10 percent highly processed foods. But if this is a ratio that you can stick with, do it. We still see it as a successful dietary change.

Let's look at an example. If you're used to going out to eat in restaurants, your typical menu choice might have been the following before trying the Paleo Diet:

- Appetizer: Deep-fried onion rings
- Main meal: Grass-fed beef burger with a bun, French fries, and wild rice
- Dessert: Full-dairy ice cream

While this might sound like a very tasty meal, it's unfortunately very close to the standard American diet ratio of 25/25/50 described above. Our first goal is to cut the highly processed foods in half and replace them with better foods. An easy way to accomplish this:

- Appetizer: Swap the onion rings for a field greens salad.
- Main meal: Keep the grass-fed beef burger but skip the bun. Keep the wild rice (which is not really a type of rice, but a grass), but replace the fries with a baked sweet potato or even sweet potato fries (cooked in avocado oil), and add a side of broccoli.
- Dessert: Go for the full-dairy ice cream because you've been good!

This now looks a lot more like the 50/25/25 breakdown, but you're still getting to eat the foods you enjoy with a few conscious swaps and additions.

In time, and as your palate changes, you can improve even further to reach the 85/10/5 goal as shown below:

- Appetizer: Field greens salad
- Main meal: Grass-fed beef burger without a bun, with wild rice, broccoli, and asparagus
- Dessert: Small scoop of full-dairy ice cream with mixed berries

While thinking of the 85/10/5 rule by volume is helpful when you are just getting started on the Paleo Diet, an easier and more healthful approach long-term is allowing three "treat" meals each week. Two can include non-Paleo unprocessed foods, while one can incorporate processed foods. Choose the approach that works for you. The ultimate goal is to reduce your processed food consumption and increase your whole natural food consumption.

Another way to start is to think about how many meals you eat each week, and divide them into 50 percent Paleo, 35 percent "mostly" Paleo, and 15 percent non-Paleo. Most people eat three meals a day, so that's 21 meals each week. If you're doing entry-level Paleo, you might want to break them down like this:

- Only Paleo foods for half your meals (11 meals/week)
- Mostly Paleo foods (that is, maybe you throw in a piece of toast or have a cookie for dessert after your salad) for 35 percent of your meals (7 meals/week)
- Non-Paleo foods for 15 percent of your meals (3 meals/week)

What About Alcohol?

Alcohol is not Paleo. Red or white wine consumed in moderation can be an enjoyable part of your 15 percent non-Paleo portion in the 85/15 Paleo Rule, but try to avoid red wine that has added sulfites, which are not healthy.

Provided you hit the 11-7-3 ratio of 11 healthiest, 7 healthy, and 3 treat meals per week, you should notice changes in how you feel within a week or two. Then, depending on your goals for health and longevity, you might want to gradually work up to a more Paleo lifestyle, perhaps eating only Paleo foods for a larger percent of your meals each week. The important thing is to find a rhythm that works for you.

To get you started—and to get you excited about trying Paleo—we've included more than 50 easy, delicious recipes for you to mix and match according to your taste buds and goals. Enjoy!

CHAPTER FIFTEEN

Delicious *and* Healthy Paleo for Life Recipes

BREAKFAST

Mushroom Omelet

A mushroom omelet is a perfect blend of simplicity and flavor, making it a great option for a busy weekday morning or a leisurely weekend brunch. We love how the sautéed mushrooms and shallots add an earthy depth to the fluffy eggs, creating a satisfying yet light meal. Regarding avidin and biotin, if biotin deficiency is a problem, or if you are on the autoimmune protocol (AIP), use only the egg yolks.

Serves 4

Ingredients

2 tablespoons + 1 teaspoon extra-virgin olive oil, divided

1 shallot, minced

8 ounces cremini mushrooms, trimmed and sliced ¼ inch thick

12 large eggs

¼ teaspoon AIP-Friendly Herbes de Provence (page 261)

2 tablespoons (or more) chopped fresh parsley, for garnish

2 green onions, trimmed and thinly sliced crosswise, for garnish

Method

1. Heat 1 tablespoon of the olive oil in a 9-inch skillet over medium-high heat. Sauté the shallot, stirring constantly, for 5 to 8 minutes, until softened. Add the mushrooms, turn the heat down to medium, and cook for 3 to 5 minutes, until browned on one side, then cook for 5 more minutes while stirring with a wooden spoon or silicone spatula. Transfer the mushrooms and shallot to a medium bowl.

2. In a large bowl, whisk the eggs; optionally, run them through a fine-mesh strainer to thoroughly combine the whites and yolks, which results in a smoother omelet. Add the Herbes de Provence. Divide the whisked eggs into 4 equal portions in 4 smaller bowls.

3. Heat 1 teaspoon of the olive oil in the same skillet over medium heat. Pour one portion of the whisked eggs into the skillet. Let them cook undisturbed for 1 minute, or until the edges start to set. Spread one-quarter of the cooked mushrooms and shallot evenly over half of the cooking eggs in the skillet. Using a spatula, gently fold the other half of the eggs over the mushroom filling. Cook for 1 minute, or until the eggs are completely set and the omelet is golden brown on the bottom. Transfer to a plate and keep warm in a low oven until ready to serve. Repeat to cook the remaining 3 omelets, using another 1 teaspoon olive oil for each.

4. Garnish the omelets with the parsley and green onions and serve hot.

Soft Scramble

A soft scramble is a meditative cooking experience as you cook the eggs low and slow. This method ensures that the eggs are creamy and tender, almost velvety in texture. Regarding avidin and biotin, if biotin deficiency is a problem, or if you are on the autoimmune protocol (AIP), use only the egg yolks.

Serves 4

Ingredients

8 large eggs
Pinch AIP-Friendly Herbes de Provence (page 261)
2 tablespoons extra-virgin olive oil, divided
Tomato or avocado slices, for serving

Method

1. In a large bowl, whisk the eggs; optionally, run them through a fine-mesh strainer to thoroughly combine the whites and yolks, which results in a smoother scramble. Add the Herbes de Provence.
2. Heat 1 tablespoon of the olive oil in a medium skillet over medium-low heat. Add half of the egg mixture to the center of the pan and allow it to fill the oil-coated skillet. When the edges of the egg start to set, use a silicone spatula to move the edges of the eggs around the outside of the pan, but do not flip them. Continue to work the eggs in a clockwise motion from outside to inside, stopping from time to time to allow the eggs to cook. Then eggs should be barely set when you take them out of the pan. Err on the side of low and slow—the total cook time will be 2 to 3 minutes. Divide the eggs between 2 plates. Cook the remaining eggs in the same manner, using the remaining 1 tablespoon oil.
3. Serve with a side of sliced tomato or avocado.

Crustless Quiche

We love how this dish is loaded with many textures and flavors, making it a great meal-prep option or a centerpiece for a weekend breakfast gathering. It can be served warm or chilled. Regarding avidin and biotin, if biotin deficiency is a problem, or if you are on the autoimmune protocol (AIP), use only the egg yolks.

Serves 4–6

Ingredients

Extra-virgin olive oil, as needed

12 large eggs

1 cup diced unrefined pork belly

1 large Japanese sweet potato, peeled and cut into small cubes

2 large portobello mushroom caps, sliced lengthwise

1 shallot, thinly sliced

1 teaspoon AIP-Friendly Herbes de Provence (page 261)

Method

1. Preheat the oven to 375°F. Lightly coat a 9 x 9-inch baking dish or quiche pan with olive oil.
2. In a large bowl, whisk the eggs; optionally, run them through a fine-mesh strainer to thoroughly combine the whites and yolks. Set aside.
3. In a large skillet, cook the pork belly over medium heat until it becomes crispy and golden brown, 3 to 5 minutes. Transfer the pork belly to a plate, leaving the rendered fat in the skillet. Add the sweet potato cubes and cook for 5 to 7 minutes, until they start to soften and get a bit of color. Add the mushrooms and shallot and cook for 5 minutes, or until everything is tender. Season with the Herbes de Provence and remove from the heat.
4. Spread the cooked sweet potato, pork belly, mushrooms, and shallot evenly in the baking dish. Pour the eggs over the top, ensuring

they cover all the ingredients. Bake for 30 to 35 minutes, or until the quiche is set and the top is golden brown. A toothpick inserted into the center should come out clean.

5. Remove the quiche from the oven and let it cool for a few minutes before slicing and serving.

Avocado Egg Bakes

Avocado lovers, this one's for you! These avocado egg bakes are as beautiful as they are delicious. If biotin deficiency is a problem, or if you are on the autoimmune protocol (AIP), use only the egg yolks.

Serves 4

Ingredients

2 ripe avocados

4 large eggs

Paprika, to taste (for AIP: omit or replace with ground turmeric)

Chopped fresh parsley or chives, for garnish

Arugula (optional), for serving

Method

1. Preheat the oven to 375°F. Line a baking dish with unbleached parchment paper.

2. Cut the avocados in half lengthwise and remove the pits. Use a spoon to scoop out a bit of avocado flesh from each half to create a larger cavity for the eggs. Place the avocado halves in the baking dish; if necessary, you can slightly trim the undersides of the avocado halves to make them more stable.

3. Carefully crack one egg into the scooped-out center of each avocado half. If the eggs are large and the avocado cavities are small, you may need to remove some of the egg whites to prevent overflow. Sprinkle with paprika.

4. Bake until the egg whites are set and the yolks are cooked to your desired level of firmness—15 minutes if you prefer runny yolks, 20 minutes for firmer yolks.
5. Garnish with additional paprika and parsley or chives and serve on a bed of arugula, if desired.

Zucchini Nest with Egg Yolk

Spiralized zucchini forms the perfect "nest" for a delicious cooked or runny egg yolk. This is a light, veggie-packed dish that's totally Paleo and a surefire way to brighten up your breakfast.

Serves 4

Ingredients

2 medium zucchinis, trimmed
4 large egg yolks
¼ teaspoon garlic powder
Extra-virgin olive oil, as needed

Method

1. Preheat the oven to 375°F. Line a rimmed baking sheet with unbleached parchment paper.
2. Use a spiralizer, julienne peeler, or mandoline slicer to create thin zucchini noodles. Take small handfuls of zucchini noodles and form them into 4 nests on the baking sheet. Create a small indentation in the center of each nest to hold the egg yolk.
3. Place an egg yolk in the center of each zucchini nest. Season the egg yolks with the garlic powder. Drizzle a little olive oil over each nest for added flavor. Bake for 10 to 15 minutes, or until the egg yolks are cooked to your desired level of firmness.
4. Serve hot.

Mushroom Egg Bites

These tasty mushroom egg bites are loaded with sautéed mushrooms, shallots, and fresh basil. You can make them the night before and then reheat them for an easy, on-the-go breakfast. Regarding avidin and biotin, if biotin deficiency is a problem, or if you are on the autoimmune protocol (AIP), use only the egg yolks.

Serves 6

Ingredients

2 tablespoons extra-virgin olive oil, divided

1–2 shallots, chopped

8 ounces mixed button and maitake mushrooms, chopped

12 large eggs

½ teaspoon garlic powder

¼ teaspoon ground black pepper (for AIP: omit or replace with extra garlic powder)

1 tablespoon water

½ cup chopped fresh basil

Method

1. Preheat the oven to 350°F. Line a muffin tin with 12 parchment paper muffin liners.

2. Heat 1 tablespoon of the olive oil in a large skillet over medium-high heat. Sauté the shallots for 5 to 8 minutes, or until softened. Transfer the shallots to a large bowl.

3. Add the mushrooms to the skillet and cook for 3 to 5 minutes, or until browned on one side, then cook for 5 more minutes while stirring with a wooden spoon or silicone spatula. Transfer the mushrooms to the bowl with the shallots and mix to combine.

4. In another large bowl, whisk the eggs; optionally, run them through a fine-mesh strainer to thoroughly combine the whites and the yolks. Add the garlic powder, pepper, remaining 1 tablespoon olive oil, and

water to the egg mixture. Mix the eggs into the mushroom and shallot mixture. Lastly, add the basil. Spoon into the prepared muffin cups. Bake for 20 to 25 minutes, or until a toothpick inserted into the center comes out clean.

5. Serve warm.

Grass-Fed Bison and Beef Breakfast Patty with Kale, Egg, and Sweet Potato Hash

This hearty breakfast brings together the best of savory, sweet, and nutritious ingredients. We love the combination of grass-fed bison and beef for the patties, paired with a sweet potato hash and kale for a balanced meal. Regarding avidin and biotin, if biotin deficiency is a problem, or if you are on the autoimmune protocol (AIP), use only the egg yolks.

Serves 4

Ingredients

Patties

8 ounces ground beef

8 ounces ground bison

1 large egg yolk

1 teaspoon garlic powder or 2 teaspoons minced garlic

1 teaspoon dried parsley flakes or 2 tablespoons chopped fresh parsley

¼ teaspoon crushed red pepper (for AIP: omit)

Sweet Potato Hash

2 medium sweet potatoes, cubed

2 medium Japanese sweet potatoes, cubed

Kale

1 tablespoon extra-virgin olive oil

2 cups chopped kale

Eggs

4 large eggs or egg yolks

Smoked paprika to taste (for AIP: omit)

Method

1. To make the patties: Combine the beef and bison in a large bowl. Add the egg yolk, garlic powder, parsley, and crushed red pepper. Mix thoroughly until the spices are evenly distributed. Form the mixture into 8 equal patties. Heat a large skillet over medium-high heat. Cook the patties for 2 to 4 minutes on each side, or until they reach your desired level of doneness. Transfer to a plate and keep warm. Reserve the fat in the skillet.

2. To make the sweet potato hash: Heat the fat remaining in the skillet over medium heat. Add the sweet potatoes and Japanese sweet potatoes and cook, stirring occasionally, for 10 to 15 minutes, until the sweet potatoes are tender and slightly crispy. Transfer to a plate and keep warm.

3. To make the kale: Add the olive oil to the same skillet and heat over medium heat. Add the kale and cook for 3 to 5 minutes, or until the kale is wilted and tender.

4. To make the eggs: In the same skillet, cook the eggs either sunny-side-up or over easy. Sprinkle with smoked paprika.

5. To serve, place 2 patties on each plate with some of the sweet potato hash and kale, and add an egg on top. Serve right away.

Banana Pancakes

These easy, kid-friendly pancakes are a wonderful way to satisfy your morning sweet tooth while keeping things Paleo. Regarding avidin and biotin, if biotin deficiency is a problem, or if you are on the autoimmune protocol (AIP), use only the egg yolks.

Serves 4

Ingredients

4 ripe bananas (for AIP: replace with ripe avocado if necessary)

4 large eggs

½ teaspoon ground cinnamon

¼ cup coconut flakes, plus extra for serving

Coconut oil as needed

Method

1. Mash the bananas in a large bowl until smooth.
2. In a large bowl, whisk the eggs; optionally, run them through a fine-mesh strainer to thoroughly combine the whites and the yolks. Add the eggs to the mashed bananas. Add the cinnamon and coconut flakes and whisk until well combined.
3. Heat a nonstick skillet or griddle over medium heat and lightly grease with coconut oil. Working in batches to avoid crowding, pour one-quarter of the pancake batter into the skillet for each pancake. Cook for 2 to 3 minutes, or until bubbles form on the surface of each pancake and the edges begin to set. Carefully flip the pancakes and cook for an additional 1 to 2 minutes, or until golden brown on both sides. Transfer to a plate. Repeat with the remaining batter, adding more coconut oil to the skillet as needed.
4. Serve the pancakes warm with additional coconut flakes.

Berry Crumble with Dairy-Free Yogurt

This berry crumble can be enjoyed during all seasons thanks to the use of frozen wild blueberries.

Note: This recipe is not AIP compliant.

Serves 4

Ingredients

4 cups frozen wild blueberries (no need to thaw)

2 tablespoons arrowroot flour/starch

1 tablespoon lemon juice

1 cup almond flour (for AIP: replace with ½ cup coconut flour)

2 tablespoons coconut oil, melted

4 pitted dates

1 teaspoon ground cinnamon

Plain dairy-free coconut yogurt (see Note), for serving

Fresh mint leaves, for garnish

> Note: Cocoyo nondairy coconut yogurt contains a proprietary blend of live and active cultures that are grown on a dairy-free medium. Coconut Cult also has a Paleo yogurt. To make your own, use organic coconut cream, organic coconut meat, organic coconut water, probiotic cultures, and a yogurt maker.

Method

1. Preheat the oven to 350°F.

2. In a large bowl, combine the blueberries, arrowroot flour, and lemon juice. Mix well until the blueberries are evenly coated. Pour the blueberry mixture into a 9 x 9-inch baking dish.

3. In a food processor, combine the almond flour, melted coconut oil, dates, and cinnamon. Pulse until the mixture is well combined and has a crumbly texture. Sprinkle the topping evenly over the blueberry filling in the baking dish. Bake for 30 to 35 minutes, or until the topping is golden brown and the filling is bubbly.

4. Allow the crumble to cool slightly before serving. To serve, add dollops of nondairy yogurt and garnish with mint.

Berries, Chocolate, and Mixed Nuts with Dairy-Free Yogurt

For a breakfast that feels like dessert, this combination of fresh berries, dark chocolate, and mixed nuts hits the mark.

Serves 4

Ingredients

1½ cups plain dairy-free coconut yogurt (see Note)
2 cups mixed fresh berries, sliced as needed
4 ounces 100% dark chocolate, chopped or shaved
1 cup mixed nuts (almonds, walnuts, pecans, hazelnuts), lightly toasted

> Note: Cocoyo nondairy coconut yogurt contains a proprietary blend of live and active cultures that are grown on a dairy-free medium. Coconut Cult also has a Paleo yogurt. To make your own, use organic coconut cream, organic coconut meat, organic coconut water, probiotic cultures, and a yogurt maker.

Method

1. Divide the nondairy yogurt evenly among four bowls. Top each with ½ cup of the mixed berries. Sprinkle dark chocolate over the berries in each bowl. Scatter ¼ cup of mixed nuts over each serving.
2. Serve right away.

Berry Cauliflower Smoothie

This smoothie is a hidden gem for those looking to sneak more veggies into their breakfasts. Cauliflower blends seamlessly with the berries, creating a creamy and nutrient-dense smoothie that's refreshing and filling. We love how the lemon juice adds a bright, tangy note, making this smoothie perfect for a quick, energizing start.

Serves 4

Ingredients

2 cups unsweetened coconut milk

1 cup coconut water

1 cup frozen cauliflower rice

2 cups frozen blueberries

1 cup frozen strawberries or mulberries

Juice of 1 lemon

Ice (optional)

1 bunch fresh mint leaves, for garnish

Method

1. In a high-powered blender (such as a Vitamix), blend all the ingredients except the mint until smooth. Add ice for desired consistency, if needed.

2. To serve, split between four glasses and serve with mint leaves on top.

Chocolate Mint Smoothie

Chocolate for breakfast can be enjoyed with this powerhouse of nutrients disguised as a smoothie.

Serves 4

Ingredients

2 cups unsweetened coconut milk

1 cup coconut water

2 bananas, sliced and frozen (for AIP: replace with ripe avocado if necessary)

1 cup frozen cauliflower rice

¼ cup cocoa powder

¼ cup frozen kale

¼ teaspoon pure peppermint oil

Ice (optional)

1 bunch fresh mint leaves, for garnish

Method

1. In a high-powered blender (such as a Vitamix), blend all the ingredients except the mint until smooth. Add ice for desired consistency, if needed.
2. To serve, split between four glasses and serve with mint leaves on top.

Unrefined Pork Belly with Figs

This elegant dish works beautifully for brunch or a special-occasion breakfast. (With a few ingredient swaps it also makes a great snack for anytime; see our recipe for Savory Date and Peach with Unrefined Pork Belly in the Snacks and Beverages section, page 257.) Uncured pork belly is best procured from an ancestral butcher. You'll need 16 toothpicks for this recipe.

Serves 4

Ingredients

8 thin slices (about the size of ordinary bacon slices) unrefined pork belly, cut in half

8 fresh or rehydrated dried Black Mission figs, cut in half

Method

1. Preheat the oven to 375°F. Line a rimmed baking sheet with unbleached parchment paper.
2. Wrap a half slice of uncured pork belly around each fig half. Secure the fig with a toothpick to hold the pork belly in place.
3. Place the wrapped figs on the prepared baking sheet. Bake for 20 to 25 minutes, turning them over halfway, until the pork belly is crispy.
4. Serve warm.

LUNCH

Avocado Citrus Salad with Mint and Grilled Fish

This refreshing salad combines the creaminess of ripe avocados with the sweetness of grapefruit and oranges, all brought together by a hint of lime juice and mint. This fresh, zesty side is perfect for a summer meal, served alongside grilled wild ruby-red rainbow trout.

Serves 4

Ingredients
Salad

2 grapefruits
2 oranges
2 blood oranges
2 ripe avocados, peeled, pitted, and thinly sliced
Juice of 1 lime
2 tablespoons extra-virgin olive oil
Ground black pepper (for AIP: omit or replace with ground ginger)
Fresh mint leaves, for serving

Trout

4 (8-ounce) trout fillets (ideally wild ruby-red rainbow trout)
Extra-virgin olive oil, for brushing
Ground ginger to taste

Method

1. To make the salad: Cut off the top and bottom of each grapefruit, orange, and blood orange, then slice off the peel and pith. Using a paring knife, cut along the membranes to release the segments. Place the segments on a platter. Add the avocados to the citrus segments. Drizzle the lime juice and olive oil over the avocado and citrus mixture. Sprinkle with black pepper. Gently toss to combine.

(Recipe continues on the next page.)

2. To make the trout: Preheat a grill or grill pan to medium-high heat. Brush the fish with olive oil and sprinkle it with ginger. Grill the fish for 4 to 5 minutes on each side, or until it is cooked through and flakes easily with a fork. The exact cooking time will depend on the thickness of the fish fillets.

3. To serve, add mint to the salad and serve with the grilled fish.

Roasted Beets with Dairy-Free Labneh

Labneh is a soft Middle Eastern cheese made from strained yogurt. In this easy but delicious lunch option, roasted red and yellow beets pair beautifully with a rich, homemade coconut-based labneh flavored with lemon and dill. This vibrant, earthy dish brings out the natural sweetness of the beets, complemented by the tangy, herb-infused labneh.

> Note: It takes at least 4 hours to drain the labneh, so you might want to do that the night before if you want to take this lunch with you to work.

Serves 4

Ingredients

Labneh

1 cup dairy-free coconut labneh or plain dairy-free coconut yogurt
¼ teaspoon ground pink peppercorns (for AIP: omit or replace with ½ teaspoon garlic powder)
1 teaspoon lemon juice
½ bunch fresh dill, chopped
Extra virgin olive oil

Beets

4 (2-inch-diameter) red beets, peeled and trimmed
2 (2-inch-diameter) yellow beets, peeled and trimmed
Extra-virgin olive oil, for drizzling

Method

1. Preheat the oven to 375°F.
2. To drain the labneh: Place a fine-mesh sieve or a colander lined with cheesecloth over a bowl. Pour the coconut labneh into the cheesecloth. Gather the edges of the cheesecloth and twist to form a bundle. Secure with a string or rubber band. Allow the yogurt to drain in the refrigerator for at least 4 hours or overnight. The longer it drains, the thicker it will become.
3. To make the beets: Place the beets on a rimmed baking sheet. Roast for 45 to 60 minutes, turning three or four times, until they are tender when pierced with a fork. Let the beets cool slightly, then cut them into wedges or slices.
4. To serve: Transfer the labneh to a bowl. Stir in the peppercorns, lemon juice, and dill. Place the labneh on a plate with the cooled beets on top. Drizzle with olive oil.

Antipasto Plate

Grilled vegetables marinated in lemon and olive oil bring a hearty, smoky flavor to this dish. Served warm or at room temperature, this makes the perfect centerpiece for a Mediterranean-inspired meal.

Serves 4

Ingredients

¼ cup extra-virgin olive oil

Juice of 1 lemon

½ teaspoon ground black pepper (for AIP: omit or replace with dried rosemary, thyme, or oregano)

2 portobello mushroom caps, sliced ½ inch thick

1 bunch asparagus, woody ends snapped off

2 zucchini, sliced lengthwise ¼-inch thick

2 yellow squash, sliced lengthwise ¼ inch thick

2 green bell peppers, seeded and quartered (for AIP: omit)

1 large white onion, sliced ½ inch thick
1 bunch kale, tough stems removed

Method

1. In a small bowl, whisk together the olive oil, lemon juice, and pepper to make the marinade. Place the mushrooms, asparagus, zucchini, yellow squash, bell peppers, onion in a large bowl or resealable plastic bag. Place the kale in a separate bowl or bag. Pour the marinade over the vegetables and kale and toss to coat evenly. Let the vegetables and kale marinate for at least 15 minutes (up to several hours if desired) in the refrigerator.
2. Preheat a grill or grill pan to medium-high heat.
3. Grill the vegetables until they are tender and have nice grill marks, turning occasionally and removing each vegetable as it is done. This should take 5 to 7 minutes for the asparagus; 8 to 10 minutes for the zucchini, yellow squash, and bell peppers; and 10 to 12 minutes for the mushrooms and onion rings. Grill the kale separately on a grill mat or basket (to prevent the leaves from falling through the grates) for 3 to 5 minutes, or until wilted and slightly crispy.
4. To serve, arrange the grilled vegetables on a large serving platter. Drizzle any remaining marinade over the top for extra flavor.

Zoodles with Bison Meatballs

Zucchini noodles (zoodles) offer a great nutrient-dense alternative to traditional pasta. These light, refreshing zoodles are a perfect contrast to the rich, savory meatballs, all topped with a simple sauce. Baking the zoodles in the oven works well to reduce moisture without making them soggy.

Serves 4

Ingredients

Zoodles

4 medium zucchinis

Meatballs

2 large egg yolks
2 tablespoons extra-virgin olive oil, divided
4 garlic cloves, minced
½ yellow bell pepper, finely diced (for AIP: omit or replace with diced zucchini)
½ cup chopped fresh parsley
1 tablespoon AIP-Friendly Italian Seasoning (page 261)
1 teaspoon onion powder
¼ teaspoon ground black pepper (for AIP: omit or replace with more AIP-Friendly Italian Seasoning)
1 pound ground grass-fed bison

Basic Pasta Sauce

2 tablespoons extra-virgin olive oil
5 garlic cloves, minced
2 (28-ounce) cans crushed San Marzano tomatoes (for AIP: replace with steamed butternut squash)
1 tablespoon AIP-Friendly Italian Seasoning (page 261)
Crushed red pepper to taste

Method

1. Preheat the oven to 350°F. Line a rimmed baking sheet with unbleached parchment paper.
2. To make the zoodles: Use a spiralizer, julienne peeler, or mandoline slicer to create thin zucchini noodles. Spread the zoodles on the baking sheet. Bake for 20 minutes, flipping the zoodles halfway through.
3. Meanwhile, to make the meatballs: Beat the egg yolks in a large bowl, then add 1 tablespoon of the olive oil, the garlic, bell pepper, parsley, Italian seasoning, onion powder, and black pepper. Add the ground bison and mix until well combined. Use a scoop to portion out 16 meatballs.

(Recipe continues on the next page.)

4. Heat the remaining 1 tablespoon olive oil in a large skillet over medium heat. Working in batches as necessary to avoid crowding, fry the meatballs, turning frequently, for 8 minutes, or until they are no longer pink on the inside. Transfer to a plate.

5. To make the sauce: Add the olive oil to the same skillet and heat over medium heat. Sauté the garlic until fragrant and slightly golden. Pour in the tomatoes and stir. Season with the Italian seasoning and crushed pepper. Simmer the sauce on low heat for 20 minutes, or until it thickens slightly, stirring occasionally. Taste and adjust the seasoning as needed. Add the meatballs and reheat briefly.

6. To serve, place one-quarter of the zoodles in each bowl and top with pasta sauce and four meatballs.

Coconut Shrimp and Avocado Ceviche

Shrimp marinated in lime juice gets a tropical twist with coconut milk and fresh coconut chunks. Combined with avocado and Persian cucumber, this ceviche is creamy, citrusy, and refreshing.

Serves 2–4

Ingredients

1 pound raw shrimp, peeled, deveined, and chopped
Juice of 4 limes
½ medium onion, finely diced
1 cup canned unsweetened coconut milk
½ cup finely chopped fresh coconut chunks
2 Persian (small, thin-skinned) cucumbers
2 ripe avocados, peeled, pitted, and diced
¼ cup chopped fresh cilantro
½ teaspoon ground black pepper (for AIP: omit or replace with grated lime zest)

Method

1. In a large bowl, combine the shrimp, lime juice, and onion. Mix well and marinate in the refrigerator for 20 to 30 minutes, or until the shrimp turns opaque in color. (This indicates that the citric acid in the lime juice has denatured the fish proteins, thus "cooking" the shrimp.)
2. Add the coconut milk, coconut chunks, and cucumbers. Stir to combine. Gently fold in the avocado and cilantro. Season with pepper and serve.

Sushi Bowl with Cauliflower Rice

This sushi-inspired bowl offers a low-carb alternative using cauliflower rice. Topped with sliced avocado, cucumber, carrots, and shrimp, it's served with a simple dressing made from apple cider vinegar and ginger for a light, satisfying meal.

Serves 4

Ingredients

1 tablespoon unsweetened apple cider vinegar

1 tablespoon grated ginger

1 garlic clove, grated

1 teaspoon honey (optional)

2 tablespoons extra-virgin olive oil

1 medium head cauliflower, riced (see Note) or 2 (10-ounce) bags frozen cauliflower rice

2 avocados, peeled, pitted, and sliced

2 Persian (small, thin-skinned) cucumbers, cut into thin strips

2 carrots, peeled and cut into thin strips

1 red bell pepper, seeded and thinly sliced (for AIP: omit or replace with zucchini)

1½ cups thinly sliced red cabbage

½ cup thinly sliced radishes

2 cups cooked shrimp or your choice of sushi-grade fish (tuna, salmon, etc.)

2 tablespoons sesame seeds (for AIP: omit)

2 sheets salt-free dried nori, cut into thin strips

1 green onion, trimmed and thinly sliced

> Note: To rice the cauliflower, cut it into florets and pulse in a food processor until it resembles rice. You can also grate the florets on the large side of a box grater.

Method

1. In a small bowl, whisk together the apple cider vinegar, ginger, garlic, and honey (if using). Set the dressing aside.
2. In a large skillet, heat the olive oil over medium heat. Add the cauliflower rice and cook, stirring occasionally, for 5 to 7 minutes, or until the cauliflower is tender.
3. Transfer the cauliflower rice to a large bowl. Arrange the avocados, cucumbers, carrots, bell pepper, cabbage, and radishes on top. Add the shrimp. Sprinkle with the sesame seeds and nori strips.
4. To serve, drizzle the dressing over the top. Garnish with the green onions.

Lamb Kebabs with Cucumber and Tomato Salad

Tender lamb kebabs seasoned with Herbes de Provence and fresh mint are grilled to perfection. Paired with a refreshing cucumber and tomato salad, this dish is a flavorful and balanced meal perfect for any season.

Serves 4

Ingredients

Lamb Kebabs

1 pound ground lamb

¼ cup almond flour

1 large egg yolk

¼ onion, grated

2 tablespoons minced fresh mint

1 garlic clove, grated

1 tablespoon AIP-Friendly Herbes de Provence (page 261)

1 tablespoon ground sumac (for AIP: omit or replace with grated lemon zest)

1 teaspoon ground cinnamon

½ teaspoon ground black pepper (for AIP: omit or replace with dried mint)

Cucumber and Tomato Salad

4 Roma tomatoes, diced (for AIP: omit or replace with peaches or Asian pears)

4 Persian (small, thin-skinned) cucumbers, diced into bite-sized pieces

⅓ cup chopped fresh dill or 4 teaspoons dried dill

2 tablespoons minced fresh mint

Extra-virgin olive oil, for drizzling

Ground black pepper to taste (for AIP: omit)

Ground sumac to taste

Method

1. To make the kebabs: Preheat a grill or grill pan to medium-high heat. If using wooden skewers, soak them in water for 30 minutes to prevent burning.

2. In a large bowl, combine all the kebab ingredients. Mix thoroughly until everything is well incorporated. Divide the mixture into 8 equal portions. Shape each portion into a long, sausage-like shape around a skewer. Grill the kebabs for 4 to 5 minutes on each side, or until the internal temperature reaches 135 to 160°F and the outside is nicely browned.

(Recipe continues on the next page.)

3. To make the salad: In a large bowl, combine the tomatoes, cucumbers, dill, and mint. Drizzle with olive oil and season with pepper and sumac to taste. Toss everything together until well mixed.
4. Arrange the lamb kebabs on a platter and serve the salad on the side.

Seaweed, Shrimp, and Veggie Rolls

Nori rolls filled with shrimp, avocado, mushrooms, and a variety of fresh vegetables make a light yet filling dish. These rolls are a convenient way to serve lunch or to have as a handy snack.

Serves 4

Ingredients

4 sheets salt-free dried nori

8 ounces cooked shrimp, sliced

1 yellow bell pepper, seeded and cut into thin strips (for AIP: omit or replace with zucchini)

1 red bell pepper, seeded and cut into thin strips (for AIP: omit or replace with zucchini)

2 celery ribs, cut into thin strips

1 carrot, peeled and cut into thin strips

2 portobello mushroom caps, sliced and cooked (see Note)

2 Persian (small, thin-skinned) cucumbers, cut into thin strips

1 avocado, peeled, pitted, and sliced into thin strips

1 bunch cilantro, stemmed

1 bunch mint, stemmed

> Note: To cook the mushrooms, sauté them in a little bit of olive oil in a small skillet over medium heat for about 5 minutes.

Method

1. Place a bamboo sushi mat on a clean surface and cover it with plastic wrap. Have a small bowl of water nearby to wet your fingers and the edge of the seaweed sheets for sealing the rolls.
2. Lay a sheet of seaweed shiny side down on the bamboo mat. Arrange a small portion of each ingredient in a horizontal line across the middle of the seaweed sheet. Starting from the edge closest to you, use the bamboo mat to begin rolling the seaweed over the filling. Press gently but firmly as you roll to keep the ingredients together. Continue rolling until the seaweed sheet is completely wrapped around the filling. Wet the edges of the seaweed sheet with a little water to seal the roll. Repeat with the remaining ingredients.
3. Serve immediately or cover and store in the refrigerator for up to 2 hours.

Thai Slaw Salad with Shrimp Skewers

This crunchy Thai-inspired slaw is made from cabbage, carrots, cucumbers, and daikon, tossed in a flavorful dressing. Grilled shrimp skewers make this a hearty yet light dish perfect for a summer BBQ.

Serves 4

Ingredients
Almond Dressing

¾ cup unsalted, additive-free almond butter (for AIP: omit or replace with tiger nut butter)
Grated zest and juice of 3 limes
2 garlic cloves, grated
1 tablespoon grated ginger
4–8 tablespoons water

Shrimp Skewers

48 medium shrimp

¼ cup almond dressing (see above)

Salad

1 cup shredded carrot

2 Persian (small, thin-skinned) cucumbers, cut into thin strips

1 red bell pepper, seeded and cut into thin strips (for AIP: omit or replace with zucchini)

1 daikon, peeled and cut into thin strips

2 celery ribs, chopped

½ head iceberg lettuce, shredded

¼ head green or red cabbage, shredded

¼ cup chopped fresh cilantro

¼ cup chopped fresh parsley

2 tablespoons chopped fresh mint

2 tablespoons unsalted sesame seeds, plus extra for garnish (for AIP: omit)

2 tablespoons unsalted pumpkin seeds (for AIP: omit)

Method

1. To make the dressing: In a food processor, pulse the almond butter, lime zest and juice, garlic, and ginger until combined. Pulse in water as needed to reach your desired thickness.

2. To make the shrimp skewers: If using wooden skewers, soak them in water for 30 minutes to prevent burning. Thread the shrimp on the skewers and arrange on a large platter or rimmed baking sheet. Drizzle with ¼ cup of the dressing, turning to coat well, and marinate at room temperature for 20 minutes.

3. Preheat a grill or grill pan to medium-high heat.

4. Grill the shrimp skewers for 2 to 3 minutes per side, or until the shrimp is pink with opaque flesh and reaches an internal temperature of 145°F. Transfer to a platter.

5. To make the salad: In a large bowl, combine the carrot, cucumbers, bell pepper, daikon, celery, iceberg lettuce, and cabbage, and toss well. Mix in the cilantro, parsley, and mint. Sprinkle the sesame seeds and pumpkin seeds over the top of the salad. Drizzle with the remaining almond dressing and toss to combine.

6. To serve, divide the salad onto four plates and place the shrimp skewers on top. Garnish with additional sesame seeds.

Veggie Stir-Fry

A mix of cabbage, bok choy, daikon, and mushrooms is stir-fried with Chinese five-spice powder. This vegetable-forward stir-fry makes for a quick, nutritious meal packed with flavor.

Serves 4

Ingredients

2 tablespoons extra-virgin olive oil
1 daikon, peeled and sliced into thin rounds
½ head green or red cabbage, shredded
1 bunch bok choy, chopped, stems and leaves reserved separately
1 cup sliced button mushrooms
1 jalapeño, seeded if desired and thinly sliced (for AIP: omit)
3 green onions, trimmed and cut crosswise into thin slices
1 teaspoon AIP-Friendly Chinese Five-Spice (page 262)
1 tablespoon apple cider vinegar
1 tablespoon black sesame seeds (AIP: omit)

Method

1. In a large wok or skillet, heat the olive oil over medium-high heat. Add the daikon and cabbage and stir-fry for 2 to 3 minutes, until they start to soften. Add the bok choy stems and mushrooms and stir-fry for 2 to 3 minutes. Add the jalapeño and green onions and stir-fry for 1 to 2 minutes. Sprinkle the Chinese five-spice over the vegetables

and stir well to coat evenly. Add the apple cider vinegar and bok choy leaves and stir-fry for 1 to 2 minutes, until the leaves just start to wilt.

2. To serve, transfer the stir-fried vegetables to a serving dish. Garnish with the black sesame seeds.

Chicken Fajitas on Jicama "Tortillas" with Cilantro Slaw

For a healthy twist on classic fajitas, grilled chicken and vegetables are seasoned with AIP-Friendly Taco Seasoning, served on thin jicama slices, and topped with a bright and tangy cilantro slaw. We love these on Taco Tuesday and throughout the week!

Serves 4

Ingredients
Cilantro Slaw

¼ head green or red cabbage, shredded
¼ bunch cilantro, chopped
½ jalapeño, seeded if desired and chopped (for AIP: omit)
1 tablespoon extra-virgin olive oil
Juice of ½ lime

Fajitas

2 pounds boneless, skinless chicken thighs, cut into ½-inch slices
2 tablespoons AIP-Friendly Taco Seasoning (page 262)
2 tablespoons extra-virgin olive oil, divided
1 onion, thinly sliced
1 green bell pepper, seeded and cut into thin strips (for AIP: omit or replace with zucchini)
1 cup sliced button mushrooms
1 jicama, thinly sliced into 12 to 16 slices (see Note)
Sesame seeds, for garnish (for AIP: omit)

> Note: Carefully use a mandoline slicer to get the thinnest slices of jicama. Some grocery stores carry pre-sliced jicama wraps.

Method

1. To make the slaw: In a large bowl, combine the cabbage, cilantro, and jalapeño. Drizzle with the olive oil and lime juice. Toss well to combine and set aside to let the flavors meld.
2. To make the fajitas: In a medium bowl, toss the chicken with the taco seasoning, ensuring each piece is well coated; set aside.
3. In a grill pan or skillet, heat 1 tablespoon of the olive oil over medium-high heat. Add the onion, bell pepper, and mushrooms and cook until softened and starting to brown, 5 to 10 minutes depending on how soft you want them. Transfer the vegetables to a large bowl.
4. Add the remaining 1 tablespoon olive oil to the skillet and heat over medium-high heat. Add the chicken and cook for 5 to 7 minutes per side, or until it reaches a temperature of 165°F and is slightly crispy.
5. To serve, arrange the jicama on a serving platter. Top with the grilled vegetables, chicken, and slaw. Garnish with sesame seeds.

Pistachio Caesar with Grilled Chicken Breast

With our Paleo take on a classic Caesar salad, a crunchy pistachio-based dressing made with olive oil and lemon pairs perfectly with grilled chicken breast.

Serves 4

Ingredients
Dressing

½ cup unsalted pistachios (for AIP: omit or replace with tiger nuts)
¼ cup extra-virgin olive oil
1 tablespoon lemon juice

1 tablespoon Dijon mustard (for AIP: omit)

1 tablespoon apple cider vinegar

1 garlic clove, grated

2–4 tablespoons water

Ground black pepper to taste (for AIP: omit)

Chicken

4 boneless, skinless chicken breasts

2 tablespoons extra-virgin olive oil

⅛ teaspoon ground black pepper (for AIP: omit)

Salad

3–4 large romaine hearts, trimmed and leaves torn

¼ cup hemp seeds (for AIP: omit or replace with 1 tablespoon grated
    lemon zest)

Method

1. Preheat a grill or grill pan over medium-high heat.
2. To make the dressing: In a food processor or blender, combine the pistachios, olive oil, lemon juice, mustard, apple cider vinegar, and garlic. Blend until smooth and creamy. If the dressing is too thick, add a little water, 1 tablespoon at a time, until you reach the desired consistency. Season with black pepper. Set aside.
3. To make the chicken: Brush the chicken with the olive oil and season with the pepper. Grill for 6 to 7 minutes on each side, or until fully cooked and the internal temperature reaches 165°F. Transfer to a cutting board and let rest for a few minutes, then slice into strips.
4. To make the salad: Place the romaine in a large bowl. Add the dressing and toss to coat evenly.
5. To serve, divide the salad between four plates. Arrange the grilled chicken strips on top of each salad. Sprinkle with the hemp seeds.

Liver and Onions

Packed with iron and nutrients, liver is often an overlooked protein source but is incredibly delicious when prepared well. The natural sweetness of caramelized onions balances the strong, earthy flavor of liver, while a touch of balsamic vinegar brightens the dish. Whether you're a long-time fan or new to liver, this recipe brings out the best of this nutrient-dense food.

Serves 4

Ingredients

1 pound grass-fed beef liver, sliced ¼ inch thick
1 tablespoon AIP-Friendly Italian Seasoning (page 261)
1 teaspoon garlic powder
1 teaspoon paprika (for AIP: omit)
⅛ teaspoon ground black pepper (for AIP: omit)
4 tablespoons extra-virgin olive oil, divided
2 large onions, thinly sliced
2 tablespoons chopped fresh parsley

Method

1. Rinse the liver under cold water and pat dry with paper towels. In a shallow dish, mix the Italian seasoning, garlic powder, paprika, and pepper. Coat each slice of liver with the spice mixture and set aside.
2. In a large skillet, heat 2 tablespoons of the olive oil over medium heat. Add the onions and cook, stirring occasionally, for 10 to 15 minutes, until they are soft and caramelized. Transfer to a plate.
3. Add the remaining 2 tablespoons olive oil to the skillet and heat over medium-high heat. Working in batches as necessary to avoid crowding, add the liver in a single layer. Cook for 2 to 3 minutes on each side, or until browned and cooked through. The liver should be slightly pink in the center but not undercooked.

(Recipe continues on the next page.)

4. Return the caramelized onions to the skillet with the liver. Stir gently to combine and heat through for 1 to 2 minutes.

5. Serve immediately, garnished with the parsley.

DINNER

Salmon en Papillote with Radicchio Salad

Experience the delicate flavors of salmon prepared en papillote—a classic French cooking technique where the fish is steamed within a parchment paper packet. This method locks in moisture and infuses the salmon with the aromatic essence of fresh dill, tarragon, and lemon slices.

Serves 4

Ingredients
Salmon

Extra-virgin olive oil, for drizzling
16 (¼-inch-thick) lemon slices (from about 2 lemons)
4 green onions, trimmed and thinly sliced
8 dill sprigs
1 pound wild Atlantic salmon, skin on, cut into 4 equal pieces
Pink peppercorns to taste, ground or crushed (for AIP: omit or replace with grated lemon zest)
8 tarragon sprigs
1 shallot, finely diced
¼ cup minced fresh parsley

Radicchio Salad

¼ cup extra-virgin olive oil
Juice of 1 lemon
⅛ teaspoon ground pink peppercorns (for AIP: omit or replace with grated lemon zest)
1 teaspoon minced shallot

1 head radicchio, shredded

½ cup diced tomatoes (for AIP: omit or replace with peach or Asian pear)

¼ cup unsalted pumpkin seeds (for AIP: omit)

Method

1. To make the salmon: Preheat the oven to 325°F. Cut out 4 parchment rectangles, each 16 inches across, then cut each into a heart shape to form parchment paper packets. Fold each heart in half down the middle, then spread the hearts open again.

2. Drizzle olive oil on each parchment heart. Place 2 lemon rounds on one side of each, then one-quarter of the green onions, 2 dill sprigs, and a piece of salmon. Sprinkle the salmon with pink peppercorns, then add 2 tarragon sprigs, one-quarter of the shallot, parsley, a final drizzle of olive oil, and 2 more lemon slices on top. Enclose each packet by folding the empty half of the heart over the filled side and pinching the sides together to seal the parchment paper. Place the packets on a rimmed baking sheet and bake for 20 minutes, or until the internal temperature reaches 145°F.

3. Meanwhile, to make the salad: In a large bowl, combine the olive oil, lemon juice, peppercorns, and shallot. Add the radicchio and toss to coat. Divide between four plates, then add the tomatoes and pumpkin seeds.

4. To serve, use scissors to carefully open the parchment packets, then transfer to plates. Serve the salmon with the salad.

Scallops with Cauliflower Puree

Scallops are not as intimidating to cook as you might think. Simply season the scallops before searing them in oil for a couple of minutes. If you prefer to make a plant-based version of this dish, you can use 6 to 8 king trumpet mushrooms, cut into 1-inch-thick rounds (about 40 "scallops").

Serves 4

Ingredients

Cauliflower Puree

1 (1½-pound) head cauliflower, trimmed and cut into florets

½ cup unsalted chicken bone broth, plus extra as needed

2 tablespoons extra-virgin olive oil

1 garlic clove, grated

Green Onion, Shallot, and Parsley Gremolata

2 green onions, trimmed and finely chopped

½ shallot, minced

3 tablespoons chopped fresh parsley

Juice of 1 lemon

3 tablespoons extra-virgin olive oil

Scallops

20 sea scallops, patted dry

1 teaspoon onion powder

1 teaspoon garlic powder

½ teaspoon paprika (for AIP: omit)

½ teaspoon ground pink peppercorns (for AIP: omit or replace with grated lemon zest)

1 tablespoon extra-virgin olive oil

Method

1. To make the cauliflower puree: Bring a large pot of water to a boil. Add the cauliflower and boil for 15 to 20 minutes, until softened. Transfer to a high-powered blender (such as a Vitamix) and add the broth, olive oil, and garlic. Puree until smooth, adding more broth as necessary to reach the desired consistency.

2. To make the gremolata: In a bowl, mix together the green onions, shallot, parsley, lemon juice, and olive oil until well combined. Set aside.

3. To make the scallops: Season the scallops with the onion powder, garlic powder, paprika, and peppercorns. Heat the oil in a large cast-iron skillet over medium-high heat. Fry the scallops for 1 to 3 minutes on each side (depending on your desired doneness), until just cooked through and lightly browned.

4. Transfer the scallops to four plates, along with a scoop of cauliflower puree and some of the gremolata drizzled on top.

Salmon and Cauliflower Rice Cakes

Transform your salmon into delectable cakes combined with nutrient-dense cauliflower rice. These salmon cakes are infused with fresh herbs like dill and parsley, offering a burst of flavor in every bite. Easy to prepare and packed with omega-3 fatty acids, these cakes make for a versatile dish—ideal for a family dinner or meal-prepping for the week.

Serves 4

Ingredients

1 pound fresh-caught salmon, skinned and cut into ¼-inch cubes

1 cup fresh or thawed frozen cauliflower rice

1 shallot, minced

2 green onions, trimmed and thinly sliced

1 large egg yolk

2 tablespoons chopped fresh parsley

1 tablespoon chopped fresh dill

1 heaping tablespoon coconut flour

1 teaspoon garlic powder

2–3 tablespoons extra-virgin olive oil, coconut oil, or avocado oil, for frying

Grated zest of 1 lemon

Method

1. In a large bowl, combine the salmon, cauliflower rice, shallot, green onions, egg yolk, parsley, dill, coconut flour, and garlic powder until well combined. Use a 2-ounce/¼-cup scoop to portion out 8 salmon cakes. Form each into a patty.
2. Heat 2 tablespoons oil in a large cast-iron skillet over medium heat. Working in batches as necessary to avoid crowding, fry the cakes for 2 minutes per side, then transfer to a plate. Add more oil as needed.
3. Garnish with lemon zest and serve right away.

Moules Marinières

This classic French dish features mussels steamed in a fragrant broth of shallots, garlic, tarragon, and a splash of lemon juice. It is sober-friendly, using bone broth instead of wine, and provides a simple yet sophisticated meal that highlights the fresh, briny flavors of the sea.

Serves 4

Ingredients

2 tablespoons extra-virgin olive oil
2 shallots, diced
4 garlic cloves, chopped
6 tarragon sprigs
4 pounds mussels, scrubbed and debearded
2 cups unsalted chicken bone broth
Juice of 2 lemons

Method

1. Heat the olive oil in a large skillet over medium-high heat. Add the shallots and garlic and sauté until the first shades of color appear, about 2 minutes. Add the tarragon, mussels, and bone broth, cover the pan, and bring to a boil. Add mussels and steam until the mussels open, about 3 to 5 minutes.

2. Discard any mussels that did not open in the cooking process. Squeeze the lemon juice into the broth and serve immediately.

Chicken and Bamboo Shoots with Garlic-Ginger Lettuce Cups

Enjoy a burst of Chinese-inspired flavors with these refreshing lettuce cups. Ground chicken is sautéed with bamboo shoots, ginger, and garlic, then served in crisp butter lettuce leaves with toppings for a delectable combination of textures and tastes.

Serves 4

Ingredients

Lime Sauce

Grated zest and juice of 1 lime
2 teaspoons honey
2 tablespoons apple cider vinegar

Veggies and Chicken

1 tablespoon extra-virgin olive oil
½ onion, diced
½ red bell pepper, diced (for AIP: omit or replace with shredded carrots)
3 tablespoons minced ginger
5 garlic cloves, grated
20 ounces ground chicken
1 (8-ounce) can sliced bamboo shoots, drained and diced, or cauliflower rice
3 tablespoons chopped fresh cilantro, plus more for garnish
2 tablespoons chopped unsalted macadamia nuts, plus more for garnish (for AIP: omit or replace with toasted coconut flakes)
Butter lettuce leaves, for serving
1 tablespoon chopped fresh mint, for garnish
Lime wedges, for serving

Method

1. To make the lime sauce: In a small bowl, whisk together the lime zest and juice, honey, and apple cider vinegar. Set aside.
2. To make the veggies and chicken: Heat the olive oil in a large skillet over medium heat. Add the onion, bell pepper, ginger, and garlic and sauté for 4 to 6 minutes, or until the vegetables are softened. Transfer to a bowl.
3. Add the chicken to the skillet and cook, breaking it apart with a spatula, for 5 to 6 minutes, until cooked through. Return the veggies to the skillet and mix in with the cooked chicken. Add the bamboo shoots and stir well. Pour the lime sauce over the chicken and vegetable mixture and cook for 2 minutes. Stir in the cilantro and macadamia nuts and cook for 2 minutes.
4. Arrange the lettuce leaves on a serving platter. Spoon the chicken and bamboo shoot mixture into each lettuce "cup." Add extra cilantro, macadamia nuts, and mint on top. Serve with lime wedges for squeezing.

Steak with Chimichurri and Portobello Mushrooms, Asparagus, and Yam Puree

This dish is perfect for a Sunday supper or any day when you're craving a hearty meal. Seared grass-fed beef pairs well with yam puree, grilled asparagus, and a savory vinegary chimichurri sauce.

Serves 4

Ingredients
Mushrooms and Asparagus

2 tablespoons extra-virgin olive oil
¼ teaspoon onion powder
¼ teaspoon garlic powder
¼ teaspoon dried parsley

4 portobello mushroom caps, optionally with gills removed

2 pounds asparagus, woody ends snapped off

Chimichurri

½ cup chopped fresh cilantro

½ cup chopped fresh parsley

¼ cup chopped fresh mint

½ jalapeño, seeded and sliced (for AIP: omit)

2 garlic cloves, grated

1 teaspoon crushed red pepper (for AIP: omit)

½ cup extra-virgin olive oil

1 tablespoon apple cider vinegar

Juice of 1 lemon

Yam Puree

2 large yams, peeled and cut into large cubes

2 tablespoons extra-virgin olive oil

¾–1 cup unsalted chicken bone broth

1–2 garlic cloves, grated

Ground black pepper to taste (for AIP: omit)

Steak

1 (2-pound) grass-fed sirloin steak

Method

1. Preheat a grill to 500°F.

2. To make the mushrooms and asparagus: In a large bowl, mix the olive oil, onion powder, garlic powder, and parsley powder. Add the mushrooms and asparagus and marinate at room temperature until ready to cook (or overnight in the refrigerator).

3. To make the chimichurri: In a food processor, blitz the cilantro, parsley, mint, jalapeño, garlic, and crushed red pepper until finely chopped. Add the oil, apple cider vinegar, and lemon juice and mix

(Recipe continues on the next page.)

together. Pour into a small bowl. Hold at room temperature until
ready to cook (or overnight in the refrigerator).

4. Meanwhile, to make the yam puree: Bring a large pot of water to a
boil. Add the yams and boil for 15 to 20 minutes, until soft. Transfer
to a high-powered blender (such as a Vitamix), add the oil and ½ cup
of the chicken bone broth, and puree until smooth. Add more broth
as needed to reach the desired thickness, but do not over overblend to
avoid a gummy puree. Remove from the blender and add the garlic
and pepper. Set aside.

5. To make the steak: Place the steak on the grill over direct heat and sear
for 3 to 7 minutes. Flip and sear for 3 to 7 minutes on the other side,
depending on your desired cooking temperature. Transfer to a cutting
board and let rest while you cook the mushrooms and asparagus.

6. Lower the grill temperature to 400°F. Remove the portobellos from
the marinade and grill gill-side down for 4 to 5 minutes. Flip and sear
for 4 to 5 minutes on the other side. Transfer to a cutting board. Place
the asparagus on the grill (perpendicular to the grill grates) or in a
grill basket. Cook by rotating every 2 minutes for a total of 8 minutes.
Transfer to a plate.

7. To serve, slice the steak and portobello mushrooms. Stack the steak
and portobello, alternating slices of each, and drizzle with chimichurri. Serve with the asparagus and yam puree.

Cauliflower Steaks with Romesco Sauce

While not AIP friendly (as written, and without substitutions), this dish
is packed with antioxidants and flavor. With substitutions as specified in
the ingredients list, it is fine for people with AIP concerns.

The mixture of roasted red peppers and lemon juice in the romesco
sauce adds a smoky, peppy flavor that pairs well with the cauliflower
"steaks," as well as with chicken or fish. You can use regular paprika, but
smoked paprika will give a deeper flavor.

Serves 4

Ingredients

Romesco Sauce

4 red bell peppers (for AIP: omit or replace with 2 cups oven-roasted butternut squash)

2 cups dry-roasted blanched almonds (for AIP: omit or replace with tiger nuts)

¼ cup extra-virgin olive oil

Juice of 1–2 lemons, divided

1 teaspoon chili powder, or more to taste (for AIP: omit)

1 teaspoon smoked paprika, or more to taste (for AIP: omit)

Cauliflower Steaks

2–3 heads (about 3 pounds) cauliflower

¼ cup extra-virgin olive oil, or as needed

Ground black pepper to taste (for AIP: omit or replace with garlic powder)

Method

1. To make the romesco sauce: Preheat the oven to 400°F.
2. Place the bell peppers on a rimmed baking sheet and roast for 20 to 25 minutes, or until the skins are charred and blistered. (You can also char them on a grill or over an open flame for 5 to 10 minutes.) Place the peppers in a large bowl. Cover with plastic wrap or a lid and let them steam for 10 minutes. Peel off the charred skins, then cut in half and remove the seeds and stems.
3. Transfer the red peppers to a food processor and add the almonds, olive oil, juice of 1 lemon, chili powder, and paprika. Pulse until the mixture is smooth and creamy. Adjust the seasoning to taste with additional chili powder or paprika and the remaining lemon juice, if desired. To thin the sauce, you can add cold water to the food processor while processing. Transfer to a bowl and set aside.
4. To make the cauliflower steaks: Preheat a grill or grill pan to medium-high heat. Remove the leaves from the cauliflower heads and trim the

stems, leaving the core intact. Slice each cauliflower head into 1-inch-thick steaks. You should get 2 or 3 steaks from each head, depending on size. Some florets will fall off, and you can grill those separately.

5. Brush both sides of the cauliflower steaks with the olive oil and season with black pepper. Grill for 5 to 10 minutes on each side, or until the steaks are tender and have nice grill marks.

6. To serve, spoon some romesco sauce on each plate, top with the grilled cauliflower steaks, and drizzle more romesco sauce on top.

Grass-Fed Beef Spring Rolls with Fresh Herbs and Dipping Sauce

Crunchy iceberg lettuce serves as the ideal vessel for thinly sliced beef, fresh herbs, and vegetables. These lettuce cups are enjoyed cold and crisp from the refrigerator, with a luscious dipping sauce.

Serves 4

Ingredients
Almond Dipping Sauce

1 garlic clove, minced

1 teaspoon grated ginger

¼ cup unsalted almond butter (for AIP: omit or replace with tiger nut butter)

1 tablespoon apple cider vinegar

2 teaspoons honey

2–4 tablespoons water

Lettuce Cups

1 (1-pound) grass-fed sirloin steak, thinly sliced (see Note)

2 portobello mushroom caps

1 head iceberg lettuce

1 large daikon radish, peeled and cut into thin strips

1 large carrot, peeled and cut into thin strips

2 Persian (small, thin-skinned) cucumbers, cut into thin strips

1 yellow bell pepper, seeded and cut into thin strips (for AIP: omit or replace with zucchini)

1 bunch fresh mint leaves

1 bunch fresh basil

1 bunch fresh cilantro

1 avocado, peeled, pitted, and cut into 16 slices

1 tablespoon black sesame seeds (for AIP: omit)

Note: Ask the butcher to slice the steak with a professional slicer to get uniformly thin strips.

Method

1. To make the dipping sauce: Place the garlic, ginger, almond butter, apple cider vinegar, and honey in a food processor and pulse to combine. Add water as needed to reach the desired consistency. Transfer to a bowl and set aside until ready to serve.

2. To make the lettuce cups: Heat a large skillet over medium-high heat. Cook the beef slices for 1 to 2 minutes on each side, or until they are browned and cooked through. Transfer to a plate and set aside to cool.

3. Add the portobello mushrooms to the skillet gill-side down and cook for 4 to 5 minutes on each side. Transfer to a cutting board and cut into ¼-inch slices.

4. To assemble the lettuce wraps, place one leaf of iceberg lettuce on a clean surface. Place a portion of the daikon radish, carrot, cucumber, and bell pepper in the lettuce "cup." Add a few leaves of mint, basil, and cilantro on top, and then two slices of avocado. Add several slices of beef and mushrooms, and sprinkle some black sesame seeds and extra herbs over the top. Repeat the process with the remaining ingredients until you make about eight cups.

5. Serve with the dipping sauce.

Grilled Chicken with Watermelon and Mint Salad

This salad is like serving summer on a platter. Refreshing watermelon, crunchy cucumber, and crisp jicama pair well with the fatty avocado. Mint and lime provide a cool flavoring, while a drizzle of olive oil brings it all together.

Serves 4

Ingredients

2 cups diced watermelon

1 cup peeled and diced jicama

2 Persian (small, thin-skinned) cucumbers, diced

1 avocado, peeled, pitted, and diced

Juice of 2 limes

Grated zest of 1 lime

3 tablespoons finely chopped fresh mint

2 tablespoons extra-virgin olive oil, plus extra for brushing

2 large boneless, skinless chicken breasts

Lime wedges, for serving

Method

1. Preheat a grill or grill pan.
2. In a large bowl, gently combine the watermelon, jicama, cucumbers, and avocado. Add the lime juice, zest, and mint. Toss everything together gently to ensure the lime juice and mint are evenly distributed. Drizzle with the olive oil, then cover and refrigerate while you cook the chicken.
3. Brush the chicken breasts with olive oil. Grill the chicken for 6 to 7 minutes on each side, or until fully cooked and the internal temperature reaches 165°F. Transfer to a cutting board and let rest for a few minutes, then slice into strips.

4. To serve, portion the watermelon salad onto plates and top with the sliced chicken. Drizzle with olive oil and serve with lime wedges for squeezing.

Mushroom Minestrone Soup

A myriad of vegetables serves as the base of this hearty soup. Mushrooms add flavor and plenty of cooking liquid. We enjoy this soup all year long.

Serves 4–8

Ingredients

2 tablespoons extra-virgin olive oil, plus more for serving
1 medium onion, finely chopped
2 carrots, peeled and finely chopped
2 celery ribs, finely chopped
3 garlic cloves, minced or sliced
1 leek, trimmed and sliced
1 green bell pepper, seeded and diced (for AIP: omit)
1 cup sliced button mushrooms
4 tomatoes, diced, or 1 (28-ounce) can no-salt-added diced tomatoes
    (for AIP: omit or replace with cooked butternut squash)
4 cups unsalted beef, chicken, or vegetable broth
2 cups filtered water
1 tablespoon AIP-Friendly Italian Seasoning (page 261)
1 teaspoon ground black pepper (for AIP: omit or replace with additional AIP-Friendly Italian Seasoning)
1 medium zucchini, diced
1 yellow squash, diced
Fresh parsley leaves, for garnish

Method

1. In a large pot, heat the olive oil over medium heat. Add the onion, carrots, and celery and sauté for 5 to 10 minutes, until the vegetables

are softened and fragrant. Add the garlic, leek, and bell pepper and cook, stirring constantly, for 3 to 4 minutes, until the leek is softened. Add the mushrooms and cook for 5 minutes, or until they start to release their moisture and become tender. Stir in the tomatoes and cook for 2 to 3 minutes to allow the flavors to meld.

2. Add the broth and water and stir to combine. Bring the soup to a boil, turn the heat down to low, and simmer for 20 minutes. Season with the Italian seasoning and black pepper. Add the zucchini and yellow squash and cook for 5 minutes.

3. To serve, ladle the soup into bowls, drizzle with olive oil, and garnish with fresh parsley.

Coconut Curry

This simple coconut curry is a great way to make curry on its own or with the addition of salmon as a protein. This soup is warming, and, with the curry powder, serves as an anti-inflammatory for the body. Use the AIP-Friendly Curry Powder if you are adhering to an AIP diet.

Serves 4

Ingredients

Curry

2 tablespoons extra-virgin olive oil

½ onion, diced

1 leek, trimmed and sliced

1 red bell pepper, seeded and diced (for AIP: omit or replace with zucchini)

1 yellow bell pepper, seeded and diced (for AIP: omit or replace with zucchini)

2 celery ribs, diced

1 large carrot, peeled and diced

1 butternut squash, peeled, seeded, and cubed

10 ounces button mushrooms, sliced

1–2 tablespoons AIP-Friendly Curry Powder (page 263) (or more to taste)
Chili powder to taste (for AIP: omit or replace with more AIP-Friendly
   Curry Powder)
3–4 makrut lime leaves
1 (13.5-ounce) can unsweetened coconut milk
3 cups unsalted chicken bone broth
Juice of 2 limes

Poached Salmon

4 cups unsalted chicken bone broth
4 (4-ounce) salmon fillets
1 lemon

Cauliflower Rice

1 medium head cauliflower
1 tablespoon coconut oil or extra-virgin olive oil
1 garlic clove, minced

To Serve

Diced avocado
Lemon slices
Fresh cilantro leaves

Method

1. To make the curry: In a large pot, heat the oil over medium heat. Add
   the onion and sauté for 3 to 4 minutes, until translucent. Add the leek
   and cook for 2 minutes. Add the bell peppers, celery, carrot, and butternut squash and cook, stirring occasionally, for 5 minutes, or until the
   vegetables start to soften. Add the mushrooms and cook for 3 minutes.
   Sprinkle in the curry powder and chili powder, stirring to coat the vegetables evenly. Add the lime leaves and pour in the coconut milk and
   bone broth. Turn the heat down to low and simmer for 20 to 25 minutes, until the butternut squash is tender and the flavors meld together.

(Recipe continues on the next page.)

2. Meanwhile, to make the salmon: Pour the bone broth in a large saucepan or deep skillet and bring it to a gentle simmer over medium heat. Carefully add the salmon fillets, ensuring they are fully submerged in the liquid. Turn the heat down to low, cover the pan, and cook for 8 to 10 minutes, until the fish is cooked through and flakes easily with a fork.

3. While the salmon is cooking, make the cauliflower rice: Remove the leaves and core from the cauliflower. Cut the cauliflower into florets and place them in a food processor. Pulse until the cauliflower is finely chopped and resembles rice. (If you don't have a food processor, you can grate the cauliflower with a box grater.) In a large skillet, heat the coconut or olive oil over medium heat. Add the garlic and sauté for 30 seconds, or until fragrant. Add the cauliflower rice and stir well to combine. Cook, stirring occasionally, for 5 to 7 minutes, until the cauliflower is tender but not mushy.

4. To serve, stir the lemon juice into the curry. Plate the salmon and cauliflower rice. Ladle the curry on top, with diced avocado, lemon slices, and cilantro.

Grass-Fed Beef and Organ Chili with Root Vegetables

Who doesn't love chili? This grass-fed beef chili boosts extra nutrition, especially B vitamins, with the addition of organ meats. This is a great recipe to cook when you want to make a meal that is savory and can stay warm in a slow cooker.

Serves 4

Ingredients

2 tablespoons extra-virgin olive oil
1 pound ground grass-fed beef
1 grass-fed beef liver, finely chopped
1 cup diced onion
1 cup diced celery

1 cup diced carrot

3 garlic cloves, grated

2 green bell peppers, seeded and diced (for AIP: omit or replace with zucchini)

2 medium Japanese sweet potatoes, peeled and diced

8 ounces mixed mushrooms, sliced

1 small beet, peeled and cubed

3 tablespoons AIP-Friendly Taco Seasoning (page 262)

1 (28-ounce) can no-salt-added crushed tomatoes (for AIP: omit or replace with butternut squash)

2 cups unsalted beef broth, plus more if desired

Crushed red pepper to taste (for AIP: omit)

Fresh parsley leaves, for garnish

1 avocado, peeled, pitted, and diced

Lime wedges, for serving

Method

1. In a large pot or Dutch oven, heat the olive oil over medium-high heat. Add the ground beef and liver and cook, breaking the meat apart with a spatula, until browned, 6 to 10 minutes. Transfer the beef and liver to a plate.

2. Add the onion, celery, and carrot to the pot and sauté for 5 to 7 minutes, until softened. Add the garlic and cook for 1 minute. Add the bell peppers, Japanese sweet potatoes, mushrooms, and beet and cook for 5 minutes, stirring occasionally. Return the browned meat to the pot. Stir in the taco seasoning and mix, ensuring everything is well coated.

3. Pour in the crushed tomatoes and beef broth. Bring the mixture to a boil, then turn the heat down and simmer for 30 to 40 minutes, until the sweet potatoes are tender and the flavors have melded together. Stir occasionally to prevent sticking and ensure even cooking. This chili is thick, so if preferred, add 2 to 3 additional cups of broth to make it more soup-like. Season with crushed red pepper to taste.

(Recipe continues on the next page.)

4. To serve, ladle the chili into bowls, garnish with parsley, and top with diced avocado, with lime wedges for squeezing.

Spaghetti Squash Bolognese

Enjoy the classic comfort of spaghetti Bolognese without the grains by replacing the pasta with tender spaghetti squash strands. The rich meat sauce is made from grass-fed beef and a medley of vegetables that deliver comfort and important longevity nutrients. The slow-simmered sauce allows flavors to meld, creating a hearty meal that's both wholesome and indulgent.

Serves 4

Ingredients
Basic Pasta Sauce

2 tablespoons extra-virgin olive oil
5 garlic cloves, minced
2 (28-ounce) cans no-salt-added crushed San Marzano tomatoes (for AIP: replace with butternut squash puree and bone broth)
1 tablespoon AIP-Friendly Italian Seasoning (page 261)
¼ teaspoon crushed red pepper (for AIP: omit)

Bolognese

1 pound 80/20 grass-fed ground beef
1 tablespoon extra-virgin olive oil
1 medium onion, diced
1 large carrot, peeled and diced
2 celery ribs, diced
6 button mushrooms, diced
1 tablespoon AIP-Friendly Italian Seasoning (page 261)

Spaghetti Squash

4 small or 2 medium-large spaghetti squash

Method

1. To make the basic pasta sauce: Heat the olive oil in a large skillet over medium heat. Add the garlic and sauté until fragrant and slightly golden, about 2 minutes. Pour in the crushed tomatoes and stir. Season with the Italian seasoning and crushed red pepper. Turn the heat down to low and simmer the sauce, stirring occasionally, for about 20 minutes or until it thickens slightly. Taste and adjust the seasoning as needed. Remove from the heat and set aside.

2. To make the Bolognese: Brown the ground beef in a large skillet on medium heat, breaking the meat apart with a spatula, until cooked through and browned, 6 to 10 minutes. Drain off the excess fat and liquid and transfer the beef to a large bowl. In the same skillet, heat the olive oil over medium-low heat. Add the onion and cook for 2 to 4 minutes, until translucent. Add the celery and mushrooms and cook about 5 minutes, then add the carrots and cook for another 5 to 10 minutes until the vegetables are as tender as you want them. Add the browned ground beef and cook for 3 minutes, then add the pasta sauce and seasoning. Turn the heat down to low and cook for 1 hour, stirring often, until the sauce has thickened and the meat is tender.

3. Meanwhile, to make the spaghetti squash: Preheat the oven to 350°F. Line a rimmed baking sheet with unbleached parchment paper.

4. Poke several holes in each spaghetti squash with a fork or knife to allow steam to escape. Place the squash on the baking sheet and bake for 60 to 75 minutes, until tender. Let them cool, then cut in half lengthwise and scoop out the seeds. Use a fork to scrape the flesh into spaghetti-like strands.

5. To serve, divide the spaghetti squash into four bowls and ladle the Bolognese on top.

Sautéed Mushrooms

Mushrooms are a versatile side dish, lending a depth of flavor and good texture to almost any main course.

Serves 4

Ingredients

3 tablespoons extra-virgin olive oil

2 shallots, finely chopped

4 garlic cloves, minced

1 tablespoon AIP-Friendly Italian Seasoning (page 261)

2 cups sliced button mushrooms

2 large portobello mushroom caps, sliced

1 cup roughly chopped maitake mushrooms

⅛ teaspoon ground black pepper (for AIP: omit or replace with more AIP-Friendly Italian Seasoning)

Method

1. In a large skillet, heat the olive oil over medium-high heat. Add the shallots and sauté for 2 minutes, or until translucent. Add the garlic and sauté for 1 minute, or until fragrant. Stir in the Italian seasoning and sauté for 30 seconds, or until fragrant. Add all the mushrooms and cook, stirring occasionally, for 10 minutes, or until the mushrooms are browned and tender.
2. Season with the black pepper and serve.

DESSERTS

Fresh Fruit Bowl

Fresh fruit is nature's candy, and you can think of chopping the fruit as a sort of moving meditation. Feel free to change up the fruits according to the season, but make sure to always include plenty of berries for their known longevity-boosting antioxidants.

Serves 4

Ingredients

1 pint strawberries, hulled and quartered

1 pint golden berries, halved

1 pint blueberries

1 pint cherries, pitted and halved

1 pear, cored and chopped

4 kiwis, peeled and chopped

Juice of 1 lemon

Arils from 1 pomegranate (for AIP: omit or replace with another seasonal fruit)

Small bunch fresh mint

Method

1. In a large bowl, combine the strawberries, golden berries, blueberries, cherries, pear, and kiwis. Add the lemon juice and toss well.
2. Sprinkle the pomegranate arils and mint leaves on top and serve.

Coconut Butter Mint Chocolate Patties

Here's our Paleo take on a classic mint candy without all the chemicals, fillers, and preservatives. These patties make for a great high-fat pre-workout snack or dessert.

Makes 8 to 12 patties

Ingredients

¼ cup melted raw organic coconut butter (such as Artisana)

1 tablespoon honey

3 fresh mint leaves, minced

1 teaspoon peppermint oil or extract

½ cup roughly chopped 100% dark chocolate

½ teaspoon coconut oil (optional)

Method

1. Line a platter or rimmed baking sheet with unbleached parchment paper. In a large bowl, mix together the coconut butter, honey, mint leaves, and mint oil until well combined. Allow the mixture to harden for a few minutes, then form into 8 to 12 patties. Place the patties on the parchment and freeze for 10 minutes, or until hard.

2. While the patties are freezing, add 1 to 2 inches of water to a small saucepan and bring to a simmer over medium-low heat. Place the dark chocolate in a heatproof glass or stainless steel bowl (or in the top of a double boiler) and set it on top of the saucepan; the bottom of the bowl should not touch the simmering water. Stir often as the steam from the simmering water melts the chocolate. Add the coconut oil if the melted chocolate is too thick. Once the chocolate is melted, set the bowl on the counter on a trivet. Use two forks to quickly dip the frozen patties, one at a time, into the melted chocolate, evenly coating each patty.

3. Set the chocolate-coated patties back on the parchment and freeze for 10 to 15 minutes before serving.

Chocolate-Dipped Strawberries

The key to the perfect chocolate-dipped strawberry is the addition of coconut oil to your chocolate. Whether you're making these for Valentine's Day or for a luscious summer evening treat, these are delicious and nutritious.

Serves 4–8

Ingredients

½ cup roughly chopped 100% dark chocolate

16 strawberries

1 teaspoon coconut oil

Method

1. Add 1 to 2 inches of water to a small saucepan and bring to a simmer over medium-low heat. Place the dark chocolate in a heatproof glass or stainless steel bowl (or in the top of a double boiler) and set it on top of the saucepan; the bottom of the bowl should not touch the simmering water. Stir often as the steam from the simmering water melts the chocolate. Add the coconut oil if the melted chocolate is too thick. Once the chocolate is melted, set the bowl on the counter on a trivet.

2. Line a large platter or rimmed baking sheet with unbleached parchment paper. Dip the strawberries into the melted chocolate, one at a time, evenly coating each berry. Set the chocolate-coated strawberries on the parchment and refrigerate for 10 to 15 minutes to harden the chocolate shell.

SNACKS AND BEVERAGES

Savory Date and Peach with Unrefined Pork Belly

This sweet and savory dish combines juicy peaches, chewy dates, and crispy unrefined pork belly for a perfect balance of flavor.

Serves 4

Ingredients

4 slices thinly cut unrefined pork belly, cut in half

8 dates, pitted

1 peach, pitted and cut into 8 slices

Method

1. Preheat the oven to 350°F. Line a rimmed baking sheet with unbleached parchment paper.
2. Wrap a half slice of pork belly around a date and peach slice and secure with a toothpick. Place on the baking sheet. Repeat with the remaining ingredients.
3. Bake for 20 to 25 minutes, flipping halfway through, until the pork belly is crispy. Make sure the date does not burn due to the caramelization process.
4. Let cool slightly before serving.

Trail Mix

Here's a simple yet satisfying Paleo trail mix made with nuts, seeds, dried fruits, and a touch of coconut—perfect for when you're on the go or need a quick energy boost!

Serves 8

Ingredients

1 cup raw almonds
1 cup raw walnuts
1 cup raw cashews
½ cup pumpkin seeds
½ cup sunflower seeds
½ cup unsweetened unsulfured dried cranberries
½ cup unsulfured unsweetened raisins
½ cup unsweetened coconut flakes
¼ cup 100% dark chocolate chips (optional)

Method

1. In a large airtight container, combine all the ingredients and toss to mix.
2. Store at room temperature for up to 2 weeks.

Mint Tea

This refreshing, caffeine-free mint tea is a simple yet invigorating beverage that you can enjoy hot or iced. Its natural flavors bring a soothing calm that's perfect for any time of day.

Serves 8

Ingredients

2 cups roughly chopped mint
2 quarts water
Lemon wedges, for serving

Method

1. Place the mint and water in a large glass pitcher with a lid or a large mason jar. Place the pitcher outside in the sun and let it steep for 5 hours.
2. Strain the mint and serve the tea in tall glasses over ice with a lemon wedge.

Hibiscus-Berry Tea

Bright, tangy, tart, and full of antioxidants, hibiscus-berry tea is a delicious, health-boosting treat.

Serves 4

Ingredients

¼ cup dried hibiscus flowers
4 cups boiling water
1 cup berries (such as blueberries or mulberries)
1 lemon

Method

1. Place the hibiscus flowers in a teapot and pour in the boiling water. Let steep for 5 to 7 minutes, depending on your preference for color and flavor, then strain out the hibiscus flowers.
2. Place the berries in a large bowl and muddle with a wooden spoon until mashed. To serve, place ¼ cup of the muddled berries in the bottom of each tall glass. Pour in the tea and add ice and a squeeze of lemon.

Hot Cocoa

Hot cocoa made with rich dark chocolate and creamy coconut milk is naturally sweet without any refined sugars or dairy. An inviting drink for a cozy moment!

Serves 4

Ingredients

4 cups canned unsweetened coconut milk
4 ounces 100% dark chocolate, roughly chopped
2¾ teaspoons honey

Method

1. Heat the coconut milk in a medium saucepan over medium-low heat until it begins to steam. Do not let it boil. Add the chocolate to the pan and stir continuously until the chocolate is completely melted and the mixture is smooth.
2. Mix in the honey and serve in mugs.

AUTOIMMUNE PROTOCOL DIET SPICE MIXTURES

If you're following the autoimmune protocol (AIP) diet, use the herbal formulas listed below. Whether you are or aren't following the AIP diet, we highly recommend buying dried herbs from top-quality organic companies like Frontier, Simply Organic, and Starwest Botanicals.

AIP-Friendly Herbes de Provence

Ingredients

2 tablespoons dried thyme
2 tablespoons dried oregano
1 tablespoon dried rosemary
1 tablespoon dried sage
1 tablespoon dried tarragon
1 tablespoon dried lavender flowers

Method

1. In a small mixing bowl, combine all the ingredients together. Store in a spice jar and label.

AIP-Friendly Italian Seasoning

Ingredients

2 tablespoons dried thyme
2 tablespoons dried oregano
2 tablespoons dried parsley
1 tablespoon dried rosemary
1 tablespoon dried marjoram
1 tablespoon dried basil

Method

1. In a small mixing bowl, combine all the ingredients together. Store in a spice jar and label.

AIP-Friendly Taco Seasoning

Ingredients

2 tablespoons dried oregano

2 tablespoons dried cilantro

2 tablespoons garlic powder

2 teaspoons onion powder

2 teaspoons ground cinnamon

2 teaspoons ground ginger

1 teaspoon ground mace

1 teaspoon dried lime zest

Method

1. In a small mixing bowl, combine all the ingredients together. Store in a spice jar and label.

AIP-Friendly Chinese Five-Spice

Ingredients

2 tablespoons ground ginger

1 tablespoon ground turmeric

1 tablespoon ground cloves

1 teaspoon ground cinnamon

1 teaspoon ground mace

Method

1. In a small mixing bowl, combine all the ingredients together. Store in a spice jar and label.

AIP-Friendly Curry Powder

Ingredients

2 tablespoons ground turmeric
2 tablespoons garlic powder
1 tablespoon ground ginger
1 tablespoon dried cilantro
1 tablespoon ground cinnamon
1 teaspoon ground cloves
1 teaspoon onion powder

Method

1. In a small mixing bowl, combine all the ingredients together. Store in a spice jar and label.

AUTOIMMUNE PROTOCOL SUBSTITUTES

Pink/black peppercorn substitutes:

Ground ginger

Chili powder substitutes:

Ground ginger
Ground turmeric

Paprika substitutes:

Ground turmeric
Saffron
Dried orange peel

Ground sumac substitutes:

Dried lemon zest

Tomato substitutes:

In sauces: roasted squashes like butternut squash, yellow squash, kabocha squash, and other winter squashes

In salads: peaches, pears, or mangoes

Oil options:

For cooking/frying, you can use coconut oil, macadamia nut oil, avocado oil, or olive oil interchangeably in recipes. Be sure to monitor smoke points.

For dressing and drizzles, freely use unheated olive oil, walnut oil, or flaxseed oil. For AIP, do not use walnut or flaxseed oils.

FOURTEEN-DAY MEAL PLANNER

Day One:

Breakfast: Mushroom Omelet
Lunch: Avocado Citrus Salad with Mint and Grilled Fish
Dinner: Salmon en Papillote with Radicchio Salad

Day Two:

Breakfast: Soft Scramble
Lunch: Zoodles with Bison Meatballs
Dinner: Grass-Fed Beef and Organ Chili with Root Vegetables

Day Three:

Breakfast: Avocado Egg Bakes
Lunch: Coconut Shrimp and Avocado Ceviche
Dinner: Chicken and Bamboo Shoots with Garlic-Ginger Lettuce Cups

Day Four:

Breakfast: Zucchini Nest with Egg Yolk
Lunch: Antipasto Plate
Dinner: Scallops with Cauliflower Puree

Day Five:

Breakfast: Grass-Fed Bison and Beef Breakfast Patty with Kale, Egg, and Sweet Potato Hash
Lunch: Sushi Bowl with Cauliflower Rice
Dinner: Grilled Chicken with Watermelon and Mint Salad

Day Six:

Breakfast: Banana Pancakes
Lunch: Thai Slaw Salad with Shrimp Skewers
Dinner: Spaghetti Squash Bolognese

Day Seven:

Breakfast: Berry Crumble with Dairy-Free Yogurt
Lunch: Lamb Kebab with Cucumber and Tomato Salad
Dinner: Steak with Chimichurri and Portobello Mushrooms, Asparagus, and Yam Puree

Day Eight:

Breakfast: Chocolate Mint Smoothie
Lunch: Seaweed, Shrimp, and Veggie Rolls
Dinner: Coconut Curry

Day Nine:

Breakfast: Mushroom Egg Bites
Lunch: Chicken Fajitas on Jicama "Tortillas" with Cilantro Slaw
Dinner: Cauliflower Steaks with Romesco Sauce

Day Ten:

Breakfast: Berries, Chocolate, and Mixed Nuts with Dairy-Free Yogurt
Lunch: Pistachio Caesar with Grilled Chicken Breast
Dinner: Grass-Fed Beef Spring Rolls with Fresh Herbs and Dipping Sauce

Day Eleven:

Breakfast: Berry Cauliflower Smoothie
Lunch: Veggie Stir-Fry
Dinner: Moules Marinières

Day Twelve:

Breakfast: Unrefined Pork Belly with Figs
Lunch: Roasted Beets with Dairy-Free Labneh
Dinner: Spaghetti Squash Bolognese with Sautéed Mushrooms

Day Thirteen:

Breakfast: Avocado Egg Bakes
Lunch: Liver and Onions
Dinner: Salmon and Cauliflower Rice Cakes

Day Fourteen:

Breakfast: Crustless Quiche
Lunch: Zoodles with Bison Meatballs
Dinner: Mushroom Minestrone Soup

Snacks (throughout the week):
- Savory Date and Peach with Unrefined Pork Belly
- Trail Mix

Desserts (rotate as desired):
- Fresh Fruit Bowl
- Coconut Butter Mint Chocolate Patties
- Chocolate-Dipped Strawberries

Beverages (rotate daily):
- Mint Tea
- Hibiscus-Berry Tea
- Hot Cocoa

ACKNOWLEDGMENTS

From Loren Cordain:

I'm grateful to Trevor Connor and Mark Smith, two of my former students who have gone on to become major leaders in the Paleo Diet movement. Their help has been enormous, especially in incorporating the most recent Paleo research and trends into this book.

I'm also happy to thank my wonderful collaborative editor, Holly Robinson, whose professionalism and talent bringing science to life in readable (and fun) prose has been essential. Thanks, too, to my literary agent, Tom Miller, who was my editor for my first three books and has been a champion of Paleo from the very beginning. I'm also grateful to the BenBella team, especially Glenn Yeffeth, Leah Wilson, and Claire Schulz, for their collaborative spirit and publishing expertise.

I'm grateful to Bruce Ames, PhD, whose brilliance and understanding greatly contributed to the synthesis of this book. Thanks also to John Speth, PhD, for his patience and his many contributions to the Paleo Diet theory; I appreciate all of his hard work.

Above all, thanks to my magnificent wife, Lorrie.

From Trevor Connor and Mark Smith:

First and foremost, we want to thank Dr. Loren Cordain, whose wisdom and guidance have helped the world learn about the optimal way to eat—the Paleo Diet, which leads to better health and longevity for all of us.

A huge special thanks to Lorrie Cordain. From reviewing the manuscript and the recipes to coordinating important details, Lorrie has been a key part of every book that Dr. Cordain has written about the Paleo Diet, and this one is no exception. Lorrie has been a major voice in the Paleo movement from the start and she has tirelessly helped to spread the word about the enormous health benefits of the diet.

We warmly thank our collaborative editor, Holly Robinson, who worked countless hours and weekends to seamlessly and professionally translate the science behind *Paleo for Life* into accessible prose. Thanks too to our development editor, Joe Rhatigan, for his editorial acumen and improvements, and our copyeditor, Karen Wise, for her excellent suggestions and attention to detail. We are also grateful to Dr. Cordain's literary agent, Tom Miller, who has been a knowledgeable and passionate project manager throughout all the stages of this book.

A huge thank you to licensed naturopathic doctor Erin Rhae Biller, ND, FAIHM, who used her extensive knowledge of nutritional science to help us create original recipes for this book that readers with any level of cooking skills can prepare while knowing that the dishes will be both delicious and health-promoting. Dr. Biller's two-week meal plan will convince any doubters that eating Paleo doesn't mean depriving yourself of yummy food at the table.

Finally, a big thank you to the Paleo Diet team—in particular, to our Chief Marketing Officer, Dave Trendler, and our Chief Content Officer, Dr. Griffin McMath. They were not directly involved in writing the book, but they were key advisors throughout, offering ideas, reviewing our writing, and helping us set an overall direction for the book. Griffin helped us keep our readers and their needs at the forefront of our thoughts, and Dave's book publishing experience was very helpful in ensuring that this book gets out to the widest possible audience.

APPENDIX

Table 1: Autoimmune Protocol: Foods to Avoid

The autoimmune protocol (AIP) is essentially a stricter version of the Paleo Diet to further eliminate problematic antinutrients from one's diet that can initiate, exacerbate, or prolong autoimmune diseases or general inflammatory conditions. Consequently, the AIP eliminates all grains, pseudo-grains (grain-like seeds), legumes, dairy products, as well as potatoes and cassava and any foods that contain non-Paleo additives.

In addition to these non-Paleo foods, there are some general Paleo food categories that should be eliminated, including all nuts and seeds, all spices made from nuts and seeds, and all nightshade plants. In addition, fruits and vegetables that contain very small seeds, such as cucumbers, can be problematic for a small percentage of people needing to follow an AIP, and may also need to be avoided. Ultimately, an individual with an autoimmune issue needs to understand that any food has the potential of being problematic; however, this table contains the most commonly identified foods.

Food Item	Notes	Food Item	Notes
Agave/Agave nectar	Some people are better avoiding raw honey too	Celery seed	
Alcohol		Chili peppers	
Allspice	Most people on AIP can consume	Chili powder	
Allulose	Some people are better avoiding raw honey too	Chinese five-spice	Usually contains star anise, peppercorns, and fennel seed
Anise seed		Chocolate	
Annatto seed		Cocona	
Ashwagandha		Coconut sugar/ nectar	Some people are better avoiding raw honey too
Bananas	All fruit for some people on AIP	Coffee	
Bell peppers		Coriander seed	
Black caraway	Aka Russian caraway/black cumin	Crushed red pepper	
Black pepper	Most people on AIP can consume	Cumin seed	
Cape gooseberries	Aka ground cherries (regular cherries are okay)	Curry powder	Usually contains coriander, cumin, fenugreek, and red pepper
Capsicums		Date paste/nectar	Some people are better avoiding raw honey too
Caraway	Most people on AIP can consume	Dill seed	
Cardamom	Most people on AIP can consume	Dried fruit	
Cayenne		Eggplant	

Food Item	Notes	Food Item	Notes
Eggs	Especially egg whites	Mustard seed	
Erythritol	Some people are better avoiding raw honey too	Naranjillas	
Fennel seed		Nut/seed butters/ flours	
Fenugreek		Nut/seed oils	Some people are better using only animal fat
Fruit juices	Some people are better avoiding raw honey too	Nutmeg	
Garam masala	Usually contains peppercorns, cumin seeds, and cardamom pods	Paprika	
Garden huckleberries	Regular huckleberries are okay	Pepinos	
Goji berries	Aka wolfberries	Pimentos	
Green peppercorns	Most people on AIP can consume	Pink peppercorns	Most people on AIP can consume
Hot peppers		Pomegranate seeds (arils)	Most people on AIP can consume
Jalapeño peppers		Poppy seed	
Juniper	Most people on AIP can consume	Poultry seasoning	Often contains pepper and nutmeg
Kutjera		Processed meats	Usually cured with nightshade spices
Maple syrup	Some people are better avoiding raw honey too	Red pepper	
Monk fruit (luo han guo)	Some people are better avoiding raw honey too	Sesame seed	

Food Item	Notes	Food Item	Notes
Star anise	Most people on AIP can consume	Vanilla bean	Most people on AIP can consume
Steak seasoning	Usually contains pepper, chili, cumin, and cayenne	White pepper	Most people on AIP can consume
Stevia		Xylitol	Some people are better avoiding raw honey too
Tamarillos		Yacon syrup	Some people are better avoiding raw honey too
Tomatillos		Yeast extract & nutritional yeast	
Tomatoes			

Table 2: Digestible Indispensable Amino Acid Score (DIAAS) and Essential Amino Acid Quantities for Certain Foods

Food	DIAAS (%)	Histidine	Isoleucine	Leucine	Lysine
Beef (skirt steak)	112	1.293	1.58	2.945	3.305
Pork (ground)		1.026	1.203	2.061	2.31
Lamb (ground)		0.784	1.194	1.925	2.186
Chicken (meat & skin)	108	0.701	1.191	1.739	1.945
Turkey (ground)		0.811	1.227	2.262	2.452
Salmon (Atlantic)		0.749	1.172	2.067	2.336
Cod (Atlantic)		0.672	1.052	1.856	2.097
Shrimp (canned)		0.485	0.974	1.681	1.813
Egg (poached)	113	0.308	0.669	1.082	0.909
Chickpeas	83	0.195	0.304	0.505	0.475
RDA 4–19 years (mg/kg/d)		14	19	42	38
RDA 19+ years (g for 70 kg person)		0.98	1.33	2.94	2.66

Note: This table outlines DIAAS and essential amino acid quantities (listed in grams per 100 grams [3.5 oz]) for select cooked animal proteins and chickpeas, and the RDA for each amino acid is listed in mg/kg/d and in grams for a 70-kilogram (154-pound) person. Shaded boxes indicate RDA is met for a 70-kilogram (154-pound) person with a 3.5-ounce serving.

Methionine (Cysteine)	Phenylalanine (Tyrosine)	Threonine	Tryptophan	Valine
0.905 (0.345)	1.351 (1.279)	1.595	0.374	1.667
0.68	1.025	1.173	0.326	1.394
0.635	1.008	1.059	0.289	1.335
0.636	0.929	0.989	0.266	1.162
0.806	1.068	1.258	0.312	1.27
0.753	0.993	1.115	0.285	1.31
0.676	0.891	1.001	0.256	1.176
0.557	0.946	0.824	0.186	0.935
0.378	0.677	0.553	0.166	0.855
0.093	0.38	0.264	0.069	0.298
19 (+ cysteine)	33 (+ tyrosine)	20	5	24
1.33	2.31	1.4	0.35	1.68

NOTES

Chapter 1

p. 8   *Drewnowski . . . published his seminal paper on the topic*   Drewnowski, Adam. 2005. "Concept of a Nutritious Food: Toward a Nutrient Density Score." *American Journal of Clinical Nutrition* 82 (4): 721–32. https://doi.org/10.1093 /ajcn/82.4.721.

Chapter 2

p. 17   *In 2006 . . . introduced the Triage Theory of Aging*   Ames, Bruce N. 2006. "Low Micronutrient Intake May Accelerate the Degenerative Diseases of Aging through Allocation of Scarce Micronutrients by Triage." *Proceedings of the National Academy of Sciences* 103 (47): 17589–94. https://doi.org/10.1073/pnas .0608757103.

p. 18   *Some of the most common deficiencies include*   Fulgoni, Victor L., Debra R. Keast, Regan L. Bailey, and Johanna Dwyer. 2011. "Foods, Fortificants, and Supplements: Where Do Americans Get Their Nutrients?" *Journal of Nutrition* 141 (10): 1847–54. https://doi.org/10.3945/jn.111.142257.

p. 18   *These important longevity nutrients include*   Ames, Bruce N. 2006. "Low Micronutrient Intake."

p. 18   *multivitamins have consistently been shown to be ineffective*   Loftfield, Erikka, Caitlin P. O'Connell, Christian C. Abnet, Barry I. Graubard, Linda M. Liao, Laura E. Beane Freeman, Jonathan N. Hofmann, Neal D. Freedman, and Rashmi Sinha. 2024. "Multivitamin Use and Mortality Risk in 3 Prospective US Cohorts." *JAMA Network Open* 7 (6): e2418729. https://doi.org/10.1001 /jamanetworkopen.2024.18729.

p. 19 *The full list of aging factors* López-Otín, Carlos, Maria A. Blasco, Linda Partridge, Manuel Serrano, and Guido Kroemer. 2013. "The Hallmarks of Aging." *Cell* 153 (6): 1194–1217. https://doi.org/10.1016/j.cell.2013.05.039.

p. 20 *scientists found viable 35,000-year-old protozoa* Yarzábal, Luis Andrés, Lenys M. Buela Salazar, and Ramón Alberto Batista-García. 2021. "Climate Change, Melting Cryosphere and Frozen Pathogens: Should We Worry . . . ?" *Environmental Sustainability* 4 (3): 489–501. https://doi.org/10.1007/s42398 -021-00184-8.

p. 20 *potentially causing damage to healthy cells and accelerating aging* Sohal, Rajindar S., and William C. Orr. 2012. "The Redox Stress Hypothesis of Aging." *Free Radical Biology and Medicine* 52 (3): 539–55. https://doi.org/10.1016 /j.freeradbiomed.2011.10.445.

p. 20 *While our mitochondria are the major natural source of ROS* Schniertshauer, Daniel, Daniel Gebhard, and Jörg Bergemann. 2018. "Age-Dependent Loss of Mitochondrial Function in Epithelial Tissue Can Be Reversed by Coenzyme Q10." *Journal of Aging Research* 2018: 1–8. https://doi.org/10.1155/2018 /6354680; Amorim, João A., Giuseppe Coppotelli, Anabela P. Rolo, Carlos M. Palmeira, Jaime M. David A. Sinclair. 2022. "Mitochondrial and Metabolic Dysfunction in Ageing and Age-Related Diseases." *Nature Reviews Endocrinology* 18 (4): 243–58. https://doi.org/10.1038/s41574-021-00626-7; Dai, Dao-Fu, Ying Ann Chiao, David J. Marcinek, Hazel H. Szeto, and Peter S. Rabinovitch. 2014. "Mitochondrial Oxidative Stress in Aging and Healthspan." *Longevity & Healthspan* 3 (1): 6. https://doi.org/10.1186/2046-2395-3-6; Gonzalez-Freire, Marta, Rafael de Cabo, Michel Bernier, Steven J. Sollott, Elisa Fabbri, Placido Navas, and Luigi Ferrucci. 2015. "Reconsidering the Role of Mitochondria in Aging." *Journals of Gerontology Series A: Biomedical Sciences and Medical Sciences* 70 (11): 1334–42. https://doi.org/10.1093/gerona/glv070.

p. 21 *This free radical theory of aging was originally proposed* Harman, Denham. 1956. "Aging: A Theory Based on Free Radical and Radiation Chemistry." *Journal of Gerontology* 11 (3): 298–300. https://doi.org/10.1093/geronj/11.3.298.

p. 21 *leakage of ROS by mitochondrial membranes represents a major player* Dai, Dao-Fu, et al. 2014. "Mitochondrial Oxidative Stress"; Gonzalez-Freire, Marta, et al. 2015. "Reconsidering the Role of Mitochondria"; Indo, Hiroko P., Hsiu-Chuan Yen, Ikuo Nakanishi, Ken-ichiro Matsumoto, Masato Tamura, Yumiko Nagano, Hirofumi Matsui, et al., 2015. "A Mitochondrial Superoxide Theory for Oxidative Stress Diseases and Aging." *Journal of Clinical Biochemistry and Nutrition* 56 (1): 1–7. https://doi.org/10.3164/jcbn.14-42; Hajam, Younis Ahmad, Raksha Rani, Shahid Yousuf Ganie, Tariq Ahmad Sheikh, Darakhshan Javaid, Syed Sanober Qadri, Sreepoorna Pramodh, et al. 2022. "Oxidative Stress in Human Pathology and Aging: Molecular Mechanisms and Perspectives." *Cells* 11 (3): 552. https://doi.org/10.3390/cells11030552.

p. 21   *if telomeres become damaged or shortened* Razgonova, Mayya P., Alexander M. Zakharenko, Kirill S. Golokhvast, Maria Thanasoula, Evangelia Sarandi, Konstantinos Nikolouzakis, Persefoni Fragkiadaki, Dimitris Tsoukalas, Demetrios A. Spandidos, and Aristidis Tsatsakis. 2020. "Telomerase and Telomeres in Aging Theory and Chronographic Aging Theory." *Molecular Medicine Reports* 22 (3): 1679–94. https://doi.org/10.3892/mmr.2020 .11274; Wang, Qi, Yiqiang Zhan, Nancy L. Pedersen, Fang Fang, and Sara Hägg. 2018. "Telomere Length and All-Cause Mortality: A Meta-Analysis." *Ageing Research Reviews* 48: 11–20. https://doi.org/10.1016/j.arr.2018.09 .002; Armanios, Mary, and Elizabeth H. Blackburn. 2012. "The Telomere Syndromes." *Nature Reviews Genetics* 13 (10): 693–704. https://doi.org/10 .1038/nrg3246; Epel, Elissa S., Elizabeth H. Blackburn, Jue Lin, Firdaus S. Dhabhar, Nancy E. Adler, Jason D. Morrow, and Richard M. Cawthon. 2004. "Accelerated Telomere Shortening in Response to Life Stress." *Proceedings of the National Academy of Sciences* 101 (49): 17312–15. https://doi.org/10.1073 /pnas.0407162101.

p. 22   *older people with shorter telomeres are at three times the risk . . . from infectious diseases* Tedone, Enzo, Ejun Huang, Ryan O'Hara, Kimberly Batten, Andrew T. Ludlow, Tsung-Po Lai, Beatrice Arosio, Daniela Mari, Woodring E. Wright, and Jerry W. Shay. 2019. "Telomere Length and Telomerase Activity in T Cells Are Biomarkers of High-Performing Centenarians." *Aging Cell* 18 (1): e12859. https://doi.org/10.1111/acel.12859; Wang and Qi. 2018. "Telomere Length and All-Cause Mortality." *Ageing Research Reviews* 48: 11–20; Armanios, Mary, and Elizabeth H. Blackburn. 2012. "The Telomere Syndromes"; Razgonova, Mayya P., Alexander M. Zakharenko, Kirill S. Golokhvast, Maria Thanasoula, Evangelia Sarandi, Konstantinos Nikolouzakis, Persefoni Fragkiadaki, Dimitris Tsoukalas, Demetrios A. Spandidos, and Aristidis Tsatsakis. 2020. "Telomerase and Telomeres in Aging Theory and Chronographic Aging Theory." *Molecular Medicine Reports* 22 (3): 1679–94. https://doi.org/10.3892 /mmr.2020.11274; Epel, Elissa S., et al. 2004. "Accelerated Telomere Shortening in Response to Life Stress"; Cawthon, R., K. Smith, E. O'Brien, A. Sivatchenko, and R. Kerber. 2003. "Association Between Telomere Length in Blood and Mortality in People Aged 60 Years or Older." *Neurology Bulletin* XXXV (3–4): 96–97. https://doi.org/10.17816/nb100175.

p. 23   *we've been aware of a phenomenon in cancer cells called the Warburg Effect* Pascale, Rosa Maria, Diego Francesco Calvisi, Maria Maddalena Simile, Claudio Francesco Feo, and Francesco Feo. 2020. "The Warburg Effect 97 Years after Its Discovery." *Cancers* 12 (10): 2819. https://doi.org/10.3390/cancers12102819.

p. 23   *not the cancer cells that directly kill the patient, but cachexia* San-Millán, Iñigo, and George A. Brooks. 2017. "Reexamining Cancer Metabolism: Lactate Production for Carcinogenesis Could Be the Purpose and Explanation of the

Warburg Effect." *Carcinogenesis* 38 (2): 119–33. https://doi.org/10.1093/carcin /bgw127.

p. 23   *Ketosis has been shown to help protect . . . [but] can speed aging in the long run*   Barrea, Luigi, Massimiliano Caprio, Dario Tuccinardi, Eleonora Moriconi, Laura Di Renzo, Giovanna Muscogiuri, Annamaria Colao, and Silvia Savastano, on Behalf of the Obesity Programs of Education, Nutrition, Research, and Assessment (OPERA) Group. 2022. "Could Ketogenic Diet 'Starve' Cancer? Emerging Evidence." *Critical Reviews in Food Science and Nutrition* 62 (7): 1800–1821. https://doi.org/10.1080/10408398.2020.1847030; Tran, Quangdon, Hyunji Lee, Chaeyeong Kim, Gyeyeong Kong, Nayoung Gong, So Hee Kwon, Jisoo Park, Seon-Hwan Kim, and Jongsun Park. 2020. "Revisiting the Warburg Effect: Diet-Based Strategies for Cancer Prevention." *BioMed Research International* 2020: 8105735. https://doi.org/10.1155/2020/8105735; Dyńka, Damian, Katarzyna Kowalcze, and Agnieszka Paziewska. 2022. "The Role of Ketogenic Diet in the Treatment of Neurological Diseases." *Nutrients* 14 (23): 5003. https://doi.org/10.3390/nu14235003; Sergeeva, Ekaterina, Tatiana Ruksha, and Yulia Fefelova. 2023. "Effects of Obesity and Calorie Restriction on Cancer Development." *International Journal of Molecular Sciences* 24 (11): 9601. https://doi.org/10.3390/ijms24119601.

p. 23   *you'll promote all stages of the cell cycle . . . and ultimately better aging*   Guo, Jun, Xiuqing Huang, Lin Dou, Mingjing Yan, Tao Shen, Weiqing Tang, and Jian Li. 2022. "Aging and Aging-Related Diseases: From Molecular Mechanisms to Interventions and Treatments." *Signal Transduction and Targeted Therapy* 7 (1): 391. https://doi.org/10.1038/s41392-022-01251-0.

p. 25   *chronic inflammation . . . linked to almost every chronic disease of aging*   Prasad, Sahdeo, Bokyung Sung, and Bharat B. Aggarwal. 2012. "Age-Associated Chronic Diseases Require Age-Old Medicine: Role of Chronic Inflammation." *Preventive Medicine* 54: S29–37. https://doi.org/10.1016/j.ypmed.2011 .11.011; Khan, S., M. Jain, V. Mathur, and S. M. A. Feroz. 2015. "Chronic Inflammation and Cancer: Paradigm on Tumor Progression, Metastasis and Therapeutic Intervention." *The Gulf Journal of Oncology* 1 (20): 86–93; Sohrab, Sayed Sartaj, Riya Raj, Amka Nagar, Susan Hawthorne, Ana Cláudia Paiva-Santos, Mohammad Amjad Kamal, Mai M. El-Daly, Esam I. Azhar, and Ankur Sharma. 2023. "Chronic Inflammation's Transformation to Cancer: A Nanotherapeutic Paradigm." *Molecules* 28 (11): 4413. https://doi.org/10.3390 /molecules28114413; Grivennikov, Sergei I., Florian R. Greten, and Michael Karin. 2010. "Immunity, Inflammation, and Cancer." *Cell* 140 (6): 883–99. https://doi.org/10.1016/j.cell.2010.01.025.

p. 25   *Chronic inflammation has also been closely linked*   Reuter, Simone, Subash C. Gupta, Madan M. Chaturvedi, and Bharat B. Aggarwal. 2010. "Oxidative Stress, Inflammation, and Cancer: How Are They Linked?" *Free Radical*

Biology and Medicine 49 (11): 1603–16. https://doi.org/10.1016/j.freeradbiomed
.2010.09.006; Papaconstantinou, John. 2019. "The Role of Signaling Pathways of Inflammation and Oxidative Stress in Development of Senescence and Aging Phenotypes in Cardiovascular Disease." *Cells* 8 (11): 1383. https://doi .org/10.3390/cells8111383; Baylis, Daniel, Georgia Ntani, Mark H. Edwards, Holly E. Syddall, David B. Bartlett, Elaine M. Dennison, Carmen Martin-Ruiz, et al. 2014. "Inflammation, Telomere Length, and Grip Strength: A 10-Year Longitudinal Study." *Calcified Tissue International* 95 (1): 54–63. https://doi.org/10.1007/s00223-014-9862-7.

p. 26　*Paleo Diet was by far the most effective diet at reducing biomarkers of inflammation*　Liang, S., J. Mijatovic, A. Li, N. Koemel, R. Nasir, C. Toniutti, K. Bell-Anderson, M. Skilton, and F. O'Leary. 2022. "Dietary Patterns and Non-Communicable Disease Biomarkers: A Network Meta-Analysis and Nutritional Geometry Approach." *Nutrients* 15 (1): 76. https://doi.org/10.3390 /nu15010076.

Chapter 3

p. 37　*Scientists have so far identified about 8,000 of these compounds*　Baião, Diego, Cyntia de Freitas, Laidson Gomes, Davi da Silva, Anna Correa, Patricia Pereira, Eduardo Aguila, and Vania Paschoalin. 2017. "Polyphenols from Root, Tubercles and Grains Cropped in Brazil: Chemical and Nutritional Characterization and Their Effects on Human Health and Diseases." *Nutrients* 9 (9): 1044. https://doi.org/10.3390/nu9091044.

p. 37　*plant foods are also rich in dietary nitrate, which can act as a substrate*　Baião, Diego dos S. 2020, "Beetroot, A Remarkable Vegetable," *Antioxidants* 9 (10): 960.

p. 38　*"a guardian of health span and gatekeeper of species longevity"*　Lewis, Kaitlyn N., James Mele, John D. Hayes, and Rochelle Buffenstein. 2010. "Nrf2, a Guardian of Healthspan and Gatekeeper of Species Longevity." *Integrative and Comparative Biology* 50 (5): 829–43. https://doi.org/10.1093/icb/icq034.

p. 38　*these 500 genes are related to almost every one of them*　Pall, Martin L., and Stephen Levine. 2015. "Nrf2, a Master Regulator of Detoxification and Also Antioxidant, Anti-Inflammatory and Other Cytoprotective Mechanisms, Is Raised by Health Promoting Factors." *Sheng Li Xue Bao [Acta Physiologica Sinica]* 67 (1): 1–18.

p. 38　*The best-known function of Nrf2 . . . heavy metals*　Pall, Martin L., and Stephen Levine. 2015. "Nrf2."

p. 38　*Nrf2 is elevated by phenolic compounds . . . [and] isothiocyanates*　Pall, Martin L., and Stephen Levine. 2015. "Nrf2."

p. 39　*Sirtuins, often called "longevity proteins," . . . epigenetic modifications*　Wątroba, Mateusz, Ilona Dudek, Marta Skoda, Aleksandra Stangret, Przemysław

Rzodkiewicz, and Dariusz Szukiewicz. 2017. "Sirtuins, Epigenetics and Longevity." *Ageing Research Reviews* 40: 11–19. https://doi.org/10.1016/j.arr.2017.08.001.

p. 39   *caloric restriction and exercise are two avenues for increasing sirtuin activation*   Ziętara, Patrycja, Marta Dziewięcka, and Maria Augustyniak. 2022. "Why Is Longevity Still a Scientific Mystery? Sirtuins—Past, Present and Future." *International Journal of Molecular Sciences* 24 (1): 728. https://doi.org/10.3390/ijms24010728.

p. 39   *the importance of NAD+ to our metabolic health*   Blanco-Vaca, Francisco, Noemi Rotllan, Marina Canyelles, Didac Mauricio, Joan Carles Escolà-Gil, and Josep Julve. 2022. "NAD+-Increasing Strategies to Improve Cardiometabolic Health?" *Frontiers in Endocrinology* 12: 815565. https://doi.org/10.3389/fendo.2021.815565; Ito, Takashi K., Tomohito Sato, Yusuke Takanashi, Zinat Tamannaa, Takuya Kitamoto, Keiichi Odagiri, and Mitsutoshi Setou. 2021. "A Single Oral Supplementation of Nicotinamide Within the Daily Tolerable Upper Level Increases Blood NAD+ Levels in Healthy Subjects." *Translational Medicine of Aging* 5: 43–51. https://doi.org/10.1016/j.tma.2021.09.001.

p. 39   *one review published in 2022 strongly criticized the "over-hype" of sirtuins*   Brenner, Charles. 2022. "Sirtuins Are Not Conserved Longevity Genes." *Life Metabolism* 1 (2): 122–33. https://doi.org/10.1093/lifemeta/loac025.

p. 39   *plant foods, which have been shown to directly activate sirtuins . . . resveratrol*   Ziętara, Patrycja, Barbara Flasz, and Maria Augustyniak. 2024. "Does Selection for Longevity in Acheta Domesticus Involve Sirtuin Activity Modulation and Differential Response to Activators (Resveratrol and Nanodiamonds)?" *International Journal of Molecular Sciences* 25 (2): 1329. https://doi.org/10.3390/ijms25021329; Zhou, Dan-Dan, Min Luo, Si-Yu Huang, Adila Saimaiti, Ao Shang, Ren-You Gan, and Hua-Bin Li. 2021. "Effects and Mechanisms of Resveratrol on Aging and Age-Related Diseases." *Oxidative Medicine and Cellular Longevity* 2021 (1): 9932218. https://doi.org/10.1155/2021/9932218; Lee, Shin-Hae, Ji-Hyeon Lee, Hye-Yeon Lee, and Kyung-Jin Min. 2019. "Sirtuin Signaling in Cellular Senescence and Aging." *BMB Reports* 52 (1): 24–34. https://doi.org/10.5483/bmbrep.2019.52.1.290; Ziętara, Patrycja, et al. 2022. "Why Is Longevity Still a Scientific Mystery?"

p. 39   *plant foods, which have been shown to directly activate sirtuins . . . curcumin*   Bańkowski, Sebastian, Miroslav Petr, Michał Rozpara, and Ewa Sadowska-Krępa. 2022. "Effect of 6-Week Curcumin Supplementation on Aerobic Capacity, Antioxidant Status and Sirtuin 3 Level in Middle-Aged Amateur Long-Distance Runners." *Redox Report* 27 (1): 186–92. https://doi.org/10.1080/13510002.2022.2123882; Izadi, Mehran, Nariman Sadri, Amirhossein Abdi, Mohammad Mahdi Raeis Zadeh, Dorsa Jalaei, Mohammad Mahdi Ghazimoradi, Sara Shouri, and Safa Tahmasebi. 2024. "Longevity and Anti-Aging Effects of Curcumin Supplementation." *GeroScience* 46 (3): 2933–50. https://doi.org/10.1007/s11357-024-01092-5; Ungurianu, Anca, Anca Zanfirescu, and Denisa Margină. 2022. "Regulation of Gene Expression Through Food—Curcumin as a Sirtuin Activity Modulator." *Plants* 11 (13): 1741. https://doi.org/10.3390/plants11131741; Grabowska, Wioleta, Ewa Sikora, and Anna Bielak-Zmijewska. 2017. "Sirtuins, a Promising Target in Slowing Down the Ageing Process." *Biogerontology* 18 (4): 447–76. https://doi .org/10.1007/s10522-017-9685-9.

p. 40   *red grapes (and the resultant red wine) have a reputation as a great source of res-veratrol, they have significantly less (79 μg/100 g) than the highest-containing foods* . . .   Xu, Yichi, Mengxue Fang, Xue Li, Du Wang, Li Yu, Fei Ma, Jun Jiang, Liangxiao Zhang, and Peiwu Li. 2024. "Contributions of Common Foods to Resveratrol Intake in the Chinese Diet." *Foods* 13 (8): 1267. https:// doi.org/10.3390/foods13081267.

p. 40   *resveratrol can be unstable once extracted*   Tian, Bingren, and Jiayue Liu. 2020. "Resveratrol: A Review of Plant Sources, Synthesis, Stability, Modification and Food Application." *Journal of the Science of Food and Agriculture* 100 (4): 1392–1404. https://doi.org/10.1002/jsfa.10152.

p. 40   *all non-Paleo plant foods have low or very low resveratrol concentrations*   Xu, Yichi, et al. 2024. "Contributions of Common Foods."

Chapter 4

p. 43   *Salty processed foods, cereals, most dairy products, legumes, meat, fish, and eggs pro-duce net acid loads*   Shariati-Bafghi, S.-E., E. Nosrat-Mirshekarlou, M. Kara-mati, and B. Rashidkhani. 2014. "Higher Dietary Acidity Is Associated with Lower Bone Mineral Density in Postmenopausal Iranian Women, Independent of Dietary Calcium Intake." *International Journal for Vitamin and Nutrition Research* 84 (3–4): 206–17. https://doi.org/10.1024/0300-9831/a000207.

p. 43   *potassium . . . has been shown to be far more effective than calcium supplements in preventing osteoporosis*   Lambert, H., L. Frassetto, J. B. Moore, D. Torg-erson, R. Gannon, P. Burckhardt, and S. Lanham-New. 2015. "The Effect of Supplementation with Alkaline Potassium Salts on Bone Metabolism: A Meta-Analysis. *Osteoporosis International* 26 (4): 1311–18. https://doi.org/10 .1007/s00198-014-3006-9; Ha, Jinwoo, Seong-Ah Kim, Kyungjoon Lim, and Sangah Shin. 2020. "The Association of Potassium Intake with Bone Mineral Density and the Prevalence of Osteoporosis Among Older Korean Adults." *Nutrition Research and Practice* 14 (1): 55–61. https://doi.org/10.4162/nrp.2020 .14.1.55.

p. 44   *the Allium genus, which has more than 1,000 accepted species*   Xie, Tiantian, Qi Wu, Han Lu, Zuomin Hu, Yi Luo, Zhongxing Chu, and Feijun Luo.

2023. "Functional Perspective of Leeks: Active Components, Health Benefits and Action Mechanisms." *Foods* 12 (17): 3225. https://doi.org/10.3390/foods12173225.

p. 44   *just a sample of the conditions treated by garlic*   Tudu, Champa Keeya, Tusheema Dutta, Mimosa Ghorai, Protha Biswas, Dipu Samanta, Patrik Oleksak, Niraj Kumar Jha, et al., 2022. "Traditional Uses, Phytochemistry, Pharmacology and Toxicology of Garlic (Allium Sativum), a Storehouse of Diverse Phytochemicals: A Review of Research from the Last Decade Focusing on Health and Nutritional Implications." *Frontiers in Nutrition* 9: 949554. https://doi.org/10.3389/fnut.2022.929554.

p. 44   *Onions, too, have been incorporated into traditional medicine*   Zhao and Xin-Xin, Fang-Jun Lin, Hang Li, Hua-Bin Li, Ding-Tao Wu, Fang Geng, Wei Ma, Yu Wang, Bao-He Miao, and Ren-You Gan. 2021. "Recent Advances in Bioactive Compounds, Health Functions, and Safety Concerns of Onion (Allium Cepa L.)." *Frontiers in Nutrition* 8: 669805. https://doi.org/10.3389/fnut.2021.669805.

p. 44   *Hippocrates prescribed onions . . . while medieval care providers relied on onions to treat everything*   Galavi, Amin, Hossein Hosseinzadeh, and Bibi Marjan Razavi. 2021. "The Effects of Allium Cepa L. (Onion) and Its Active Constituents on Metabolic Syndrome: A Review." *Iranian Journal of Basic Medical Sciences* 24 (1): 3–16. https://doi.org/10.22038/ijbms.2020.46956.10843.

p. 44   The Compendium of Materia Medica . . . *describes how cooked leek roots*   Wang, Huaijian, Ying Tian, Hao Tan, Mengru Zhou, Miao Li, Yuchen Zhi, Yanbin Shi, and Xuefeng Li. 2023. "Research and Application of Leek Roots in Medicinal Field." *Chinese Herbal Medicines* 15 (3): 391–97. https://doi.org/10.1016/j.chmed.2023.05.002.

p. 45   *In garlic, probably the most beneficial are the sulfur-containing compounds*   El-Saadony, Mohamed T., Ahmed M. Saad, Sameh A. Korma, Heba M. Salem, Taia A. Abd El-Mageed, Samar Sami Alkafaas, Mohamed I. Elsalahaty, et al. 2024. "Garlic Bioactive Substances and Their Therapeutic Applications for Improving Human Health: A Comprehensive Review." *Frontiers in Immunology* 15: 1277074. https://doi.org/10.3389/fimmu.2024.1277074.

p. 45   *Onions and leeks are especially rich sources*   Xie, Tiantian, Qi Wu, Han Lu, Zuomin Hu, Yi Luo, Zhongxing Chu, and Feijun Luo. 2023. "Functional Perspective of Leeks: Active Components, Health Benefits and Action Mechanisms." *Foods* 12 (17): 3225. https://doi.org/10.3390/foods12173225.

p. 45   Allium *vegetables may have anticarcinogenic, . . . protecting cardiovascular health*   Xie, Tiantian, et al. 2023. "Functional Perspective of Leeks."

p. 45   *aged garlic extract has been shown to decrease reactive oxygen species*   Ansary, Johura, Tamara Yuliett Forbes-Hernández, Emilio Gil, Danila Cianciosi, Jiaojiao Zhang, Maria Elexpuru-Zabaleta, Jesus Simal-Gandara, Francesca

Giampieri, and Maurizio Battino. 2020. "Potential Health Benefit of Garlic Based on Human Intervention Studies: A Brief Overview." *Antioxidants* 9 (7): 619. https://doi.org/10.3390/antiox9070619.

p. 45   *onions' powerful potential as an antioxidant, including its ability to upregulate Nrf2*   Ezeorba, Timothy, Prince Chidike, Arinze Linus Ezugwu, Ifeoma Felicia Chukwuma, Emeka Godwin Anaduaka, and Chibuike C. Udenigwe. 2024. "Health-Promoting Properties of Bioactive Proteins and Peptides of Garlic (Allium Sativum)." *Food Chemistry* 435: 137632. https://doi.org/10.1016/j.foodchem.2023.137632; Mounir, Rafik, Walaa A. Alshareef, Eman A. El Gebaly, Alaadin E. El-Haddad, Abdallah M. Said Ahmed, Osama G. Mohamed, Eman T. Enan, et al. 2023. "Unlocking the Power of Onion Peel Extracts: Antimicrobial and Anti-Inflammatory Effects Improve Wound Healing Through Repressing Notch-1/NLRP3/Caspase-1 Signaling." *Pharmaceuticals* 16 (10): 1379. https://doi.org/10.3390/ph16101379.

p. 45   *garlic's potential to exert anti-inflammatory effects*   Ezeorba, Chidike, et al. 2024. "Health-Promoting Properties of Bioactive Proteins."

p. 46   *Leeks have also demonstrated anti-inflammatory activities*   Xie, Tiantian, et al. 2023. "Functional Perspective of Leeks."

p. 46   *a study where people with moderately elevated cholesterol were given garlic extract*   Ansary, Johura, et al. 2020. "Potential Health Benefit of Garlic."

p. 46   *supplementing your diet with onion may significantly reduce systolic blood pressure*   Hejazi, Najmeh, Hamid Ghalandari, Mehran Nouri, and Moein Askarpour. 2023. "Onion Supplementation and Health Metabolic Parameters: A Systematic Review and Meta-Analysis of Randomized Controlled Trials." *Clinical Nutrition ESPEN* 58: 1–13. https://doi.org/10.1016/j.clnesp.2023.08.032.

p. 46   *consuming garlic powder is linked to lowering those factors and protecting heart health*   El-Saadony, Mohamed T., et al. 2024. "Garlic Bioactive Substances."

p. 46   *garlic can significantly reduce the risk of... myocardial infarction*   Ansary, Johura, et al. 2020. "Potential Health Benefit of Garlic."

p. 46   *animals fed high-cholesterol or high-fat diets experience decreased levels of total cholesterol*   Zhao, Xin-Xin, et al. 2021. "Recent Advances in Bioactive Compounds."

p. 46   *leek roots have proven effective in promoting blood circulation*   Xie, Tiantian, et al. 2023. "Functional Perspective of Leeks."

p. 46   *Garlic can help prevent cancer. It has been shown ... in multiple studies*   Ansary, Johura, et al. 2020. "Potential Health Benefit of Garlic."

p. 46   *the association between consuming Alliums and a lower risk of breast, colorectal, and liver cancer*   Xie, Tiantian, et al. 2023. "Functional Perspective of Leeks."

p. 47   *in vitro studies have linked garlic's sulfur-containing compounds*   El-Saadony, Mohamed T., et al. 2024. "Garlic Bioactive Substances."

p. 47   *Fresh onion consumption has been associated with improving insulin sensitivity and fasting blood glucose*   Zhao, Xin-Xin, et al. 2021. "Recent Advances in Bioactive Compounds."

p. 47   *Human breast cancer cells treated with leek extract*   Xie, Tiantian, et al. 2023. "Functional Perspective of Leeks."

p. 47   Allium *vegetables can help protect us against metabolic syndrome*   Galavi, Amin, et al. 2021. "The Effects of Allium Cepa L. (Onion)."

p. 47   *people consuming 100 mg of raw crushed garlic twice a day for a month*   Ansary, Johura, et al. 2020. "Potential Health Benefit of Garlic."

p. 47   *onions and their bioactive compounds . . . act as powerful antioxidants*   Galavi, Amin, et al. 2021. "The Effects of Allium Cepa L. (Onion)."

p. 48   *overweight or obese women with knee osteoarthritis also experienced less pain*   Ansary, Johura, et al. 2020. "Potential Health Benefit of Garlic."

p. 48   *people with type 2 diabetes were able to reduce their blood glucose*   Ansary, Johura, et al. 2020. "Potential Health Benefit of Garlic."

p. 48   *garlic prevented pancreatic cell damage*   El-Saadony, Mohamed T., et al. 2024. "Garlic Bioactive Substances."

p. 48   *blood glucose levels declined in diabetic rats*   Zhao, Xin-Xin, et al. 2021. "Recent Advances in Bioactive Compounds."

p. 48   *garlic ethanol extract had an important neuroprotective effect*   El-Saadony, Mohamed T., et al. 2024. "Garlic Bioactive Substances."

p. 48   *neuroprotective effects of onion consumption against brain issues*   Zhao, Xin-Xin, et al. 2021. "Recent Advances in Bioactive Compounds."

p. 49   *sulforaphane can prevent cancer cells from growing and even kill them*   Mordecai, James, Saleem Ullah, and Irshad Ahmad. 2023. "Sulforaphane and Its Protective Role in Prostate Cancer: A Mechanistic Approach." *International Journal of Molecular Sciences* 24 (8): 6979. https://doi.org/10.3390/ijms24086979.

p. 49   *Sulforaphane . . . has an 80 percent bioavailability*   Wang, Xiang, Xinxin Chen, Wenqian Zhou, Hongbo Men, Terigen Bao, Yike Sun, Quanwei Wang, et al. 2022. "Ferroptosis Is Essential for Diabetic Cardiomyopathy and Is Prevented by Sulforaphane via AMPK/NRF2 Pathways." *Acta Pharmaceutica Sinica B* 12 (2): 708–22. https://doi.org/10.1016/j.apsb.2021.10.005.

p. 49   *It is 14 times more powerful*   Mordecai, James, et al. 2023. "Sulforaphane and Its Protective Role."

p. 50   *has a renal protective effect in kidney disease*   Liebman, Scott E., and Thu H. Le. 2021. "Eat Your Broccoli: Oxidative Stress, NRF2, and Sulforaphane in Chronic Kidney Disease." *Nutrients* 13 (1): 266. https://doi.org/10.3390/nu13010266.

p. 50   *helps regulate glucose in people with type 2 diabetes*   Mahn, Andrea, and Antonio Castillo. 2021. "Potential of Sulforaphane as a Natural Immune

System Enhancer: A Review." *Molecules* 26 (3): 752. https://doi.org/10.3390/molecules26030752.

p. 50   *Animal studies have also highlighted how this humble compound has the potential to lower uric acid*   Wang, Xiang, et al. 2022. "Ferroptosis Is Essential for Diabetic Cardiomyopathy."

p. 50   *sulforaphane may prolong overall lifespan*   Russo, Maria, Carmela Spagnuolo, Gian Luigi Russo, Krystyna Skalicka-Woźniak, Maria Daglia, Eduardo Sobarzo-Sánchez, Seyed Fazel Nabavi, and Seyed Mohammad Nabavi. 2018. "Nrf2 Targeting by Sulforaphane: A Potential Therapy for Cancer Treatment." *Critical Reviews in Food Science and Nutrition* 58 (8): 1391–1405. https://doi.org/10.1080/10408398.2016.1259983; Lewis, Kaitlyn N., James Mele, John D. Hayes, and Rochelle Buffenstein. 2010. "Nrf2, a Guardian of Healthspan and Gatekeeper of Species Longevity." *Integrative and Comparative Biology* 50 (5): 829–43. https://doi.org/10.1093/icb/icq034; Qi, Zhimin, Huihui Ji, Monika Le, Hanmei Li, Angela Wieland, Sonja Bauer, Li Liu, Michael Wink, and Ingrid Herr. 2021. "Sulforaphane Promotes C. Elegans Longevity and Healthspan via DAF-16/DAF-2 Insulin/IGF-1 Signaling." *Aging (Albany NY)* 13 (2): 1649–70. https://doi.org/10.18632/aging.202512; Otoo, Raymond A., and Antiño R. Allen. 2023. "Sulforaphane's Multifaceted Potential: From Neuroprotection to Anticancer Action." *Molecules* 28 (19): 6902. https://doi.org/10.3390/molecules28196902; Chen, Mangmang, Lipeng Huang, Yangxun Lv, Liubing Li, and Qirong Dong. 2021. "Sulforaphane Protects Against Oxidative Stress-Induced Apoptosis via Activating SIRT1 in Mouse Osteoarthritis." *Molecular Medicine Reports* 24 (2): 612. https://doi.org/10.3892/mmr.2021.12251.

p. 52   *most important longevity action of betanin is its ability to scavenge reactive oxygen species*   Chen, Mangmang, et al. 2021. "Sulforaphane Protects Against Oxidative Stress-Induced Apoptosis."

p. 52   *betanin can help reduce the risk of some cancers*   Baião, Diego dos S., Davi V. T. da Silva, and Vania M. F. Paschoalin. 2020. "Beetroot, a Remarkable Vegetable: Its Nitrate and Phytochemical Contents Can Be Adjusted in Novel Formulations to Benefit Health and Support Cardiovascular Disease Therapies." *Antioxidants* 9 (10): 960. https://doi.org/10.3390/antiox9100960.

p. 52   *giving betanin extract helped stop skin and lung tumors in mice*   Chen, Mangmang, et al. 2021. "Sulforaphane Protects Against Oxidative Stress-Induced Apoptosis." *Molecular Medicine Reports* 24 (2): 612.

p. 52   *when nitrate comes from food sources, it triggers the body to produce nitric oxide*   Milton-Laskibar, Iñaki, J. Alfredo Martínez, and María P. Portillo. 2021. "Current Knowledge on Beetroot Bioactive Compounds: Role of Nitrate and Betalains in Health and Disease." *Foods* 10 (6): 1314. https://doi.org/10.3390/foods10061314.

p. 52   *Ascorbic acid has also been shown to regulate collagen synthesis*   Baião, Diego dos S., et al. 2020. "Beetroot, a Remarkable Vegetable."

p. 53   *beetroot nitrate can lead to improved blood flow and decreased blood pressure*   Chen, Mangmang, et al. 2021. "Sulforaphane Protects Against Oxidative Stress-Induced Apoptosis"; Milton-Laskibar, Iñaki, et al. 2021. "Current Knowledge on Beetroot."

p. 53   *betanin in beets has an antidiabetic role*   Baião, Diego dos S., et al. 2020. "Beetroot, a Remarkable Vegetable."

p. 53   *beets have the potential to keep your organs healthier*   Baião, Diego dos S., et al. 2020."Beetroot, a Remarkable Vegetable."

p. 53   *beet juice increased enzyme activity and prevented systemic liver damage*   Chen, Liping, Yuankang Zhu, Zijing Hu, Shengjie Wu, and Chengtao Jin. 2021. "Beetroot as a Functional Food with Huge Health Benefits: Antioxidant, Antitumor, Physical Function, and Chronic Metabolomics Activity." *Food Science & Nutrition* 9 (11): 6406–20. https://doi.org/10.1002/fsn3.2577.

p. 53   *in a clinical study with nonsmoking adults diagnosed with coronary artery disease*   Milton-Laskibar, Iñaki, et al. 2021. "Current Knowledge on Beetroot."

p. 53   *one wide-ranging review of studies supporting the impact of beet consumption on cognitive health*   Chen, Liping, et al. 2021. "Beetroot as a Functional Food."

p. 54   *Seaweed has a long history of serving not only as human food, but as medicine*   Lopez-Santamarina, Aroa, Jose Manuel Miranda, Alicia del Carmen Mondragon, Alexandre Lamas, Alejandra Cardelle-Cobas, Carlos Manuel Franco, and Alberto Cepeda. 2020. "Potential Use of Marine Seaweeds as Prebiotics: A Review." *Molecules* 25 (4): 1004. https://doi.org/10.3390/molecules25041004.

p. 54   *There are about 25,000 different species of seaweed . . . about three-quarters of their biomass*   Zang, Liqing, Maedeh Baharlooeian, Masahiro Terasawa, Yasuhito Shimada, and Norihiro Nishimura. 2023. "Beneficial Effects of Seaweed-Derived Components on Metabolic Syndrome via Gut Microbiota Modulation." *Frontiers in Nutrition* 10: 1173225. https://doi.org/10.3389/fnut.2023.1173225.

p. 54   *nutritional foods rich in dietary fiber, minerals, protein, and vitamins*   Guerrero-Wyss, Marion, Caroline Yans, Arturo Boscán-González, Pablo Duran, Solange Parra-Soto, and Lissé Angarita. 2023. "Durvillaea Antarctica: A Seaweed for Enhancing Immune and Cardiometabolic Health and Gut Microbiota Composition Modulation." *International Journal of Molecular Sciences* 24 (13): 10779. https://doi.org/10.3390/ijms241310779.

p. 54   *potential of seaweed polysaccharides to have therapeutic effects on the metastasis of various cancers*   Liu, Tingting, Qing Li, Xu Xu, Guoxia Li, Chengwang Tian, and Tiejun Zhang. 2022. "Molecular Mechanisms of Anti-Cancer Bioactivities of Seaweed Polysaccharides." *Chinese Herbal Medicines* 14 (4): 528–34. https://doi.org/10.1016/j.chmed.2022.02.003.

p. 55   *polysaccharides in seaweeds may have powerful antiviral potential* Jabeen, Mehwish, Mélody Dutot, Roxane Fagon, Bernard Verrier, and Claire Monge. 2021. "Seaweed Sulfated Polysaccharides Against Respiratory Viral Infections." *Pharmaceutics* 13 (5): 733. https://doi.org/10.3390/pharmaceutics13050733.

p. 55   *polyphenols and proteins from all seaweed varieties are being widely studied* Tanna, Bhakti, Sonam Yadav, Manish Kumar Patel, and Avinash Mishra. 2024. "Metabolite Profiling, Biological and Molecular Analyses Validate the Nutraceutical Potential of Green Seaweed Acrosiphonia Orientalis for Human Health." *Nutrients* 16 (8): 1222. https://doi.org/10.3390/nu16081222.

p. 55   *scientists are especially focused on extracting and studying* fucoidans Liu, Ting-Ting, et al. 2022. "Molecular Mechanisms of Anti-Cancer Bioactivities."

p. 55   *brown seaweed is a great source of omega-3 polyunsaturated fatty acids* Zang, Liqing, et al. 2023. "Beneficial Effects of Seaweed."

p. 55   *potential therapeutic effects of rhamnan sulfate in green algae* Zang, Liqing, et al. 2023. "Beneficial Effects of Seaweed."

p. 56   *polysaccharides in algae have wonderful potential as therapeutic agents for treating IBD* Liyanage, N. M., D. P. Nagahawatta, Thilina U. Jayawardena, and You-Jin Jeon. 2023. "The Role of Seaweed Polysaccharides in Gastrointestinal Health: Protective Effect against Inflammatory Bowel Disease." *Life* 13 (4): 1026. https://doi.org/10.3390/life13041026. ·

p. 56   *nutrients in seaweed . . . have the potential to act as prebiotics* Guerrero-Wyss, Marion, et al. 2023. "Durvillaea Antarctica."

p. 57   *Methylation patterns can change as we age, and this contributes* Wang, Kang, Huicong Liu, Qinchao Hu, Lingna Wang, Jiaqing Liu, Zikai Zheng, Weiqi Zhang, Jie Ren, Fangfang Zhu, and Guang-Hui Liu. 2022. "Epigenetic Regulation of Aging: Implications for Interventions of Aging and Diseases." *Signal Transduction and Targeted Therapy* 7 (1): 374. https://doi.org/10.1038/s41392 -022-01211-8.

p. 57   *it has been associated with an increased risk of some forms of cancer* Pieroth, Renee, Stephanie Paver, Sharon Day, and Carolyn Lammersfeld. 2018. "Folate and Its Impact on Cancer Risk." *Current Nutrition Reports* 7 (3): 70–84. https://doi .org/10.1007/s13668-018-0237-y.

p. 57   *Oxalate can cause several health problems* Ermer, Theresa, Lama Nazzal, Maria Clarissa Tio, Sushrut Waikar, Peter S. Aronson, and Felix Knauf. 2023. "Oxalate Homeostasis." *Nature Reviews Nephrology* 19 (2): 123–38. https://doi.org /10.1038/s41581-022-00643-3.

p. 57   *What may be more important here is our magnesium-to-calcium ratio* Takasaki, E. 1972. "The Magnesium:Calcium Ratio in the Concentrated Urines of Patients with Calcium Oxalate Calculi." *Investigative Urology* 10 (2): 147–50; Rattan, V., S. K. Thind, R. K. Jethi, and R. Nath. 1993. "Intestinal Absorption of Calcium and Oxalate in Magnesium-Deficient Rats." *Magnesium Research*

6 (1): 3–10; Zimmermann, Diana J., Susanne Voss, Gerd E. von Unruh, and Albrecht Hesse. 2005. "Importance of Magnesium in Absorption and Excretion of Oxalate." *Urologia Internationalis* 74 (3): 262–67. https://doi.org/10 .1159/000083560; Ogawa, Yoshihide, Kazumi Yamaguchi, and Makoto Morozumi. 1990. "Effects of Magnesium Salts in Preventing Experimental Oxalate Urolithiasis in Rats." *The Journal of Urology* 144 (2): 385–89. https:// doi.org/10.1016/s0022-5347(17)39466-1.

p. 59   *Antinutrients can exert their negative influence via several mechanisms*   López-Moreno, M., M. Garcés-Rimón, and M. Miguel. 2022. "Antinutrients: Lectins, Goitrogens, Phytates and Oxalates, Friends or Foe?" *Journal of Functional Foods* 89: 104938. https://doi.org/10.1016/j.jff.2022.104938; Petroski, Weston, and Deanna M. Minich. 2020. "Is There Such a Thing as 'Anti-Nutrients'? A Narrative Review of Perceived Problematic Plant Compounds." *Nutrients* 12 (10): 2929. https://doi.org/10.3390/nu12102929.

p. 59   *The prevalence of autoimmune diseases has increased significantly*   Miller, Frederick W. 2023. "The Increasing Prevalence of Autoimmunity and Autoimmune Diseases: An Urgent Call to Action for Improved Understanding, Diagnosis, Treatment, and Prevention." *Current Opinion in Immunology* 80: 102266. https://doi.org/10.1016/j.coi.2022.102266.

p. 60   *the flip side is that these antinutrients can be beneficial for some people*   López-Moreno, M., et al. 2022. "Antinutrients."

Chapter 5

p. 62   *a diet rich in fruit can protect us*   Figueira, José A., Priscilla Porto-Figueira, Cristina Berenguer, Jorge A. M. Pereira, and José S. Câmara. 2021. "Evaluation of the Health-Promoting Properties of Selected Fruits." *Molecules* 26 (14): 4202. https://doi.org/10.3390/molecules26144202.

p. 62   *in one recent cross-sectional study involving 1,346 participants*   Bouayed, Jaouad, and Farhad Vahid. 2024. "Carotenoid Pattern Intake and Relation to Metabolic Status, Risk and Syndrome, and Its Components—Divergent Findings from the ORISCAV-LUX-2 Survey." *British Journal of Nutrition*, 1–17. https:// doi.org/10.1017/s0007114524000758.

p. 63   *greater consumption of fruit and vegetables is linked to a lower risk of chronic diseases*   Blumfield, Michelle, Hannah Mayr, Nienke De Vlieger, Kylie Abbott, Carlene Starck, Flavia Fayet-Moore, and Skye Marshall. 2022. "Should We 'Eat a Rainbow'? An Umbrella Review of the Health Effects of Colorful Bioactive Pigments in Fruits and Vegetables." *Molecules* 27 (13): 4061. https://doi .org/10.3390/molecules27134061.

p. 63   *a 2024 Chinese study of 13,738 adults*   Li, Huiqi, Li-Ting Sheng, Aizhen Jin, An Pan, and Woon-Puay Koh. 2024. "Association Between Consumption of

Fruits and Vegetables in Midlife and Depressive Symptoms in Late Life: The Singapore Chinese Health Study." *The Journal of Nutrition, Health and Aging* 28 (6): 100275. https://doi.org/10.1016/j.jnha.2024.100275.

p. 63 *About 78 percent of adults around the world suffer a nutrient gap* Blumfield, Michelle, et al. 2022. "Should We 'Eat a Rainbow'?"

p. 64 *In a 2022 meta-analysis published in* Molecules Blumfield, Michelle, et al. 2022. "Should We 'Eat a Rainbow'?"

p. 64 *researchers have focused on anthocyanins' health benefits and longevity properties* Bolling, Bradley W. 2023. "Anthocyanins and Health: Are Fruit and Vegetable Dietary Recommendations Outdated in the Context of Ultraprocessed Foods?" *Nutrition Research* 115: 61–62. https://doi.org/10.1016/j.nutres .2023.05.013; Mattioli, Roberto, Antonio Francioso, Luciana Mosca, and Paula Silva. 2020. "Anthocyanins: A Comprehensive Review of Their Chemical Properties and Health Effects on Cardiovascular and Neurodegenerative Diseases." *Molecules* 25 (17): 3809. https://doi.org/10.3390/molecules25173809; Cerletti, Chiara, Amalia De Curtis, Francesca Bracone, Cinzia Digesù, Alessio G. Morganti, Licia Iacoviello, Giovanni de Gaetano, and Maria Benedetta Donati. 2017. "Dietary Anthocyanins and Health: Data from FLORA and ATHENA EU Projects." *British Journal of Clinical Pharmacology* 83 (1): 103–6. https://doi.org/10.1111/bcp.12943; DiNicolantonio, James J., Mark F. McCarty, Simon Iloki Assanga, Lidianys Lewis Lujan, and James H. O'Keefe. 2022. "Ferulic Acid and Berberine, via Sirt1 and AMPK, May Act as Cell Cleansing Promoters of Healthy Longevity." *Open Heart* 9 (1): e001801. https://doi.org /10.1136/openhrt-2021-001801; Li, Daotong, Pengpu Wang, Yinghua Luo, Mengyao Zhao, and Fang Chen. 2017. "Health Benefits of Anthocyanins and Molecular Mechanisms: Update from Recent Decade." *Critical Reviews in Food Science and Nutrition* 57 (8): 1729–41. https://doi.org/10.1080/10408398 .2015.1030064.

p. 64 *Anthocyanins have also been attributed to reducing obesity-induced inflammation* Ngamsamer, Chanya, Jintana Sirivarasai, and Nareerat Sutjarit. 2022. "The Benefits of Anthocyanins Against Obesity-Induced Inflammation." *Biomolecules* 12 (6): 852. https://doi.org/10.3390/biom12060852.

p. 65 *a diet including fruits is associated with a reduced risk of cardiovascular disease* Kelly, Rebecca K., Tammy Y. N. Tong, Cody Z. Watling, Andrew Reynolds, Carmen Piernas, Julie A. Schmidt, Keren Papier, Jennifer L. Carter, Timothy J. Key, and Aurora Perez-Cornago. 2023. "Associations Between Types and Sources of Dietary Carbohydrates and Cardiovascular Disease Risk: A Prospective Cohort Study of UK Biobank Participants." *BMC Medicine* 21 (1): 34. https://doi.org/10.1186/s12916-022-02712-7.

p. 66 *Fruit and Sugar Content [table]* USDA. "FoodData Central Food Search." Accessed October 2024. https://fdc.nal.usda.gov/food-search.

p. 70   *one 2021 study . . . demonstrated that giving the animals coconut water* Dai, Yanan, Li Peng, Xiaohua Zhang, Qingjing Wu, Jie Yao, Qiu Xing, Yunyan Zheng, Xiaobo Huang, Shaomei Chen, and Qing Xie. 2021. "Effects of Coconut Water on Blood Sugar and Retina of Rats with Diabetes." *PeerJ* 9: e10667. https://doi.org/10.7717/peerj.10667.

p. 70   *Scientists are also examining the potential of coconut water to lower blood pressure* Hewlings, Susan. 2020. "Coconuts and Health: Different Chain Lengths of Saturated Fats Require Different Consideration." *Journal of Cardiovascular Development and Disease* 7 (4): 59. https://doi.org/10.3390/jcdd7040059.

p. 73   *this may provide important protection against Alzheimer's disease* Sandupama, Poorni, Dilusha Munasinghe, and Madhura Jayasinghe. 2022. "Coconut Oil as a Therapeutic Treatment for Alzheimer's Disease: A Review." *Journal of Future Foods* 2 (1): 41–52. https://www.sciencedirect.com/science/article/pii/S2772566922000295.

p. 74   *Alzheimer's is also characterized by insulin insensitivity in the brain* Janoutová, Jana, Ondřej Machaczka, Anna Zatloukalová, and Vladimír Janout. 2022. "Is Alzheimer's Disease a Type 3 Diabetes? A Review." *Central European Journal of Public Health* 30 (3): 139–43. https://doi.org/10.21101/cejph.a7238.

p. 74   *a multifactorial approach to Alzheimer's that includes diet, exercise, and reducing stress* Toups, Kat, Ann Hathaway, Deborah Gordon, Henrianna Chung, Cyrus Raji, Alan Boyd, Benjamin D. Hill, et al. 2022. "Precision Medicine Approach to Alzheimer's Disease: Successful Pilot Project." *Journal of Alzheimer's Disease* 88 (4): 1411–21. https://doi.org/10.3233/jad-215707; Rao, Rammohan V., Kaavya G. Subramaniam, Julie Gregory, Aida L. Bredesen, Christine Coward, Sho Okada, Lance Kelly, and Dale E. Bredesen. 2023. "Rationale for a Multi-Factorial Approach for the Reversal of Cognitive Decline in Alzheimer's Disease and MCI: A Review." *International Journal of Molecular Sciences* 24 (2): 1659. https://doi.org/10.3390/ijms24021659; Bredesen, Dale E., Edwin C. Amos, Jonathan Canick, Mary Ackerley, Cyrus Raji, Milan Fiala, and Jamila Ahdidan. 2016. "Reversal of Cognitive Decline in Alzheimer's Disease." *Aging (Albany NY)* 8 (6): 1250–58. https://doi.org/10.18632/aging.100981.

p. 75   *In one small pilot study with 44 people* Klimova, Blanka, Michal Novotny, Petr Schlegel, and Martin Valis. 2021. "The Effect of Mediterranean Diet on Cognitive Functions in the Elderly Population." *Nutrients* 13 (6): 2067. https://doi.org/10.3390/nu13062067.

p. 75   *in another Sri Lankan study* Fernando, Malika G., Renuka Silva, W. M. A. D. Binosha Fernando, H. Asita de Silva, A. Rajitha Wickremasinghe, Asoka S. Dissanayake, Hamid R. Sohrabi, Ralph N. Martins, and Shehan S. Williams. 2023. "Effect of Virgin Coconut Oil Supplementation on Cognition of Individuals with Mild-to-Moderate Alzheimer's Disease in Sri Lanka (VCO-AD Study): A Randomized Placebo-Controlled Trial." *Journal of Alzheimer's Disease* 96 (3): 1195–206. https://doi.org/10.3233/jad-230670.

p. 76   *various studies demonstrating that avocado intake may help improve glucose/insulin homeostasis*   Senn, MacKenzie K., Mark O. Goodarzi, Gautam Ramesh, Matthew A. Allison, Mariaelisa Graff, Kristin L. Young, Gregory A. Talavera, et al. 2023. "Associations Between Avocado Intake and Measures of Glucose and Insulin Homeostasis in Hispanic Individuals with and without Type 2 Diabetes: Results from the Hispanic Community Health Study/Study of Latinos (HCHS/SOL)." *Nutrition, Metabolism and Cardiovascular Diseases* 33 (12): 2428–39. https://doi.org/10.1016/j.numecd.2023.08.002.

p. 76   *another 2022 comprehensive meta-analysis and systematic review*   James-Martin, Genevieve, Paige G. Brooker, Gilly A. Hendrie, and Welma Stonehouse. 2024. "Avocado Consumption and Cardiometabolic Health: A Systematic Review and Meta-Analysis." *Journal of the Academy of Nutrition and Dietetics* 124 (2): 233-248.e4. https://doi.org/10.1016/j.jand.2022.12.008.

p. 76   *For one 2021 study, researchers surveyed 2,886 adults*   Cheng, Feon W., Nikki A. Ford, and Matthew K. Taylor. 2021. "US Older Adults That Consume Avocado or Guacamole Have Better Cognition Than Non-Consumers: National Health and Nutrition Examination Survey 2011–2014." *Frontiers in Nutrition* 8: 746453. https://doi.org/10.3389/fnut.2021.746453.

p. 77   *green bananas helped correct testicular dysfunction in diabetic rats*   Apostolopoulos, Vasso, Juliana Antonipillai, Kathy Tangalakis, John F. Ashton, and Lily Stojanovska. 2017. "Let's Go Bananas! Green Bananas and Their Health Benefits." *PRILOZI* 38 (2): 147–51. https://doi.org/10.1515/prilozi-2017-0033.

p. 77   *berry consumption was associated with a 10 to 17 percent decreased risk of short sleep*   Zhang, Li, Joshua E. Muscat, Penny M. Kris-Etherton, Vernon M. Chinchilli, Julio Fernandez-Mendoza, Laila Al-Shaar, and John P. Richie. 2023. "Berry Consumption and Sleep in the Adult US General Population: Results from the National Health and Nutrition Examination Survey 2005–2018." *Nutrients* 15 (24): 5115. https://doi.org/10.3390/nu15245115.

p. 78   *black raspberries and strawberries exhibit anticancer effects against esophageal cancer*   Shi, Ni, and Tong Chen. 2022. "Chemopreventive Properties of Black Raspberries and Strawberries in Esophageal Cancer Review." *Antioxidants* 11 (9): 1815. https://doi.org/10.3390/antiox11091815.

p. 78   *dietary flavonoids . . . have been associated with a decrease in subjective cognitive decline*   Yeh, Tian-Shin, Changzheng Yuan, Alberto Ascherio, Bernard A. Rosner, Walter C. Willett, and Deborah Blacker. 2021. "Long-Term Dietary Flavonoid Intake and Subjective Cognitive Decline in US Men and Women." *Neurology* 97 (10): e1041–56. https://doi.org/10.1212/wnl.0000000000012454.

p. 78 *the Clery strawberry, has been shown to have anti-candida activity* Cairone, Francesco, Giovanna Simonetti, Anastasia Orekhova, Maria Antonietta Casadei, Gokhan Zengin, and Stefania Cesa. 2021. "Health Potential of Clery Strawberries: Enzymatic Inhibition and Anti-Candida Activity Evaluation." *Molecules* 26 (6): 1731. https://doi.org/10.3390/molecules26061731.

p. 78 *Another dietary antioxidant, fisetin . . . has attracted interest in preventing cancer* Qaed, Eskandar, Bandar Al-Hamyari, Ahmed Al-Maamari, Abdullah Qaid, Haneen Alademy, Marwan Almoiliqy, Jean Claude Munyemana, et al. 2023. "Fisetin's Promising Antitumor Effects: Uncovering Mechanisms and Targeting for Future Therapies." *Global Medical Genetics* 10 (03): 205–20. https://doi.org/10.1055/s-0043-1772219.

p. 78 *Fisetin has also been shown to activate sirtuins* Zhou, Qing, Chao Zhu, Anwu Xuan, Junyou Zhang, Zhenbiao Zhu, Liang Tang, and Dike Ruan. 2023. "Fisetin Regulates the Biological Effects of Rat Nucleus Pulposus Mesenchymal Stem Cells Under Oxidative Stress by Sirtuin-1 Pathway." *Immunity, Inflammation and Disease* 11 (5): e865. https://doi.org/10.1002/iid3.865; Wang, Xuezhong, Xuyang Li, Jianlin Zhou, Zheng Lei, and Xiaoming Yang. 2024. "Fisetin Suppresses Chondrocyte Senescence and Attenuates Osteoarthritis Progression by Targeting Sirtuin 6." *Chemico-Biological Interactions* 390: 110890. https://doi.org/10.1016/j.cbi.2024.110890.

p. 79 *the procyanidin and polyphenol content of coffee fruit can protect your brain* Grabska-Kobyłecka, Izabela, Piotr Szpakowski, Aleksandra Król, Dominika Książek-Winiarek, Andrzej Kobyłecki, Andrzej Głąbiński, and Dariusz Nowak. 2023. "Polyphenols and Their Impact on the Prevention of Neurodegenerative Diseases and Development." *Nutrients* 15 (15): 3454. https://doi.org/10.3390/nu15153454; Ruan, Wenli, Shuoheng Shen, Yang Xu, Na Ran, and Heng Zhang. 2021. "Mechanistic Insights into Procyanidins as Therapies for Alzheimer's Disease: A Review." *Journal of Functional Foods* 86: 104683. https://doi.org/10.1016/j.jff.2021.104683.

p. 80 *"Pomegranates: A Nutritional and Medicinal Powerhouse."* Vibha, Maheshwari, Rajawat Anjay Kumar, and Parashar Amit. 2024. "Pomegranates: A Nutritional and Medicinal Powerhouse." *International Journal of Scientific Research and Engineering Trends.* https://ijsret.com/wp-content/uploads/2024/03/IJSRET_V10_issue2_197.pdf.

p. 80 *a wide variety of studies with people who have type 2 diabetes demonstrate that pomegranates can* Silva, Vanessa, Adriana Silva, Jessica Ribeiro, Alfredo Aires, Rosa Carvalho, Joana S. Amaral, Lillian Barros, Gilberto Igrejas, and Patrícia Poeta. 2023. "Screening of Chemical Composition, Antimicrobial and Antioxidant Activities in Pomegranate, Quince, and Persimmon Leaf, Peel, and Seed: Valorization of Autumn Fruits By-Products for a One Health Perspective."

Antibiotics 12 (7): 1086. https://doi.org/10.3390/antibiotics12071086; Kandylis, Panagiotis, and Evangelos Kokkinomagoulos. 2020. "Food Applications and Potential Health Benefits of Pomegranate and Its Derivatives." *Foods.* https://doi.org/10.3390/foods9020122.

Chapter 6

p. 83   *dental calculus found on the Red Lady's teeth showed that she had eaten mushrooms* Straus, Lawrence G., Manuel R. González Morales, Jose Miguel Carretero, and Ana Belen Marín-Arroyo. 2015. "'The Red Lady of El Mirón'. Lower Magdalenian Life and Death in Oldest Dryas Cantabrian Spain: An Overview." *Journal of Archaeological Science* 60: 134–37. https://doi.org/10.1016/j.jas.2015.02.034.

p. 84   *Scientists have been studying the carbohydrates derived from mushrooms* Kumar, Krishan, Rahul Mehra, Raquel P. F. Guiné, Maria João Lima, Naveen Kumar, Ravinder Kaushik, Naseer Ahmed, Ajar Nath Yadav, and Harish Kumar. 2021. "Edible Mushrooms: A Comprehensive Review on Bioactive Compounds with Health Benefits and Processing Aspects." *Foods* 10 (12): 2996. https://doi.org/10.3390/foods10122996.

p. 84   *mushroom lectins . . . can bind to cell surface carbohydrates and act as antitumor warriors* Singh, Ram Sarup, Amandeep Kaur Walia, and John F. Kennedy. 2020. "Mushroom Lectins in Biomedical Research and Development." *International Journal of Biological Macromolecules* 151: 1340–50. https://doi.org/10.1016/j.ijbiomac.2019.10.180.

p. 84   *ergosterol, which has demonstrated antimicrobial, antioxidant, anticancer, antidiabetic, and antineurodegenerative effects* Rangsinth, Panthakarn, Rajasekharan Sharika, Nattaporn Pattarachotanant, Chatrawee Duangjan, Chamaiphron Wongwan, Chanin Sillapachaiyaporn, Sunita Nilkhet, et al. 2023. "Potential Beneficial Effects and Pharmacological Properties of Ergosterol, a Common Bioactive Compound in Edible Mushrooms." *Foods* 12 (13): 2529. https://doi.org/10.3390/foods12132529.

p. 85   *Mushrooms Improve Lipid Profiles* Kumar, Kirshan, et al. 2021. "Edible Mushrooms."

p. 85   *Mushrooms Decrease Cancer Risk* Ba, Djibril M., Paddy Ssentongo, Robert B. Beelman, Joshua Muscat, Xiang Gao, and John P. Richie. 2021. "Higher Mushroom Consumption Is Associated with Lower Risk of Cancer: A Systematic Review and Meta-Analysis of Observational Studies." *Advances in Nutrition* 12 (5): 1691–704. https://doi.org/10.1093/advances/nmab015.

p. 86   *Mushrooms Support a Healthier Immune System* Case, Sarah, Tara O'Brien, Anna E. Ledwith, Shilong Chen, Cian J.H. Horneck Johnson, Emer E.

Hackett, Michele O'Sullivan, et al. 2024. "β-Glucans from Agaricus Bisporus Mushroom Products Drive Trained Immunity." *Frontiers in Nutrition* 11. https://doi.org/10.3389/fnut.2024.1346706.

p. 86   *Mushrooms Protect Brain Health*   Yang, Yun, Danni Zhu, Ran Qi, Yanchun Chen, Baihe Sheng, and Xinyu Zhang. 2024. "Association Between Intake of Edible Mushrooms and Algae and the Risk of Cognitive Impairment in Chinese Older Adults." *Nutrients.* https://doi.org/10.3390/nu16050637; Apparoo, Yasaaswini, Chia Wei Phan, Umah Rani Kuppusamy, and Eric Wei Chiang Chan. 2024. "Potential Role of Ergothioneine Rich Mushroom as Anti-Aging Candidate Through Elimination of Neuronal Senescent Cells." *Brain Research* 1824: 148693. https://doi.org/10.1016/j.brainres.2023.148693.

p. 86   *Two of the most powerful nutrients in mushrooms*   Samuel, Priscilla, Menelaos Tsapekos, Nuria de Pedro, Ann G. Liu, J. Casey Lippmeier, and Steven Chen. 2022. "Ergothioneine Mitigates Telomere Shortening Under Oxidative Stress Conditions." *Journal of Dietary Supplements* 19 (2): 212–25. https://doi.org/10.1080/19390211.2020.1854919; Kalaras, Michael D., John P. Richie, Ana Calcagnotto, and Robert B. Beelman. 2017. "Mushrooms: A Rich Source of the Antioxidants Ergothioneine and Glutathione." *Food Chemistry* 233: 429–33. https://doi.org/10.1016/j.foodchem.2017.04.109.

p. 87   *It also plays a key role in preventing the potentially damaging shortening of telomeres*   Samuel, Priscilla, et al. 2022. "Ergothioneine Mitigates Telomere Shortening."

p. 87   *ergothioneine is known as the longevity vitamin in some research circles*   Roda, Elisa, Daniela Ratto, Fabrizio De Luca, Anthea Desiderio, Martino Ramieri, Lorenzo Goppa, Elena Savino, Maria Grazia Bottone, Carlo Alessandro Locatelli, and Paola Rossi. 2022. "Searching for a Longevity Food, We Bump into Hericium Erinaceus Primordium Rich in Ergothioneine: The 'Longevity Vitamin' Improves Locomotor Performances During Aging." *Nutrients* 14 (6): 1177. https://doi.org/10.3390/nu14061177; Apparoo, Yasaaswini, et al. 2024. "Potential Role of Ergothioneine."

p. 87   *senescent cells are those that . . . don't die off when they should, potentially causing damage*   Pucci, Bruna, Margaret Kasten, and Antonio Giordano. 2000. "Cell Cycle and Apoptosis." *Neoplasia* 2 (4): 291–99. https://doi.org/10.1038/sj.neo.7900101; Childs, Bennett G., Darren J. Baker, James L. Kirkland, Judith Campisi, and Jan M. van Deursen. 2014. "Senescence and Apoptosis: Dueling or Complementary Cell Fates?" *EMBO Reports* 15 (11): 1139–53. https://doi.org/10.15252/embr.201439245.

p. 87   *Emerging research demonstrates that glutathione promotes*   Al-Temimi, Anfal Alwan, Aum-El-Bashar Al-Mossawi, Sawsan A. Al-Hilifi, Sameh A. Korma, Tuba Esatbeyoglu, João Miguel Rocha, and Vipul Agarwal. 2023. "Glutathione for Food and Health Applications with Emphasis on Extraction,

Identification, and Quantification Methods: A Review." *Metabolites* 13 (4): 465. https://doi.org/10.3390/metabo13040465.

p. 87   *In one particularly exciting animal study*   Kumar, P., O. W. Osahon, and R. V. Sekhar. 2023. "GlyNAC (Glycine and N-Acetylcysteine) Supplementation in Old Mice Improves Brain Glutathione Deficiency, Oxidative Stress, Glucose Uptake, Mitochondrial Dysfunction, Genomic Damage, Inflammation and Neurotrophic Factors to Reverse Age-Associated Cognitive Decline: Implications for Improving Brain Health in Aging." *Antioxidants (Basel)* 12 (5): 1042. https://doi.org/10.3390/antiox12051042.

p. 87   *Scientists are now studying the benefits of glutathione supplements*   Dludla, P. V., K. Ziqubu, S. E. Mabhida, S. E. Mazibuko-Mbeje, S. Hanser, B. B. Nkambule, A. K. Basson, C. Pheiffer, L. Tiano, and A. P. Kengne. 2023. "Dietary Supplements Potentially Target Plasma Glutathione Levels to Improve Cardiometabolic Health in Patients with Diabetes Mellitus: A Systematic Review of Randomized Clinical Trials." *Nutrients* 15 (4): 944. https://doi.org/10.3390/nu15040944.

p. 89   *a skin rash called "shiitake dermatitis"*   Boels, D., A. Landreau, C. Bruneau, R. Garnier, C. Pulce, M. Labadie, L. de Haro, and P. Harry. 2014. "Shiitake Dermatitis Recorded by French Poison Control Centers—New Case Series with Clinical Observations." *Clinical Toxicology* 52 (6): 625–28. https://doi.org/10.3109/15563650.2014.923905; Corazza, M., S. Zauli, M. Ricci, A. Borghi, M. Pedriali, L. Mantovani, and A. Virgili. 2015. "Shiitake Dermatitis: Toxic or Allergic Reaction?" *Journal of the European Academy of Dermatology and Venereology* 29 (7): 1449–51. https://doi.org/10.1111/jdv.12505.

p. 89   *contain a biotin-binding avidin-like protein*   Takakura, Yoshimitsu, Kozue Sofuku, Masako Tsunashima, and Shigeru Kuwata. 2016. "Lentiavidins: Novel Avidin-like Proteins with Low Isoelectric Points from Shiitake Mushroom (Lentinula Edodes)." *Journal of Bioscience and Bioengineering* 121 (4): 420–23. https://doi.org/10.1016/j.jbiosc.2015.09.003.

p. 90   *potential for mushroom poisoning and even myocardial infarction*   Leonard, James B., Bruce Anderson, and Wendy Klein-Schwartz. 2018. "Does Getting High Hurt? Characterization of Cases of LSD and Psilocybin-Containing Mushroom Exposures to National Poison Centers Between 2000 and 2016." *Journal of Psychopharmacology* 32 (12): 1286–94. https://doi.org/10.1177/0269881118793086; Borowiak, Krzysztof S., Kazimierz Ciechanowski, and Piotr Waloszczyk. 1998. "Psilocybin Mushroom (Psilocybe Semilanceata) Intoxication with Myocardial Infarction." *Journal of Toxicology: Clinical Toxicology* 36 (1–2): 47–49. https://doi.org/10.3109/15563659809162584.

p. 91   *It has been associated with various inflammatory conditions*   Talapko, Jasminka, Martina Juzbašić, Tatjana Matijević, Emina Pustijanac, Sanja Bekić, Ivan Kotris, and Ivana Škrlec. 2021. "Candida Albicans—The Virulence Factors and Clinical Manifestations of Infection." *Journal of Fungi* 7 (2): 79. https://doi.org/10.3390/jof7020079.

p. 91 Candida albicans *has been linked to poor aging* Parambath, Sarika, Aiken Dao, Hannah Yejin Kim, Shukry Zawahir, Ana Alastruey Izquierdo, Evelina Tacconelli, Nelesh Govender, et al. 2024. "Candida Albicans—A Systematic Review to Inform the World Health Organization Fungal Priority Pathogens List." *Medical Mycology* 62 (6): myae045. https://doi.org/10.1093/mmy/myae045.

p. 91 *A recent review of candida provided several suggestions, including eating* diallyl disulfides *(DADS)* Hu, Wanchao, Liou Huang, Ziyang Zhou, Liping Yin, and Jianguo Tang. 2022. "Diallyl Disulfide (DADS) Ameliorates Intestinal Candida Albicans Infection by Modulating the Gut Microbiota and Metabolites and Providing Intestinal Protection in Mice." *Frontiers in Cellular and Infection Microbiology* 11: 743454. https://doi.org/10.3389/fcimb.2021.743454.

p. 91 *Taking* Trachyspermom ammi *and* tryptophan *can also help* Peng, Ziyao, Jiali Zhang, Meng Zhang, Liping Yin, Ziyang Zhou, Cuiting Lv, Zetian Wang, and Jianguo Tang. 2024. "Tryptophan Metabolites Relieve Intestinal Candida Albicans Infection by Altering the Gut Microbiota to Reduce IL-22 Release from Group 3 Innate Lymphoid Cells of the Colon Lamina Propria." *Food & Function*. https://doi.org/10.1039/d4fo00432a.

Chapter 7

p. 96 *"spices and herbs are the treasure house of useful bioactive compounds"* Singh, Neetu, and Surender Singh Yadav. 2022. "A Review on Health Benefits of Phenolics Derived from Dietary Spices." *Current Research in Food Science* 5: 1508–23. https://doi.org/10.1016/j.crfs.2022.09.009.

p. 96 *Many researchers are now looking at the value of phytochemicals* Kumar, Ashwani, Nirmal P, Mukul Kumar, Anina Jose, Vidisha Tomer, Emel Oz, Charalampos Proestos, et al. 2023. "Major Phytochemicals: Recent Advances in Health Benefits and Extraction Method." *Molecules* 28 (2): 887. https://doi.org/10.3390/molecules28020887; Guan, Ruirui, Quyet Van Le, Han Yang, Dangquan Zhang, Haiping Gu, Yafeng Yang, Christian Sonne, et al. 2021. "A Review of Dietary Phytochemicals and Their Relation to Oxidative Stress and Human Diseases." *Chemosphere* 271: 129499. https://doi.org/10.1016/j.chemosphere.2020.129499.

p. 97 *many of them are rich in polyphenols* Singh, Neetu, and Surender Singh Yadav. 2022. "A Review on Health Benefits of Phenolics."

p. 97 *diabetes and oxidative stress are inextricably connected* Yaribeygi, Habib, Thozhukat Sathyapalan, Stephen L. Atkin, and Amirhossein Sahebkar. 2020. "Molecular Mechanisms Linking Oxidative Stress and Diabetes

Mellitus." *Oxidative Medicine and Cellular Longevity* 2020: 8609213. https://doi.org/10.1155/2020/8609213; Darenskaya, M. A., L. I. Kolesnikova, and S. I. Kolesnikov. 2021. "Oxidative Stress: Pathogenetic Role in Diabetes Mellitus and Its Complications and Therapeutic Approaches to Correction." *Bulletin of Experimental Biology and Medicine* 171 (2): 179–89. https://doi.org/10.1007/s10517-021-05191-7.

p. 97   *adding herbs and spices to a balanced, diverse diet supported better immune responses*   Isbill, Jonathan, Jayanthi Kandiah, and Natalie Kružliaková. 2020. "Opportunities for Health Promotion: Highlighting Herbs and Spices to Improve Immune Support and Well-Being." *Integrative Medicine (Encinitas, Calif.)* 19 (5): 30–42.

p. 99   *Researchers have confirmed the beneficial antibacterial properties of basil*   Prasongdee, Panita, Kakanang Posridee, Anant Oonsivilai, and Ratchadaporn Oonsivilai. 2024. "A Culinary and Medicinal Gem: Exploring the Phytochemical and Functional Properties of Thai Basil." *Foods* 13 (4): 632. https://doi.org/10.3390/foods13040632.

p. 99   *basil might be beneficial in protecting against Alzheimer's and other neurodegenerative disorders*   Razazan, Atefeh, Prashantha Karunakar, Sidharth P. Mishra, Shailesh Sharma, Brandi Miller, Shalini Jain, and Hariom Yadav. 2021. "Activation of Microbiota Sensing—Free Fatty Acid Receptor 2 Signaling Ameliorates Amyloid-β Induced Neurotoxicity by Modulating Proteolysis-Senescence Axis." *Frontiers in Aging Neuroscience* 13: 735933. https://doi.org/10.3389/fnagi.2021.735933.

p. 99   *compounds in basil can lower blood pressure and lipid levels*   Hong, Seong Jun, Da-Som Kim, Jookyeong Lee, Chang Guk Boo, Moon Yeon Youn, Brandy Le, Jae Kyeom Kim, and Eui-Cheol Shin. 2022. "Inhalation of Low-dose Basil (Ocimum Basilicum) Essential Oil Improved Cardiovascular Health and Plasma Lipid Markers in High Fat Diet-induced Obese Rats." *Journal of Food Science* 87 (6): 2450–62. https://doi.org/10.1111/1750-3841.16196.

p. 99   *In examining 11 meta-analyses from 235 different papers*   Li, Zhongyu, Yang Wang, Qing Xu, Jinxin Ma, Xuan Li, Jiaxing Yan, Yibing Tian, Yandong Wen, and Ting Chen. 2023. "Berberine and Health Outcomes: An Umbrella Review." *Phytotherapy Research* 37 (5): 2051–66. https://doi.org/10.1002/ptr.7806.

p. 99   *Berberine also has proven neuroprotective effects*   Gasmi, Amin, Farah Asghar, Saba Zafar, Petro Oliinyk, Oksana Khavrona, Roman Lysiuk, Massimiliano Peana, et al. 2024. "Berberine: Pharmacological Features in Health, Disease and Aging." *Current Medicinal Chemistry* 31 (10): 1214–34. https://doi.org/10.2174/0929867330666230207112539; Dehau, Tessa, Marc Cherlet, Siska Croubels, Michiel Van De Vliet, Evy Goossens, and Filip Van Immerseel. 2023. "Berberine-Microbiota Interplay: Orchestrating Gut Health Through

Modulation of the Gut Microbiota and Metabolic Transformation into Bioactive Metabolites." *Frontiers in Pharmacology* 14: 1281090. https://doi.org/10.3389/fphar.2023.1281090.

p. 99 *One of the oldest and most popular spices, black pepper* Newerli-Guz, Joanna, and Maria Śmiechowska. 2022. "Health Benefits and Risks of Consuming Spices on the Example of Black Pepper and Cinnamon." *Foods* 11 (18): 2746. https://doi.org/10.3390/foods11182746.

p. 100 *piperine can effectively inhibit the growth of breast cancer and pancreatic cancer stem cells* Gökalp, Faik. 2016. "A Study on Piperine, Active Compound of Black Pepper." *Akademik Platform Mühendislik ve Fen Bilimleri Dergisi* 4 (3). https://doi.org/10.21541/apjes.66230; Samykutty, Abhilash, Aditya Vittal Shetty, Gajalakshmi Dakshinamoorthy, Mary Margaret Bartik, Gary Leon Johnson, Brian Webb, Guoxing Zheng, Aoshuang Chen, Ramaswamy Kalyanasundaram, and Gnanasekar Munirathinam. 2013. "Piperine, a Bioactive Component of Pepper Spice Exerts Therapeutic Effects on Androgen Dependent and Androgen Independent Prostate Cancer Cells." *PLoS ONE* 8 (6): e65889. https://doi.org/10.1371/journal.pone.0065889.

p. 100 *Piperine also has anticonvulsant effects* Gökalp, Faik. 2016. "A Study on Piperine."

p. 100 *it can stimulate the stomach to produce more digestive fluids* Rosca, Adrian Eugen, Mara Ioana Iesanu, Carmen Denise Mihaela Zahiu, Suzana Elena Voiculescu, Alexandru Catalin Paslaru, and Ana-Maria Zagrean. 2020. "Capsaicin and Gut Microbiota in Health and Disease." *Molecules* 25 (23): 5681. https://doi.org/10.3390/molecules25235681.

p. 100 *Animal studies have shown that consuming capsaicin helps* Szallasi, Arpad. 2022. "Dietary Capsaicin: A Spicy Way to Improve Cardio-Metabolic Health?" *Biomolecules* 12 (12): 1783. https://doi.org/10.3390/biom12121783.

p. 101 *studies showing an association between spicy food intake and longevity* Shen, Jie, Jianying Shan, Xiang Zhu, Peijing Yang, Dake Zhang, Boying Liang, Motao Li, Xiaohui Zang, and Zhuoping Dai. 2020. "Sex Specific Effects of Capsaicin on Longevity Regulation." *Experimental Gerontology* 130: 110788. https://doi.org/10.1016/j.exger.2019.110788.

p. 101 *people who regularly eat chili peppers appear to live longer* Szallasi, Arpad. 2022. "Dietary Capsaicin."

p. 101 *a study in the United States with 16,179 adults* Chopan, Mustafa, and Benjamin Littenberg. 2017. "The Association of Hot Red Chili Pepper Consumption and Mortality: A Large Population-Based Cohort Study." *PLoS ONE* 12 (1): e0169876. https://doi.org/10.1371/journal.pone.0169876.

p. 101 *eugenol, another powerful antioxidant that has been linked to reduced inflammation* Haro-González, José Nabor, Gustavo Adolfo Castillo-Herrera, Moisés Martínez-Velázquez, and Hugo Espinosa-Andrews. 2021. "Clove Essential

Oil (Syzygium Aromaticum L. Myrtaceae): Extraction, Chemical Composition, Food Applications, and Essential Bioactivity for Human Health." *Molecules* 26 (21): 6387. https://doi.org/10.3390/molecules26216387.

p. 102 *one systematic review of 109 randomized controlled trials using ginger* Anh, Nguyen Hoang, Sun Jo Kim, Nguyen Phuoc Long, Jung Eun Min, Young Cheol Yoon, Eun Goo Lee, Mina Kim, et al. 2020. "Ginger on Human Health: A Comprehensive Systematic Review of 109 Randomized Controlled Trials." *Nutrients* 12 (1): 157. https://doi.org/10.3390/nu12010157.

p. 102 *in an umbrella review of orally consumed ginger and human health* Crichton, Megan, Alexandra R. Davidson, Celia Innerarity, Wolfgang Marx, Anna Lohning, Elizabeth Isenring, and Skye Marshall. 2022. "Orally Consumed Ginger and Human Health: An Umbrella Review." *The American Journal of Clinical Nutrition* 115 (6): 1511–27. https://doi.org/10.1093/ajcn/nqac035.

p. 102 *scientists are conducting studies on ginseng* Ahmad, Syed Sayeed, Khurshid Ahmad, Ye Chan Hwang, Eun Ju Lee, and Inho Choi. 2023. "Therapeutic Applications of Ginseng Natural Compounds for Health Management." *International Journal of Molecular Sciences* 24 (24): 17290. https://doi.org/10.3390/ijms242417290.

p. 103 *In one 2022 paper, researchers looked at the association of ginseng consumption* Pradhan, Pranoti, Wanqing Wen, Hui Cai, Yu-Tang Gao, Gong Yang, Xiao-ou Shu, and Wei Zheng. 2022. "Association of Ginseng Consumption with All-Cause and Cause-Specific Mortality: Shanghai Women's Health Study." *Journal of Epidemiology* 32 (10): 469–75. https://doi.org/10.2188/jea.je20210393.

p. 103 *Chinese researchers culled 19 meta-analyses from 1,233 scientific papers* Li, Zhongyu, Yang Wang, Qing Xu, Jinxin Ma, Xuan Li, Yibing Tian, Yandong Wen, and Ting Chen. 2023. "Ginseng and Health Outcomes: An Umbrella Review." *Frontiers in Pharmacology* 14: 1069268. https://doi.org/10.3389/fphar.2023.1069268.

p. 103 *inhaling or applying peppermint essential oil greatly reduced migraine symptoms* Koren, Laura de Oliveira, Vanessa Bordenowsky Pereira Lejeune, Darciane Favero Baggio, Fernanda Mariano Ribeiro da Luz, and Juliana Geremias Chichorro. 2024. "Effect of Peppermint Essential Oil (Mentha Piperita L.) in Migraine-like Responses in Female Rats." *Headache Medicine* 15 (2): 78–85. https://doi.org/10.48208/headachemed.2024.17.

p. 103 *in a study in which people were given either a nasal application of peppermint oil or lidocaine* Rafieian-Kopaei, Mahmood, Ali Hasanpour-Dehkordi, Zahra Lorigooini, Fatemeh Deris, Kamal Solati, and Faezeh Mahdiyeh. 2019. "Comparing the Effect of Intranasal Lidocaine 4% with Peppermint Essential Oil Drop 1.5% on Migraine Attacks: A Double-Blind Clinical Trial." *International Journal of Preventive Medicine* 10 (1): 121. https://doi.org/10.4103/ijpvm.IJPVM_530_17.

p. 104   *one recent overarching review of nutmeg's biological and pharmacological activi-*
ties   Ashokkumar, Kaliyaperumal, Jesus Simal-Gandara, Muthusamy Muru-
gan, Mannananil Krishnankutty Dhanya, and Arjun Pandian. 2022. "Nutmeg
(Myristica Fragrans Houtt.) Essential Oil: A Review on Its Composition, Biological, and Pharmacological Activities." *Phytotherapy Research* 36 (7): 2839–
51. https://doi.org/10.1002/ptr.7491.

p. 104   *one wide-ranging review of the nutritional health benefits of wild thyme*   Jalil,
Banaz, Ivo Pischel, Björn Feistel, Cynthia Suarez, Andressa Blainski, Ralf
Spreemann, René Roth-Ehrang, and Michael Heinrich. 2024. "Wild Thyme
(Thymus Serpyllum L.): A Review of the Current Evidence of Nutritional and
Preventive Health Benefits." *Frontiers in Nutrition* 11: 1380962. https://doi
.org/10.3389/fnut.2024.1380962.

p. 104   *in a study using orange thyme*   Silva, Amélia M., Luís M. Félix, Isabel Teix-
eira, Carlos Martins-Gomes, Judith Schäfer, Eliana B. Souto, Dario J. Santos,
Mirko Bunzel, and Fernando M. Nunes. 2021. "Orange Thyme: Phytochemical Profiling, in Vitro Bioactivities of Extracts and Potential Health Benefits."
Food Chemistry: X 12: 100171. https://doi.org/10.1016/j.fochx.2021.100171.

p. 105   *which can help regulate several essential factors in the metabolic pathway of lipids*   El-Saadony, Mohamed T., Tao Yang, Sameh A. Korma, Mahmoud
Sitohy, Taia A. Abd El-Mageed, Samy Selim, Soad K. Al Jaouni, et al.
2023. "Impacts of Turmeric and Its Principal Bioactive Curcumin on Human
Health: Pharmaceutical, Medicinal, and Food Applications: A Comprehensive Review." *Frontiers in Nutrition* 9: 1040259. https://doi.org/10.3389/fnut
.2022.1040259.

p. 105   *Curcumin has been used for centuries in traditional Chinese and Indian Ayurvedic
medicines*   Porro, Chiara, and Maria Antonietta Panaro. 2023. "Recent Prog-
ress in Understanding the Health Benefits of Curcumin." *Molecules* 28 (5):
2418. https://doi.org/10.3390/molecules28052418.

p. 106   *one of the most extensive reviews examining studies conducted on the effects of
curcumin on metabolic syndrome*   Jabczyk, Marzena, Justyna Nowak, Bar-
tosz Hudzik, and Barbara Zubelewicz-Szkodzińska. 2021. "Curcumin in
Metabolic Health and Disease." *Nutrients* 13 (12): 4440. https://doi.org/10
.3390/nu13124440.

p. 106   *scientists point to curcumin's potential to lower the level of proteins associated with
the aging process*   Izadi, Mehran, Nariman Sadri, Amirhossein Abdi, Moham-
mad Mahdi Raeis Zadeh, Dorsa Jalaei, Mohammad Mahdi Ghazimoradi,
Sara Shouri, and Safa Tahmasebi. 2024. "Longevity and Anti-Aging Effects
of Curcumin Supplementation." *GeroScience* 46 (3): 2933–50. https://doi.org
/10.1007/s11357-024-01092-5.

Chapter 8

p. 109   *bread is one of the biggest sources of salt in the Western diet*   Pashaei, Mitra, Leila Zare, Elham Khalili Sadrabad, Amin Hosseini Sharif Abad, Neda Mollakhalili-Meybodi, and Abdol-Samad Abedi. 2022. "The Impacts of Salt Reduction Strategies on Technological Characteristics of Wheat Bread: A Review." *Journal of Food Science and Technology* 59 (11): 4141–51. https://doi.org/10.1007/s13197-021-05263-6.

p. 111   *two studies published in 2014*   Pfister, Roman, Guido Michels, Stephen J. Sharp, Robert Luben, Nick J. Wareham, and Kay-Tee Khaw. 2014. "Estimated Urinary Sodium Excretion and Risk of Heart Failure in Men and Women in the EPIC-Norfolk Study." *European Journal of Heart Failure* 16 (4): 394–402. https://doi.org/10.1002/ejhf.56; O'Donnell, Martin, Andrew Mente, Sumathy Rangarajan, Matthew J. McQueen, Xingyu Wang, Lisheng Liu, Hou Yan, et al. 2014. "Urinary Sodium and Potassium Excretion, Mortality, and Cardiovascular Events." *New England Journal of Medicine* 371 (7): 612–23. https://doi.org/10.1056/nejmoa1311889.

p. 112   *in 2016, they analyzed data from a larger study tracking 3,126 subjects*   Cook, Nancy R., Lawrence J. Appel, and Paul K. Whelton. 2014. "Lower Levels of Sodium Intake and Reduced Cardiovascular Risk." *Circulation* 129 (9): 981–89. https://doi.org/10.1161/circulationaha.113.006032.

p. 113   *Too Much Sodium Increases Inflammation*   Wu, Chuan, Nir Yosef, Theresa Thalhamer, Chen Zhu, Sheng Xiao, Yasuhiro Kishi, Aviv Regev, and Vijay Kuchroo. 2013. "Induction of Pathogenic Th17 Cells by Inducible Salt Sensing Kinase SGK1." *Nature* 496 (7446): 513–17. https://doi.org/10.1038/nature11984; O'Shea, John J., and Russell G. Jones. 2013. "Rubbing Salt in the Wound." *Nature* 496 (7446): 437–39. https://doi.org/10.1038/nature11959; Kleinewietfeld, Markus, Arndt Manzel, Jens Titze, Heda Kvakan, Nir Yosef, Ralf A. Linker, Dominik N. Muller, and David A. Hafler. 2013. "Sodium Chloride Drives Autoimmune Disease by the Induction of Pathogenic TH17 Cells." *Nature* 496 (7446): 518–22. https://doi.org/10.1038/nature11868; Zhou, Xin, Ling Zhang, Wen-Jie Ji, Fei Yuan, Zhao-Zeng Guo, Bo Pang, Tao Luo, et al. 2013. "Variation in Dietary Salt Intake Induces Coordinated Dynamics of Monocyte Subsets and Monocyte-Platelet Aggregates in Humans: Implications in End Organ Inflammation." *PLoS ONE* 8 (4): e60332. https://doi.org/10.1371/journal.pone.0060332.

p. 113   *Too Much Sodium Increases the Chance of Heart Disease*   Dmitrieva, Natalia I., and Maurice B. Burg. 2015. "Elevated Sodium and Dehydration Stimulate Inflammatory Signaling in Endothelial Cells and Promote Atherosclerosis." *PLoS ONE* 10 (6): e0128870. https://doi.org/10.1371/journal.pone.0128870; Cook, Nancy, et al. 2014. "Lower Levels of Sodium Intake"; Dickinson,

Kacie M., Peter M. Clifton, Louise M. Burrell, P. Hugh R. Barrett, and Jennifer B. Keogh. 2014. "Postprandial Effects of a High Salt Meal on Serum Sodium, Arterial Stiffness, Markers of Nitric Oxide Production and Markers of Endothelial Function." *Atherosclerosis* 232 (1): 211–16. https://doi.org/10.1016/j.atherosclerosis.2013.10.032; Aaron, Kristal J., and Paul W. Sanders. 2013. "Role of Dietary Salt and Potassium Intake in Cardiovascular Health and Disease: A Review of the Evidence." *Mayo Clinic Proceedings* 88 (9): 987–95. https://doi.org/10.1016/j.mayocp.2013.06.005; Wild, Johannes, Oliver Soehnlein, Barbara Dietel, Katharina Urschel, Christoph D. Garlichs, and Iwona Cicha. 2014. "Rubbing Salt into Wounded Endothelium: Sodium Potentiates Proatherogenic Effects of TNF-? Under Non-Uniform Shear Stress." *Thrombosis and Haemostasis* 112 (01): 183–95. https://doi.org/10.1160/th13-11-0908; Edwards, David G., and William B. Farquhar. 2015. "Vascular Effects of Dietary Salt." *Current Opinion in Nephrology and Hypertension* 24 (1): 8–13. https://doi.org/10.1097/mnh.0000000000000089.

p. 113　*Too Much Sodium Can Contribute to Cancer*　Ge, Sheng, Xiaohui Feng, Li Shen, Zhanying Wei, Qiankun Zhu, and Juan Sun. 2012. "Association Between Habitual Dietary Salt Intake and Risk of Gastric Cancer: A Systematic Review of Observational Studies." *Gastroenterology Research and Practice* 2012: 808120. https://doi.org/10.1155/2012/808120; Amara, Suneetha, and Venkataswarup Tiriveedhi. 2017. "Inflammatory Role of High Salt Level in Tumor Microenvironment (Review)." *International Journal of Oncology* 50 (5): 1477–81. https://doi.org/10.3892/ijo.2017.3936; Jansson, B. 1996. "Potassium, Sodium, and Cancer: A Review." *Journal of Environmental Pathology, Toxicology and Oncology: Official Organ of the International Society for Environmental Toxicology and Cancer* 15 (2–4): 65–73.

p. 113　*Increasing Potassium While Reducing Sodium Can Reverse Negative Health Effects*　Zhao, Xin, Yan Zhang, Xiaolin Zhang, Yi Kang, Xiaoxiang Tian, Xiaozeng Wang, Junyin Peng, Zhiming Zhu, and Yaling Han. 2017. "Associations of Urinary Sodium and Sodium to Potassium Ratio with Hypertension Prevalence and the Risk of Cardiovascular Events in Patients with Prehypertension." *Journal of Clinical Hypertension* 19 (12): 1231–39. https://doi.org/10.1111/jch.13104; Okayama, Akira, Nagako Okuda, Katsuyuki Miura, Tomonori Okamura, Takehito Hayakawa, Hiroshi Akasaka, Hirofumi Ohnishi, et al. 2016. "Dietary Sodium-to-Potassium Ratio as a Risk Factor for Stroke, Cardiovascular Disease and All-Cause Mortality in Japan: The NIPPON DATA80 Cohort Study." *BMJ Open* 6 (7): e011632. https://doi.org/10.1136/bmjopen-2016-011632; Granchi, Donatella, Renata Caudarella, Claudio Ripamonti, Paolo Spinnato, Alberto Bazzocchi, Annamaria Massa, and Nicola Baldini. 2018. "Potassium Citrate Supplementation Decreases the Biochemical Markers of Bone Loss in a Group of Osteopenic Women: The

Results of a Randomized, Double-Blind, Placebo-Controlled Pilot Study."
Nutrients 10 (9): 1293. https://doi.org/10.3390/nu10091293; Cook, Nancy, et
al. 2014. "Lower Levels of Sodium Intake."

Chapter 9

p. 116   *evidence of humans eating olives and using olive trees for fuel 100,000 years*
ago   Marquer, L., T. Otto, E. Ben Arous, E. Stoetzel, E. Campmas, A.
Zazzo, O. Tombret, et al. 2022. "The First Use of Olives in Africa Around
100,000 Years Ago." *Nature Plants* 8 (3): 204–8. https://doi.org/10.1038
/s41477-022-01109-x.

p. 116   *olive oil being produced as early as 2500 BCE*   Albini, A., F. Albini, P. Cor-
radino, L. Dugo, L. Calabrone, and D. M. Noonan. 2023. "From Antiquity
to Contemporary Times: How Olive Oil By-Products and Waste Water Can
Contribute to Health." *Frontiers in Nutrition* 10: 1254947. https://www.ncbi
.nlm.nih.gov/pmc/articles/PMC10615083/.

p. 117   *hydroxytyrosol, oleocanthal, and oleuropein, all of which help give olive oil its poten-*
tial to increase lifespan   Millman, Jasmine F., Shiki Okamoto, Taiki Teruya,
Tsugumi Uema, Shinya Ikematsu, Michio Shimabukuro, and Hiroaki Masu-
zaki. 2021. "Extra-Virgin Olive Oil and the Gut-Brain Axis: Influence on Gut
Microbiota, Mucosal Immunity, and Cardiometabolic and Cognitive Health."
Nutrition Reviews 79 (12): 1362–74. https://doi.org/10.1093/nutrit/nuaa148.

p. 118   *the brine stimulates the microbial activity for fermentation and also reduces the bit-*
terness   Rocha, Janete, Nuno Borges, and Olívia Pinho. 2020. "Table Olives
and Health: A Review." *Journal of Nutritional Science* 9: e57. https://doi.org/10
.1017/jns.2020.50; Lanza, Barbara, and Paolino Ninfali. 2020. "Antioxidants
in Extra Virgin Olive Oil and Table Olives: Connections between Agriculture
and Processing for Health Choices." *Antioxidants* 9 (1): 41. https://doi.org/10
.3390/antiox9010041.

p. 118   *oleic acid, which can help support the body's immune response*   Flynn, Mary M.,
Audrey Tierney, and Catherine Itsiopoulos. 2023. "Is Extra Virgin Olive
Oil the Critical Ingredient Driving the Health Benefits of a Mediterranean
Diet? A Narrative Review." *Nutrients* 15 (13): 2916. https://doi.org/10.3390
/nu15132916.

p. 118   *These powerful antioxidants are linked to treating and preventing inflammation*
Bilal, R.M., C. Liu, H. Zhao, Y. Wang, M. R. Farag, M. Alagawany, F. U. Has-
san, et al. 2021. "Olive Oil: Nutritional Applications, Beneficial Health Aspects
and Its Prospective Application in Poultry Production." *Frontiers in Pharmacol-*
ogy 12: 723040. https://www.ncbi.nlm.nih.gov/pmc/articles/PMC8424077/.

p. 118   *EVOO consumption is linked to lower rates of cardiovascular disease and all-cause*
mortality   Martínez-González, Miguel A., Carmen Sayón-Orea, Vanessa

Bullón-Vela, Maira Bes-Rastrollo, Fernando Rodríguez-Artalejo, María José Yusta-Boyo, and Marta García-Solano. 2022. "Effect of Olive Oil Consumption on Cardiovascular Disease, Cancer, Type 2 Diabetes, and All-Cause Mortality: A Systematic Review and Meta-Analysis." *Clinical Nutrition* 41 (12): 2659–82. https://doi.org/10.1016/j.clnu.2022.10.001; Xia, Meng, Yi Zhong, Yongquan Peng, and Cheng Qian. 2022. "Olive Oil Consumption and Risk of Cardiovascular Disease and All-Cause Mortality: A Meta-Analysis of Prospective Cohort Studies." *Frontiers in Nutrition* 9: 1041203. https://doi.org/10.3389/fnut.2022.1041203.

p. 119   *one large cohort study in Italy involving 22,892 men and women*   Ruggiero, Emilia, Augusto Di Castelnuovo, Simona Costanzo, Simona Esposito, Amalia De Curtis, Mariarosaria Persichillo, Chiara Cerletti, et al. 2024. "Olive Oil Consumption Is Associated with Lower Cancer, Cardiovascular and All-Cause Mortality Among Italian Adults: Prospective Results from the Moli-Sani Study and Analysis of Potential Biological Mechanisms." *European Journal of Clinical Nutrition*, 1–10. https://doi.org/10.1038/s41430-024-01442-8.

p. 119   *scientists see the potential of oleocanthal as a naturally occurring nonsteroidal anti-inflammatory drug (NSAID)*   Bilal, R. M., et al. 2021. "Olive Oil: Nutritional Applications."

p. 119   *one study demonstrated that 25 middle-aged participants consuming 10 to 20 g of EVOO daily*   Martínez-Zamora, Lorena, Rocío Peñalver, Gaspar Ros, and Gema Nieto. 2021. "Olive Tree Derivatives and Hydroxytyrosol: Their Potential Effects on Human Health and Its Use as Functional Ingredient in Meat." *Foods* 10 (11): 2611. https://doi.org/10.3390/foods10112611.

p. 120   *EVOO can help lower the risk of stroke by boosting endothelial function*   Zhao, Weiwei, Huizhen Wei, Jun Lu, Wenjun Sha, Dusang Sun, Ting Pan, and Tao Lei. 2023. "Tyrosol Attenuates Lipopolysaccharideinduced Inflammation in HUVECs to Promote Vascular Health Against Atheroscleros Challenge." *Experimental and Therapeutic Medicine* 25 (5): 240. https://doi.org/10.3892/etm.2023.11939.

p. 120   *lowering the aggregation of platelets*   Flynn, Mary M., et al. 2023. "Is Extra Virgin Olive Oil the Critical Ingredient."

p. 120   *In one study, 3,042 Greek men and women*   Millman, Jasmine F., et al. 2021. "Extra-Virgin Olive Oil and the Gut-Brain Axis."

p. 120   *EVOO has a lipid-lowering effect*   Zupo, Roberta, Fabio Castellana, Pasquale Crupi, Addolorata Desantis, Mariangela Rondanelli, Filomena Corbo, and Maria Lisa Clodoveo. 2023. "Olive Oil Polyphenols Improve HDL Cholesterol and Promote Maintenance of Lipid Metabolism: A Systematic Review and Meta-Analysis of Randomized Controlled Trials." *Metabolites* 13 (12): 1187. https://doi.org/10.3390/metabo13121187.

p. 120   *Oleic acid, the primary fatty acid in EVOO, can help maintain healthy glucose lev-els*   Millman, Jasmine F., et al. 2021. "Extra-Virgin Olive Oil and the Gut-Brain Axis."

p. 120   *in a 2024 meta-analysis of randomized clinical trials*   Morvaridzadeh, Mojgan, Alan A. Cohen, Javad Heshmati, Mehdi Alami, Hicham Berrougui, Nada Zoubdane, Ana Beatriz Pizarro, and Abdelouahed Khalil. 2024. "Effect of Extra Virgin Olive Oil on Anthropometric Indices, Inflammatory and Cardiometabolic Markers: A Systematic Review and Meta-Analysis of Randomized Clinical Trials." *Journal of Nutrition* 154 (1): 95–120. https://doi.org/10.1016/j.tjnut.2023.10.028.

p. 120   *Laboratory studies have also shown that oleuropein inhibits the growth of cancer cells*   Bilal, R. M., et al. 2021. "Olive Oil: Nutritional Applications."

p. 121   *olive oil is being studied as a tool to treat and even cure multiple sclerosis*   Bilal, R. M., et al. 2021. "Olive Oil: Nutritional Applications."

p. 121   *EVOO or its specific phenolic compounds can reduce the accumulation of plaque deposits in the brain*   Millman, Jasmine F., et al. 2021. "Extra-Virgin Olive Oil and the Gut-Brain Axis."

p. 121   *EVOO can also support the health of the mucus lining of the intestines*   Millman, Jasmine F., et al. 2021. "Extra-Virgin Olive Oil and the Gut-Brain Axis."

p. 122   *the greatest single factor responsible for elevating the ratio of dietary omega-6 to omega-3*   DiNicolantonio, James J, and James O'Keefe. 2021. "The Importance of Maintaining a Low Omega-6/Omega-3 Ratio for Reducing the Risk of Autoimmune Diseases, Asthma, and Allergies." *Missouri Medicine* 118 (5): 453–59.

Chapter 10

p. 126   *researchers are exploring the association between consuming chocolate and a decreased risk of many chronic diseases*   Martin, María Ángeles, and Sonia Ramos. 2021. "Impact of Cocoa Flavanols on Human Health." *Food and Chemical Toxicology* 151: 112121. https://doi.org/10.1016/j.fct.2021.112121.

p. 127   *The first people to recognize the benefits of consuming chocolate*   Clark, Caitlin. 2021. "Chocolate's Secret Ingredient Is Fermenting Microbes." *Scientific American*. https://www.scientificamerican.com/article/chocolates-secret-ingredient-is-fermenting-microbes/.

p. 127   *The Mayans cultivated . . . medicinal purposes*   Sarıtaş, Sümeyye, Hatice Duman, Burcu Pekdemir, João Miguel Rocha, Fatih Oz, and Sercan Karav. 2024. "Functional Chocolate: Exploring Advances in Production and Health Benefits." *International Journal of Food Science & Technology* 59 (8): 5303–25. https://doi.org/10.1111/ijfs.17312.

p. 127 *Cacao first appeared . . . digestion and elimination* Dillinger, Teresa L., Patricia Barriga, Sylvia Escárcega, Martha Jimenez, Diana Salazar Lowe, and Louis E. Grivetti. 2000. "Food of the Gods: Cure for Humanity? A Cultural History of the Medicinal and Ritual Use of Chocolate." *Journal of Nutrition* 130 (8): 2057S-72S. https://doi.org/10.1093/jn/130.8.2057s.

p. 128 *"three of the longest-lived women were all great consumers of chocolate"* Jeune, Bernard, Jean-Marie Robine, Robert Young, Bertrand Desjardins, Axel Skytthe, and James W. Vaupel. 2010. "Supercentenarians." *Demographic Research Monographs*, 285–323. https://doi.org/10.1007/978-3-642-11520-2_16.

p. 129 *natural fermentation . . . is a critical part of what gives cacao its health benefits* Clark, Caitlin. 2021. "Chocolate's Secret Ingredient."

p. 129 *The quality and flavor of chocolate are dependent* Sarıtaş, Sümeyye, et al. 2024. "Functional Chocolate."

p. 129 *White chocolate has no cocoa solids at all, which means it's . . . devoid of most of the beneficial phenols* Sarıtaş, Sümeyye, et al. 2024. "Functional Chocolate."

p. 130 *Frequently manufacturers then add milk, sugar, and other ingredients* Kababie-Ameo, Rebeca, Griselda Mericia Rabadán-Chávez, Natalia Vázquez-Manjarrez, and Gabriela Gutiérrez-Salmeán. 2022. "Potential Applications of Cocoa (Theobroma Cacao) on Diabetic Neuropathy: Mini-Review." *Frontiers in Bioscience-Landmark* 27 (2): 57. https://doi.org/10.31083/j.fbl2702057.

p. 129 *Cocoa beans are composed of 33 to 62 percent cocoa butter* Sarıtaş, Sümeyye, et al. 2024. "Functional Chocolate."

p. 130 *Cacao . . . contains about 300 natural components and a surprising mix of beneficial nutrients* Martin, María Ángeles, and Sonia Ramos. 2021. "Impact of Cocoa Flavanols."

p. 130 *essential physiological functions such as reproduction and growth* Jonscher, Karen R., Winyoo Chowanadisai, and Robert B. Rucker. 2021. "Pyrroloquinoline-Quinone Is More Than an Antioxidant: A Vitamin-like Accessory Factor Important in Health and Disease Prevention." *Biomolecules* 11 (10): 1441. https://doi.org/10.3390/biom11101441.

p. 130 *protecting the brain from neurodegenerative diseases targeting metabolism* Canovai, Alessio, and Pete A. Williams. 2025. "Pyrroloquinoline Quinone: A Potential Neuroprotective Compound for Neurodegenerative Diseases Targeting Metabolism." *Neural Regeneration Research* 20 (1): 41–53. https://doi.org/10.4103/nrr.nrr-d-23-01921.

p. 131 *scientists are now suggesting it acts more like an essential vitamin* Jonscher, Karen R., et al. 2021. "Pyrroloquinoline-Quinone."

p. 131 *PQQ was indeed a new vitamin* Kasahara, Takaoki, and Tadafumi Kato. 2003. "A New Redox-Cofactor Vitamin for Mammals." *Nature* 422 (6934): 832. https://doi.org/10.1038/422832a.

p. 131   *in 2018 Dr. Bruce Ames agreed*   Ames, Bruce N. 2018. "Prolonging Healthy
         Aging: Longevity Vitamins and Proteins." *Proceedings of the National Academy
         of Sciences* 115 (43): 10836–44. https://doi.org/10.1073/pnas.1809045115.

p. 131   *PQQ has even been linked to slowing down the aging process*   Ishak, Nur
         Syafiqah Mohamad, Midori Kikuchi, and Kazuto Ikemoto. 2024. "Dietary
         Pyrroloquinoline Quinone Hinders Aging Progression in Male Mice and
         D-Galactose-Induced Cells." *Frontiers in Aging* 5: 1351860. https://doi
         .org/10.3389/fragi.2024.1351860; Xue, Qi, Jie Li, Ran Qin, Mingying Li,
         Yiping Li, Jing Zhang, Rong Wang, David Goltzman, Dengshun Miao, and
         Renlei Yang. 2024. "Nrf2 Activation by Pyrroloquinoline Quinone Inhibits
         Natural Aging-related Intervertebral Disk Degeneration in Mice." *Aging Cell*
         23 (8): e14202. https://doi.org/10.1111/acel.14202.

p. 131   *Laboratory studies conducted on everything from fungi to mice*   Jonscher, Karen
         R., et al. 2021. "Pyrroloquinoline-Quinone."

p. 131   *research shows that PQQ has great promise in protecting us against the neurodegen-
         eration*   Jonscher, Karen R., et al. 2021. "Pyrroloquinoline-Quinone."

p. 131   *PQQ supplementation can help slow the osteoporosis*   Li, Jie, Jing Zhang, Qi Xue,
         Boyang Liu, Ran Qin, Yiping Li, Yue Qiu, et al. 2023. "Pyrroloquinoline
         Quinone Alleviates Natural Aging-related Osteoporosis via a Novel MCM3-
         Keap1-Nrf2 Axis-mediated Stress Response and Fbn1 Upregulation." *Aging
         Cell* 22 (9): e13912. https://doi.org/10.1111/acel.13912.

p. 131   *dark chocolate) can help people better perform continuous, challenging cognitive
         tasks*   Sasaki, Akihiro, Kei Mizuno, Yusuke Morito, Chisato Oba, Kentaro
         Nakamura, Midori Natsume, Kyosuke Watanabe, Emi Yamano, and Yasuy-
         oshi Watanabe. 2024. "The Effects of Dark Chocolate on Cognitive Perfor-
         mance during Cognitively Demanding Tasks: A Randomized, Single-Blinded,
         Crossover, Dose-Comparison Study." *Heliyon* 10 (2): e24430. https://doi.org
         /10.1016/j.heliyon.2024.e24430.

p. 131   *a 2024 study with older adults experiencing mild cognitive decline*   Baltic, Ned-
         eljkovic, Todorovic, N., Ranisavljev, M., Korovljev, et al. 2024. "The Impact
         of Six-Week Dihydrogen-Pyrroloquinoline Quinone Supplementation on
         Mitochondrial Biomarkers, Brain Metabolism, and Cognition in Elderly Indi-
         viduals with Mild Cognitive Impairment: A Randomized Controlled Trial."
         Journal of Nutrition, Health and Aging 28 (8): 100287. https://doi.org/10.1016
         /j.jnha.2024.100287.

p. 132   *residue from a black drink that contained theobromine, caffeine, and ursolic
         acid*   Crown, Patricia L., Thomas E. Emerson, Jiyan Gu, W. Jeffrey Hurst,
         Timothy R. Pauketat, and Timothy Ward. 2012. "Ritual Black Drink Con-
         sumption at Cahokia." *Proceedings of the National Academy of Sciences* 109 (35):
         13944–49. https://doi.org/10.1073/pnas.1208404109.

p. 132   *they act on the central nervous system's adenosine receptors*   Crown, Patricia L., et al. 2012. "Ritual Black Drink Consumption."

p. 132   *Theobromine has other benefits as well. For instance, methylxanthines*   Samanta, S., T. Sarkar, R. Chakraborty, M. Rebezov, M. A. Shariati, M. Thiruvengadam, and K. R. R. Rengasamy. 2022. "Dark Chocolate: An Overview of Its Biological Activity, Processing, and Fortification Approaches." *Current Research in Food Science* 5: 1916–43. https://doi.org/10.1016/j.crfs.2022.10.017.

p. 132   *studies examining the use of theobromine to suppress cough in both humans and guinea pigs*   Crown, Patricia L., et al. 2012. "Ritual Black Drink Consumption."

p. 133   *humans have relied on fermentation since around 8000 BCE to help produce and preserve food*   Cuamatzin-García, Leonel, Paola Rodríguez-Rugarcía, Elie Girgis El-Kassis, Georgina Galicia, María de Lourdes Meza-Jiménez, Ma. del Rocío Baños-Lara, Diego Salatiel Zaragoza-Maldonado, and Beatriz Pérez-Armendáriz. 2022. "Traditional Fermented Foods and Beverages from Around the World and Their Health Benefits." *Microorganisms* 10 (6): 1151. https://doi.org/10.3390/microorganisms10061151.

p. 133   *might have developed a taste for fermented foods even earlier*   Amato, K. R., E.K. Mallott, A. Maia, A., and M. L. Savo Sardaro. 2021. "Predigestion as an Evolutionary Impetus for Human Use of Fermented Food." *Current Anthropology* 62 (S24). https://doi.org/10.1086/715238.

p. 133   *early humans developed two specific gene variants associated with increased fermented food consumption*   Amato, K. R., et al. 2021. "Predigestion as an Evolutionary Impetus."

p. 133   *"food made through desired microbial growth and enzymatic conversions of food components"*   Valentino, Vincenzo, Raffaele Magliulo, Dominic Farsi, Paul D. Cotter, Orla O'Sullivan, Danilo Ercolini, and Francesca De Filippis. 2024. "Fermented Foods, Their Microbiome and Its Potential in Boosting Human Health." *Microbial Biotechnology* 17 (2): e14428. https://doi.org/10.1111/1751-7915.14428.

p. 134   *The microorganisms most often used in fermented foods*   Clark, Caitlin, 2021. "Chocolate's Secret Ingredient."

p. 134   *Consuming probiotic fermented foods is associated*   Ibrahim, Salam A., Philip J. Yeboah, Raphael D. Ayivi, Abdulhakim S. Eddin, et al. 2023. "A Review and Comparative Perspective on Health Benefits of Probiotic and Fermented Foods." *International Journal of Food Science & Technology* 58 (10): 4948–64. https://doi.org/10.1111/ijfs.16619.

p. 134   *when researchers screened*   Hill, Colin, Daniel J. Tancredi, Christopher J. Cifelli, Joanne L. Slavin, Jaime Gahche, Maria L. Marco, Robert Hutkins, Victor L. Fulgoni, Daniel Merenstein, and Mary Ellen Sanders. 2023. "Positive Health Outcomes Associated with Live Microbe Intake from Foods, Including Fermented Foods, Assessed Using the NHANES Database." *Journal of Nutrition*

153 (4): 1143–49. https://doi.org/10.1016/j.tjnut.2023.02.019; Valentino, Vincenzo, et al. 2024. "Fermented Foods."

p. 134 *our Paleolithic ancestors would have regularly eaten meat that was starting to go rancid* Speth, John D. 2017. "Putrid Meat and Fish in the Eurasian Middle and Upper Paleolithic: Are We Missing a Key Part of Neanderthal and Modern Human Diet?" *Paleo Anthropology*: 44–72.

p. 134 *fermented fish products from this region that are recognized for their probiotic diversity* Narzary, Yutika, Sandeep Das, Arvind Kumar Goyal, Su Shiung Lam, Hemen Sarma, and Dolikajyoti Sharma. 2021. "Fermented Fish Products in South and Southeast Asian Cuisine: Indigenous Technology Processes, Nutrient Composition, and Cultural Significance." *Journal of Ethnic Foods* 8 (1): 33. https://doi.org/10.1186/s42779-021-00109-0.

p. 135 *vitamin K1 (phylloquinone), which is synthesized in algae, plants, and some bacteria* Simes, Dina C., Carla S. B. Viegas, Nuna Araújo, and Catarina Marreiros. 2019. "Vitamin K as a Powerful Micronutrient in Aging and Age-Related Diseases: Pros and Cons from Clinical Studies." *International Journal of Molecular Sciences* 20 (17): 4150. https://doi.org/10.3390/ijms20174150.

p. 135 *The other is vitamin K2 (menaquinone), which is divided further . . . combatting chronic disease* Gast, G. C. M., N. M. de Roos, I. Sluijs, M. L. Bots, J. W. J. Beulens, J. M. Geleijnse, J. C. Witteman, D. E. Grobbee, P. H. M. Peeters, and Y. T. van der Schouw. 2009. "A High Menaquinone Intake Reduces the Incidence of Coronary Heart Disease." *Nutrition, Metabolism and Cardiovascular Diseases* 19 (7): 504–10. https://doi.org/10.1016/j.numecd.2008.10.004.

p. 135 *we can get them in only three ways* Fenn, Kathrin, Philip Strandwitz, Eric J. Stewart, Eric Dimise, Sarah Rubin, Shreya Gurubacharya, Jon Clardy, and Kim Lewis. 2017. "Quinones Are Growth Factors for the Human Gut Microbiota." *Microbiome* 5 (1): 161. https://doi.org/10.1186/s40168-017-0380-5.

p. 136 *the typical Western diet is low or deficient in total menaquinones* Walther, Barbara, J. Philip Karl, Sarah L. Booth, and Patrick Boyaval. 2013. "Menaquinones, Bacteria, and the Food Supply: The Relevance of Dairy and Fermented Food Products to Vitamin K Requirements." *Advances in Nutrition* 4 (4): 463–73. https://doi.org/10.3945/an.113.003855.

p. 136 *menaquinones make up a major class of growth factors* Fenn, Kathrin, et al. 2017. "Quinones Are Growth Factors."

p. 136 *Vitamin K2 has also shown its effectiveness as an anti-inflammatory* Simes, Dina C., Carla S. B. Viegas, Nuna Araújo, and Catarina Marrieros. 2020. "Vitamin K as a Diet Supplement with Impact in Human Health: Current Evidence in Age-Related Diseases." *Nutrients* 12 (1): 138. https://doi.org/10.3390/nu12010138; Simes, Dina C., et al. 2019. "Vitamin K as a Powerful Micronutrient."

p. 136   *In one study conducted with 564 postmenopausal women in the Netherlands*   Beulens, J. W., M. L. Bots, F. Atsma, M. L. Bartelink, M. Prokop, J. M. Geleijnse, J. C. Witteman, D. E. Grobbee, and Y. T. van der Schouw. 2009. "High Dietary Menaquinone Intake Is Associated with Reduced Coronary Calcification." *Atherosclerosis.* https://doi.org/10.1016/j.atherosclerosis.2008.07.010.

p. 136   *In another Netherlands study with 4,807 men and women*   Geleijnse, J. M., C. Vermeer, D. E. Grobbee, L. J. Schurgers, M. H. Knapen, I. M. van der Meer, A. Hofman, and J. C. Witteman. 2004. "Dietary Intake of Menaquinone Is Associated with a Reduced Risk of Coronary Heart Disease: The Rotterdam Study." *Journal of Nutrition* 134 (11): 3100–5. https://doi.org/10.1093/jn/134.11.3100.

p. 136   *in a study with 6,759 women*   Ma, Ming-ling, Zi-jian Ma, Yi-lang He, Hao Sun, Bin Yang, Bin-jia Ruan, Wan-da Zhan, Shi-xuan Li, Hui Dong, and Yong-xiang Wang. 2022. "Efficacy of Vitamin K2 in the Prevention and Treatment of Postmenopausal Osteoporosis: A Systematic Review and Meta-Analysis of Randomized Controlled Trials." *Frontiers in Public Health* 10: 979649. https://doi.org/10.3389/fpubh.2022.979649; Simes, Dina C., et al. 2019. "Vitamin K as a Powerful Micronutrient."

p. 137   *One study, published in 2021, followed 91,891 people*   Zhong, Guo-Chao, Tian-Yang Hu, Peng-Fei Yang, Yang Peng, Jing-Jing Wu, Wei-Ping Sun, Long Cheng, and Chun-Rui Wang. 2021. "Chocolate Consumption and All-Cause and Cause-Specific Mortality in a US Population: A Post Hoc Analysis of the PLCO Cancer Screening Trial." *Aging.* https://www.ncbi.nlm.nih.gov/pmc/articles/PMC8351724/.

p. 138   *Another study, this one published in 2023, included 84,709 postmenopausal women*   Sun, Yangbo, Buyun Liu, Linda G. Snetselaar, Robert B. Wallace, Aladdin H. Shadyab, Guo-Chong Chen, James M. Shikany, JoAnn E. Manson, and Wei Bao. 2023. "Chocolate Consumption in Relation to All-Cause and Cause-Specific Mortality in Women: The Women's Health Initiative." *Journal of the Academy of Nutrition and Dietetics.* https://doi.org/10.1016/j.jand.2022.12.007.

p. 138   *cacao is also directly associated with supporting heart health*   Razola-Díaz, María del Carmen, María José Aznar-Ramos, Vito Verardo, Sonia Melgar-Locatelli, Estela Castilla-Ortega, and Celia Rodríguez-Pérez. 2023. "Exploring the Nutritional Composition and Bioactive Compounds in Different Cocoa Powders." *Antioxidants* 12 (3): 716. https://doi.org/10.3390/antiox12030716.

p. 138   *researchers noticed the heart-protective effects of chocolate among the Kuna people*   Samanta, S., et al. 2022. "Dark Chocolate."

p. 138   *consuming cacao products can lower your risk of cardiovascular disease*   Martin, María Ángeles, and Sonia Ramos. 2021. "Impact of Cocoa Flavanols."

p. 138   *One meta-analysis was conducted on the association of chocolate with cardiometabolic disorders*   Tan, Terence Yew Chin, Xin Yi Lim, Julie Hsiao Hui Yeo, Shaun Wen Huey Lee, and Nai Ming Lai. 2021. "The Health Effects of Chocolate and Cocoa: A Systematic Review." *Nutrients* 13 (9): 2909. https://doi.org/10 .3390/nu13092909.

p. 138   *a study published in 2024 demonstrated*   Yang, Juntao, Jiedong Zhou, Jie Yang, Haifei Lou, Bingjie Zhao, Jufang Chi, and Weiliang Tang. 2024. "Dark Chocolate Intake and Cardiovascular Diseases: A Mendelian Randomization Study." *Scientific Reports* 14 (1): 968. https://doi.org/10.1038/s41598-023 -50351-6.

p. 138   *Researchers in Japan also showed a link*   Matsumoto, Chisa, Hirofumi Tomiyama, Kazutaka Kimura, Kazuki Shiina, Masanori Kamei, Hiroyuki Inagaki, Taishirou Chikamori, and Akira Yamshina. 2020. "Modulation of Blood Pressure-Lowering Effects of Dark Chocolate According to an Insulin Sensitivity-Randomized Crossover Study." *Hypertension Research* 43 (6): 575–78. https://doi.org/10.1038/s41440-020-0395-3.

p. 138   *Many investigations worldwide have looked at the relationship*   Martin, María Ángeles, and Sonia Ramos. 2021. "Impact of Cocoa Flavanols."

p. 139   *Laboratory studies both in vitro and with animals have demonstrated*   Pérez-Cano, Francisco J., Malen Massot-Cladera, Àngels Franch, Cristina Castellote, and Margarida Castell. 2013. "The Effects of Cocoa on the Immune System." *Frontiers in Pharmacology* 4: 71. https://doi.org/10.3389/fphar.2013 .00071.

p. 139   *theobromine and caffeine, both of which act as stimulants on the brain*   Samanta, S., et al. 2022. "Dark Chocolate."

p. 139   *polyphenols in cacao can activate intracellular pathways*   Razola-Díaz, María del Carmen, et al. 2023. "Exploring the Nutritional Composition."

p. 139   *cacao and its flavonoids can help protect against neurodegenerative diseases*   Kababie-Ameo, Rebeca, et al. 2022. "Potential Applications of Cocoa."

p. 139   *Researchers believe there are two possible mechanisms of action*   Martin, María Ángeles, and Sonia Ramos. 2021. "Impact of Cocoa Flavanols."

p. 140   *menaquinones have been shown to help protect bone health*   Palermo, Andrea, Dario Tuccinardi, Luca D'Onofrio, Mikiko Watanabe, Daria Maggi, Anna Rita Maurizi, Valentina Greto, et al. 2017. "Vitamin K and Osteoporosis: Myth or Reality?" *Metabolism* 70: 57–71. https://doi.org/10.1016/j.metabol .2017.01.032; Ma, Ming-ling, et al. 2022. "Efficacy of Vitamin K2."

p. 140   *a menaquinone deficiency . . . can increase the deposition of calcium*   Gast, G. C. M., et al. 2009. "A High Menaquinone Intake"; Millar, Sophie A., Hinal Patel, Susan I. Anderson, Timothy J. England, and Saoirse E. O'Sullivan. 2017. "Osteocalcin, Vascular Calcification, and Atherosclerosis: A

Systematic Review and Meta-Analysis." *Frontiers in Endocrinology* 8: 183. https://doi.org/10.3389/fendo.2017.00183; Aaseth, Jan O., Urban Alehagen, Trine Baur Opstad, and Jan Alexander. 2023. "Vitamin K and Calcium Chelation in Vascular Health." *Biomedicines* 11 (12): 3154. https://doi.org/10.3390/biomedicines11123154.

Part III Introduction

p. 145   *"Historical and clinical data suggest"* O'Hearn, Amber. 2020. "Can a Carnivore Diet Provide All Essential Nutrients?" *Current Opinion in Endocrinology, Diabetes & Obesity* 27 (5): 312–16. https://doi.org/10.1097/med.0000000000000576.

p. 146   *the carnivore diet may be extremely beneficial in the short term* Norwitz, Nicholas G., Michelle Hurn, and Fernando Espi Forcen. 2023. "Animal-Based Ketogenic Diet Puts Severe Anorexia Nervosa into Multi-Year Remission: A Case Series." *Journal of Metabolic Health* 6 (1): 8. https://doi.org/10.4102/jir.v6i1.84; Lennerz, Belinda S., Jacob T. Mey, Owen H. Henn, and David S. Ludwig. 2021. "Behavioral Characteristics and Self-Reported Health Status among 2029 Adults Consuming a 'Carnivore Diet.'" *Current Developments in Nutrition* 5 (12): nzab133. https://doi.org/10.1093/cdn/nzab133; Norwitz, Nicholas G., and Adrian Soto-Mota. 2024. "Case Report: Carnivore–Ketogenic Diet for the Treatment of Inflammatory Bowel Disease: A Case Series of 10 Patients." *Frontiers in Nutrition* 11: 1467475. https://doi.org/10.3389/fnut.2024.1467475; Yar, Nadia, Lawrance T. Mukona, Kim Nguyen, Linette Nalbandyan, Lorraine Mukona, Guinda St. Fleur, Norman L. Lamberty, et al. 2022. "Consuming an All-Meat Ketogenic Diet for the Long-Term Management of Candida Vulvovaginitis and Vaginal Hidradenitis Suppurativa: A 47-Month Follow-Up Case Report." *Cureus* 14 (10): e30510. https://doi.org/10.7759/cureus.30510.

Chapter 11

p. 149   *studies suggesting that red meat is to blame for everything* Farvid, Maryam S., Elkhansa Sidahmed, Nicholas D. Spence, Kingsly Mante Angua, Bernard A. Rosner, and Junaidah B. Barnett. 2021. "Consumption of Red Meat and Processed Meat and Cancer Incidence: A Systematic Review and Meta-Analysis of Prospective Studies." *European Journal of Epidemiology* 36 (9): 937–51. https://doi.org/10.1007/s10654-021-00741-9; Chan, Doris S. M., Rosa Lau, Dagfinn Aune, Rui Vieira, Darren C. Greenwood, Ellen Kampman, and Teresa Norat. 2011. "Red and Processed Meat and Colorectal Cancer

Incidence: Meta-Analysis of Prospective Studies." *PloS One* 6 (6): e20456. https://doi.org/10.1371/journal.pone.0020456; Willett, W. C., M. J. Stampfer, G. A. Colditz, B. A. Rosner, and F. E. Speizer. 1990. "Relation of Meat, Fat, and Fiber Intake to the Risk of Colon Cancer in a Prospective Study Among Women." *The New England Journal of Medicine* 323 (24): 1664–72. https://doi.org/10.1056/nejm199012133232404.

p. 149   *One of the most alarming studies*   Chao, Ann, Michael J. Thun, Cari J. Connell, Marjorie L. McCullough, Eric J. Jacobs, W. Dana Flanders, Carmen Rodriguez, Rashmi Sinha, and Eugenia E. Calle. 2005. "Meat Consumption and Risk of Colorectal Cancer." *JAMA* 293 (2): 172–82. https://doi.org/10.1001/jama.293.2.172.

p. 149   *Another study, published in 2019, linked*   Esfandiar, Zohre, Firoozeh Hosseini-Esfahani, Parvin Mirmiran, Ali-Siamak Habibi-Moeini, and Fereidoun Azizi. 2019. "Red Meat and Dietary Iron Intakes Are Associated with Some Components of Metabolic Syndrome: Tehran Lipid and Glucose Study." *Journal of Translational Medicine* 17 (1): 313. https://doi.org/10.1186/s12967-019-2059-0.

p. 149   *And in 2024, a group of researchers published*   Li, Chunxiao, Tom R. P. Bishop, Fumiaki Imamura, Stephen J. Sharp, Matthew Pearce, Soren Brage, Ken K. Ong, et al. 2024. "Meat Consumption and Incident Type 2 Diabetes: An Individual-Participant Federated Meta-Analysis of 1.97 Million Adults with 100,000 Incident Cases from 31 Cohorts in 20 Countries." *The Lancet Diabetes & Endocrinology* 12 (9): 619–30. https://doi.org/10.1016/s2213-8587(24)00179-7.

p. 150   *a group of researchers reviewed all published observational studies*   Wang, Yumin, Tyler Pitre, Joshua D. Wallach, Russell J. de Souza, Tanvir Jassal, Dennis Bier, Chirag J. Patel, and Dena Zeraatkar. 2024. "Grilling the Data: Application of Specification Curve Analysis to Red Meat and All-Cause Mortality." *Journal of Clinical Epidemiology* 168: 111278. https://doi.org/10.1016/j.jclinepi.2024.111278.

p. 150   *particularly since the 1980s, when fat became the boogeyman*   Siegel, Rebecca L., Stacey A. Fedewa, William F. Anderson, Kimberly D. Miller, Jiemin Ma, Philip S. Rosenberg, and Ahmedin Jemal. 2017. "Colorectal Cancer Incidence Patterns in the United States, 1974–2013." *Journal of the National Cancer Institute* 109 (8): djw322. https://doi.org/10.1093/jnci/djw322.

p. 151   *Red meat consumption has been declining*   Daniel, Carrie R., Amanda J. Cross, Corinna Koebnick, and Rashmi Sinha. 2011. "Trends in Meat Consumption in the USA." *Public Health Nutrition* 14 (4): 575–83. https://doi.org/10.1017/s1368980010002077.

p. 152   *the differences in the fatty acid profiles were staggering*   Cordain, L., B. A. Watkins, G. L. Florant, M. Kelher, L. Rogers, and Y. Li. 2002. "Fatty Acid

Analysis of Wild Ruminant Tissues: Evolutionary Implications for Reducing Diet-Related Chronic Disease." *European Journal of Clinical Nutrition* 56 (3): 181–91. https://doi.org/10.1038/sj.ejcn.1601307.

p. 152 *ultra-processed foods . . . are associated with most chronic diseases* Lane, Melissa M., Elizabeth Gamage, Shutong Du, Deborah N. Ashtree, Amelia J. McGuinness, Sarah Gauci, Phillip Baker, et al. 2024. "Ultra-Processed Food Exposure and Adverse Health Outcomes: Umbrella Review of Epidemiological Meta-Analyses." *BMJ* 384: e077310. https://doi.org/10.1136/bmj-2023-077310; Asensi, Marta Tristan, Antonia Napoletano, Francesco Sofi, and Monica Dinu. 2023. "Low-Grade Inflammation and Ultra-Processed Foods Consumption: A Review." *Nutrients* 15 (6): 1546. https://doi.org/10.3390/nu15061546; Levy, Renata Bertazzi, Mayra Figueiredo Barata, Maria Alvim Leite, and Giovanna Calixto Andrade. 2023. "How and Why Ultra-Processed Foods Harm Human Health." *Proceedings of the Nutrition Society* 83 (1): 1–8. https://doi.org/10.1017/s0029665123003567.

p. 152 *researchers are starting to make the distinction between processed and unprocessed meats* McAfee, A. J., E. M. McSorley, G. J. Cuskelly, A. M. Fearon, B. W. Moss, J. A. M. Beattie, J. M. W. Wallace, M. P. Bonham, and J. J. Strain. 2011. "Red Meat from Animals Offered a Grass Diet Increases Plasma and Platelet N-3 PUFA in Healthy Consumers." *British Journal of Nutrition* 105 (1): 80–89. https://doi.org/10.1017/s0007114510003090; Micha, Renata, Sarah K. Wallace, and Dariush Mozaffarian. 2010. "Red and Processed Meat Consumption and Risk of Incident Coronary Heart Disease, Stroke, and Diabetes Mellitus." *Circulation* 121 (21): 2271–83. https://doi.org/10.1161/circulationaha.109.924977; Lescinsky, Haley, Ashkan Afshin, Charlie Ashbaugh, Catherine Bisignano, Michael Brauer, Giannina Ferrara, Simon I. Hay, et al. 2022. "Health Effects Associated with Consumption of Unprocessed Red Meat: A Burden of Proof Study." *Nature Medicine* 28 (10): 2075–82. https://doi.org/10.1038/s41591-022-01968-z.

p. 153 *"the anaerobic breakdown of undigested protein in the colon by microbiota"* Kim, Eunjung, Desire Coelho, and François Blachier. 2013. "Review of the Association Between Meat Consumption and Risk of Colorectal Cancer." *Nutrition Research* 33 (12): 983–94. https://doi.org/10.1016/j.nutres.2013.07.018.

p. 153 *many researchers refer to the putrefaction process* Windey, Karen, Vicky De Preter, and Kristin Verbeke. 2012. "Relevance of Protein Fermentation to Gut Health." *Molecular Nutrition & Food Research* 56 (1): 184–96. https://doi.org/10.1002/mnfr.201100542.

p. 153 *One 2024 study showed that consuming just 30 grams per day of leafy vegetables* Donghia, Rossella, Rossella Tatoli, Angelo Campanella, Francesco Cuccaro, Caterina Bonfiglio, and Gianluigi Giannelli. 2024. "Adding a Leafy Vegetable Fraction to Diets Decreases the Risk of Red Meat Mortality in

MASLD Subjects: Results from the MICOL Cohort." *Nutrients* 16 (8): 1207. https://doi.org/10.3390/nu16081207.

p. 153 *most studies "used levels of meat or meat components well in excess"* Turner, Nancy D., and Shannon K. Lloyd. 2017. "Association Between Red Meat Consumption and Colon Cancer: A Systematic Review of Experimental Results." *Experimental Biology and Medicine* 242 (8): 813–39. https://doi.org/10.1177/1535370217693117.

p. 154 *A high-quality protein has a good profile of both* Berrazaga, Insaf, Valérie Micard, Marine Gueugneau, and Stéphane Walrand. 2019. "The Role of the Anabolic Properties of Plant- versus Animal-Based Protein Sources in Supporting Muscle Mass Maintenance: A Critical Review." *Nutrients* 11 (8): 1825. https://doi.org/10.3390/nu11081825.

p. 155 *Do Your Protein Needs Change as You Age?* Bauer, Jürgen, Gianni Biolo, Tommy Cederholm, Matteo Cesari, Alfonso J. Cruz-Jentoft, John E. Morley, Stuart Phillips, et al. 2013. "Evidence-Based Recommendations for Optimal Dietary Protein Intake in Older People: A Position Paper from the PROT-AGE Study Group." *Journal of the American Medical Directors Association* 14 (8): 542–59. https://doi.org/10.1016/j.jamda.2013.05.021.

p. 155 *DIAAS (digestible indispensable amino acid score) protein quality rating* Marinangeli, Christopher P. F., and James D. House. 2017. "Potential Impact of the Digestible Indispensable Amino Acid Score as a Measure of Protein Quality on Dietary Regulations and Health." *Nutrition Reviews* 75 (8): 658–67. https://doi.org/10.1093/nutrit/nux025.

p. 157 *In a comprehensive analysis of 229 hunter-gatherer diets* Cordain, L., J. B. Miller, S. B. Eaton, N. Mann, S. H. Holt, and J. D. Speth. 2000. "Plant-Animal Subsistence Ratios and Macronutrient Energy Estimations in Worldwide Hunter-Gatherer Diets." *American Journal of Clinical Nutrition* 71 (3): 682–92. https://doi.org/10.1093/ajcn/71.3.682.

p. 157 *discovery of fossils in Africa of butchered animals* Cordain, L., B. A. Watkins, and N. J. Mann. 2001. "Fatty Acid Composition and Energy Density of Foods Available to African Hominids." *World Review of Nutrition and Dietetics* 90: 144–61. https://doi.org/10.1159/000059813.

p. 158 *today's humans, like our Paleo ancestors, benefit* Leroy, Frédéric, Nick W. Smith, Adegbola T. Adesogan, Ty Beal, Lora Iannotti, Paul J. Moughan, and Neil Mann. 2023. "The Role of Meat in the Human Diet: Evolutionary Aspects and Nutritional Value." *Animal Frontiers: The Review Magazine of Animal Agriculture* 13 (2): 11–18. https://doi.org/10.1093/af/vfac093; Cordain, L., et al. 2001. "Fatty Acid Composition."

p. 158 *it's simply not possible for older adults to consume adequate protein on a vegan diet* Tong, Tammy Y. N., Paul N. Appleby, Miranda E. G. Armstrong, Georgina K. Fensom, Anika Knuppel, Keren Papier, Aurora Perez-Cornago,

Ruth C. Travis, and Timothy J. Key. 2020. "Vegetarian and Vegan Diets and Risks of Total and Site-Specific Fractures: Results from the Prospective EPIC-Oxford Study." *BMC Medicine* 18 (1): 353. https://doi.org/10.1186/s12916-020-01815-3; Mahalle, Namita, Mohan V. Kulkarni, Mahendra K. Garg, and Sadanand S. Naik. 2013. "Vitamin B12 Deficiency and Hyperhomocysteinemia as Correlates of Cardiovascular Risk Factors in Indian Subjects with Coronary Artery Disease." *Journal of Cardiology* 61 (4): 289–94. https://doi.org/10.1016/j.jjcc.2012.11.009; Domić, Jacintha, Pol Grootswagers, Luc J. C. van Loon, and Lisette C. P. G. M. de Groot. 2022. "Perspective: Vegan Diets for Older Adults? A Perspective On the Potential Impact On Muscle Mass and Strength." *Advances in Nutrition* 13 (3): 712–25. https://doi.org/10.1093/advances/nmac009.

p. 159 *a study published in 2023 using data from 1,570 adults* Groenendijk, Inge, Pol Grootswagers, Aurelia Santoro, Claudio Franceschi, Alberto Bazzocchi, Nathalie Meunier, et al. 2023. "Protein Intake and Bone Mineral Density: Cross-Sectional Relationship and Longitudinal Effects in Older Adults." *Journal of Cachexia, Sarcopenia and Muscle* 14 (1): 116–25. https://doi.org/10.1002/jcsm.13111.

p. 159 *one recent study examining the emerging evidence on how dietary protein intake influences the muscles* Campbell, Wayne W., Nicolaas E. P. Deutz, Elena Volpi, and Caroline M. Apovian. 2023. "Nutritional Interventions: Dietary Protein Needs and Influences on Skeletal Muscle of Older Adults." *Journals of Gerontology Series A* 78: 67–72. https://doi.org/10.1093/gerona/glad038.

p. 160 *Animal Protein Promotes Improved Kidney Function* Cheng, Yu, Guanghao Zheng, Zhen Song, Gan Zhang, Xuepeng Rao, and Tao Zeng. 2024. "Association Between Dietary Protein Intake and Risk of Chronic Kidney Disease: A Systematic Review and Meta-Analysis." *Frontiers in Nutrition* 11: 1408424. https://doi.org/10.3389/fnut.2024.1408424.

p. 160 *researchers examined the association between life expectancy and meat consumption* You, Wenpeng, Renata Henneberg, Arthur Saniotis, Yanfei Ge, and Maciej Henneberg. 2022. "Total Meat Intake Is Associated with Life Expectancy: A Cross-Sectional Data Analysis of 175 Contemporary Populations." *International Journal of General Medicine* 15: 1833–51. https://doi.org/10.2147/ijgm.s333004.

p. 160 *When the folate cycle doesn't function properly* Guieu, Régis, Jean Ruf, and Giovanna Mottola. 2022. "Hyperhomocysteinemia and Cardiovascular Diseases." *Annales de Biologie Clinique* 80 (1): 7–14. https://doi.org/10.1684/abc.2021.1694; McNulty, Helene, Kristina Pentieva, Leane Hoey, and Mary Ward. 2008. "Homocysteine, B-Vitamins and CVD." *Proceedings of the Nutrition Society* 67 (2): 232–37. https://doi.org/10.1017/s0029665108007076.

p. 161   *researchers have generally pointed to the prevalent high levels of homocyste-*
ine Kumar, Jitender, Gaurav Garg, Elayanambi Sundaramoorthy, P. Veer-
endra Prasad, Ganesan Karthikeyan, Lakshmy Ramakrishnan, Saurabh
Ghosh, and Shantanu Sengupta. 2009. "Vitamin B12 Deficiency Is Associated
with Coronary Artery Disease in an Indian Population." *Clinical Chemistry
and Laboratory Medicine* 47 (3): 334–38. https://doi.org/10.1515/cclm.2009
.074; Mahalle, Namita, Mohan V. Kulkarni, Mahendra K. Garg, and Sadanand S. Naik. 2013. "Vitamin B12 Deficiency and Hyperhomocysteinemia as
Correlates of Cardiovascular Risk Factors in Indian Subjects with Coronary
Artery Disease." *Journal of Cardiology* 61 (4): 289–94. https://doi.org/10.1016
/j.jjcc.2012.11.009; Woo, Kam S., Timothy C. Y. Kwok, and David S. Celer-
majer. 2014. "Vegan Diet, Subnormal Vitamin B-12 Status and Cardiovascular
Health." *Nutrients* 6 (8): 3259–73. https://doi.org/10.3390/nu6083259.

p. 161   *even vegans who eat high amounts of B6* Waldmann, A., B. Dörr, J. W. Kos-
chizke, C. Leitzmann, and A. Hahn. 2006. "Dietary Intake of Vitamin B6 and
Concentration of Vitamin B6 in Blood Samples of German Vegans." *Public
Health Nutrition* 9 (6): 779–84. https://doi.org/10.1079/phn2005895.

p. 161   *the form of omega-3 fatty acids found in most plant foods is the essential fatty acid
ALA* Lane, Katie E., Megan Wilson, Teuta G. Hellon, and Ian G. Davies.
2022. "Bioavailability and Conversion of Plant Based Sources of Omega-3
Fatty Acids—a Scoping Review to Update Supplementation Options for
Vegetarians and Vegans." *Critical Reviews in Food Science and Nutrition* 62
(18): 4982–97. https://doi.org/10.1080/10408398.2021.1880364; Wald-
mann, A., J. W. Koschizke, C. Leitzmann, and A. Hahn. 2005. "German
Vegan Study: Diet, Life-Style Factors, and Cardiovascular Risk Profile."
Annals of Nutrition and Metabolism 49 (6): 366–72. https://doi.org/10.1159
/000088888.

p. 161   *vegans who do not supplement with taurine are usually deficient* Laidlaw, S.
A., T. D. Shultz, J. T. Cecchino, and J. D. Kopple. 1988. "Plasma and Urine
Taurine Levels in Vegans." *American Journal of Clinical Nutrition* 47 (4):
660–63. https://doi.org/10.1093/ajcn/47.4.660; McCarty, Mark F. 2004. "A
Taurine-Supplemented Vegan Diet May Blunt the Contribution of Neutro-
phil Activation to Acute Coronary Events." *Medical Hypotheses* 63 (3): 419–25.
https://doi.org/10.1016/j.mehy.2004.03.040.

p. 161   *Taurine deficiency can contribute to many adverse health effects* Bhat, Mujtaba
Aamir, Khurshid Ahmad, Mohd Sajjad Ahmad Khan, Mudasir Ahmad Bhat,
Ahmad Almatroudi, Safikur Rahman, and Arif Tasleem Jan. 2020. "Expedi-
tion into Taurine Biology: Structural Insights and Therapeutic Perspective of
Taurine in Neurodegenerative Diseases." *Biomolecules* 10 (6): 863. https://doi
.org/10.3390/biom10060863.

p. 161 *taurine and vitamin B12 are important for maintaining our vision* García-Ayuso, Diego, Johnny Di Pierdomenico, Ana Martínez-Vacas, Manuel Vidal-Sanz, Serge Picaud, and María P. Villegas-Pérez. 2023. "Taurine: A Promising Nutraceutic in the Prevention of Retinal Degeneration." *Neural Regeneration Research* 19 (3): 606–10. https://doi.org/10.4103/1673-5374.380820.

p. 162 *signs point to vegans being at risk of age-related macular degeneration* Roda, Matilde, Natalie di Geronimo, Marco Pellegrini, and Costantino Schiavi. 2020. "Nutritional Optic Neuropathies: State of the Art and Emerging Evidences." *Nutrients* 12 (9): 2653. https://doi.org/10.3390/nu12092653.

p. 162 *That Goes for Taurine, Too* Tong, Tammy, et al. 2020. "Vegetarian and Vegan Diets"; Mahalle, Namita, et al. 2013. "Vitamin B12 Deficiency"; Domić, Jacintha, et al. 2022. "Perspective: Vegan Diets for Older Adults?"; Groenendijk, Inge, et al. 2023. "Protein Intake and Bone Mineral Density"; Campbell, Wayne W., et al. 2023. "Nutritional Interventions"; Cheng, Yu, et al. 2024. "Association Between Dietary Protein Intake and Risk of Chronic Kidney Disease."

p. 162 *What About Plant-Based Meat Substitutes?* Pham, Toan, Scott Knowles, Emma Bermingham, Julie Brown, Rina Hannaford, David Cameron-Smith, and Andrea Braakhuis. 2022. "Plasma Amino Acid Appearance and Status of Appetite Following a Single Meal of Red Meat or a Plant-Based Meat Analog: A Randomized Crossover Clinical Trial." *Current Developments in Nutrition* 6 (5): 6005013. https://doi.org/10.1093/cdn/nzac082.

p. 162 *Each American eats about 100.6 pounds* Connolly, G., and W. W. Campbell. 2023. "Poultry Consumption and Human Cardiometabolic Health-Related Outcomes: A Narrative Review." *Nutrients* 15 (16): 3550. https://doi.org/10.3390/nu15163550.

p. 163 *research on the health benefits of eating poultry is marred* Connolly, G., and W. W. Campbell. 2023. "Poultry Consumption."

p. 163 *Chicken provides up to 31 grams of protein* Connolly, G., and W. W. Campbell. 2023. "Poultry Consumption."

p. 163 *unprocessed chicken and other poultry meats provide many essential nutrients* Connolly, G., and W. W. Campbell. 2023. "Poultry Consumption."

p. 164 *how much they produce is partly determined by the amount of available CoQ10* Scialo, Filippo, and Alberto Sanz. 2021. "Coenzyme Q Redox Signalling and Longevity." *Free Radical Biology and Medicine* 164: 187–205. https://doi.org/10.1016/j.freeradbiomed.2021.01.018.

p. 164 *CoQ10 has been shown to reduce mortality* Mantle, David, and Iain Hargreaves. 2019. "Coenzyme Q10 and Degenerative Disorders Affecting Longevity: An Overview." *Antioxidants* 8 (2): 44. https://doi.org/10.3390/antiox8020044.

p. 166 *male longevity in Okinawa has declined dramatically* Hokama, Tomiko, and Colin Binns. 2008. "Declining Longevity Advantage and Low Birthweight in Okinawa." *Asia-Pacific Journal of Public Health* 20 Suppl: 95–101.

p. 166   *Pigs were traditionally the most important domesticated food animals*   Lee, Sanghee, and Hyekyung Hyun. 2018. "Pork Food Culture and Sustainability on Islands Along the Kuroshio Current: Resource Circulation and Ecological Communities on Okinawa and Jeju." *Island Studies Journal* 13 (1). https://doi .org/10.24043/001c.83918.

p. 166   *Pork is so high because pigs tend to eat*   Fu, Xueyan, Xiaohua Shen, Emily G. Finnan, David B. Haytowitz, and Sarah L. Booth. 2016. "Measurement of Multiple Vitamin K Forms in Processed and Fresh-Cut Pork Products in the U.S. Food Supply." *Journal of Agricultural and Food Chemistry* 64 (22): 4531–35. https://doi.org/10.1021/acs.jafc.6b00938.

Chapter 12

p. 170   *hunter-gatherers typically preferred eating large animals*   Cordain, L., J. B. Miller, S. B. Eaton, N. Mann, S. H. Holt, and J. D. Speth. "Plant-Animal Subsistence Ratios and Macronutrient Energy Estimations in Worldwide Hunter-Gatherer Diets." *American Journal of Clinical Nutrition* 71(3): 682–92. https://doi.org/10.1093/ajcn/71.3.682

p. 171   *our earliest human ancestors also enjoyed eggs*   Demarchi, Beatrice, Josefin Stiller, Alicia Grealy, Meaghan Mackie, Yuan Deng, Tom Gilbert, Julia Clarke, et al. 2022. "Ancient Proteins Resolve Controversy over the Identity of Genyornis Eggshell." *Proceedings of the National Academy of Sciences* 119 (43): e2109326119. https://doi.org/10.1073/pnas.2109326119.

p. 171   *In one 2023 study, researchers followed 617 men and 898 women*   Kritz-Silverstein, Donna, and Ricki Bettencourt. 2023. "The Longitudinal Association of Egg Consumption with Cognitive Function in Older Men and Women: The Rancho Bernardo Study." *Nutrients* 16 (1): 53. https://doi.org/10.3390 /nu16010053.

p. 171   *scientists speculate that it might have to do with the choline*   Wallace, Taylor C. 2018. "A Comprehensive Review of Eggs, Choline, and Lutein on Cognition Across the Life-Span." *Journal of the American College of Nutrition* 37 (4): 269–85. https://doi.org/10.1080/07315724.2017.1423248.

p. 171   *scientists are just beginning to study as a nutrient that is essential*   Zeisel, Steven H. 2012. "Dietary Choline Deficiency Causes DNA Strand Breaks and Alters Epigenetic Marks on DNA and Histones." *Mutation Research/Fundamental and Molecular Mechanisms of Mutagenesis* 733 (1–2): 34–38. https://doi.org/10 .1016/j.mrfmmm.2011.10.008.

p. 172   *the average choline intake in adults is far below adequate intake levels*   Zeisel, Steven H., and Kerry-Ann da Costa. 2009. "Choline: An Essential Nutrient for Public Health." *Nutrition Reviews* 67 (11): 615–23. https://doi.org/10.1111 /j.1753-4887.2009.00246.x.

p. 172   *Recommended daily values for choline . . . meet these guidelines*   Wallace, Taylor C., and Victor L. Fulgoni. 2017. "Usual Choline Intakes Are Associated with Egg and Protein Food Consumption in the United States." *Nutrients* 9 (8): 839. https://doi.org/10.3390/nu9080839.

p. 172   *Young women have less need for dietary sources*   Zeisel, Steven H. 2012. "Dietary Choline Deficiency."

p. 172   *choline deficiency has been associated with DNA strand breaks*   Zeisel, Steven H. 2012. "Dietary Choline Deficiency."

p. 172   *A choline deficiency even impairs folate metabolism*   Zeisel, Steven H. 2007. "Gene Response Elements, Genetic Polymorphisms and Epigenetics Influence the Human Dietary Requirement for Choline." *IUBMB Life* 59 (6): 380–87. https://doi.org/10.1080/15216540701468954.

p. 172   *one 2024 Chinese study followed 1,887 older adults*   Huang, Feifei, Fangxu Guan, Xiaofang Jia, Jiguo Zhang, Chang Su, Wenwen Du, Yifei Ouyang, et al. 2024. "Dietary Choline Intake Is Beneficial for Cognitive Function and Delays Cognitive Decline: A 22-Year Large-Scale Prospective Cohort Study from China Health and Nutrition Survey." *Nutrients* 16 (17): 2845. https://doi.org/10.3390/nu16172845.

p. 172   *up to 25 percent of your daily requirement*   Wallace, Taylor C., and Victor L. Fulgoni. 2017. "Usual Choline Intakes."

p. 172   *a study exploring the best ways to meet our daily requirements*   Wilcox, Jennifer, Sarah M. Skye, Brett Graham, Allyson Zabell, Xinmin S. Li, Lin Li, Shamanthika Shelkay, et al. 2021. "Dietary Choline Supplements, but Not Eggs, Raise Fasting TMAO Levels in Participants with Normal Renal Function: A Randomized Clinical Trial." *American Journal of Medicine* 134 (9): 1160-1169. e3. https://doi.org/10.1016/j.amjmed.2021.03.016.

p. 175   *"Eating Eggs Is Not Associated with Cardiovascular Disease"*   Shaughnessy, Allen F. 2021. "Eating Eggs Is Not Associated with Cardiovascular Disease." *American Family Physician* 103 (11): 695.

p. 176   *one major study of 177,000 people*   Dehghan, Mahshid, Andrew Mente, Sumathy Rangarajan, et al. 2020. "Association of Egg Intake with Blood Lipids, Cardiovascular Disease, and Mortality in 177,000 People in 50 Countries." *American Journal of Clinical Nutrition* 111 (4): 795-803. https://doi.org/10.1093/ajcn/nqz348.

p. 176   *2021 research paper by Japanese scientists*   Sugano, Michihiro, and Ryosuke Matsuoka. 2021. "Nutritional Viewpoints on Eggs and Cholesterol." *Foods* 10 (3): 494. https://doi.org/10.3390/foods10030494.

p. 177   *Eating a diet high in omega-3 fatty acids and low in omega-6 fatty acids leads*   Gupta, Ruby, Ramakrishnan Lakshmy, Ransi Ann Abraham, Kolli Srinath Reddy, Panniyammakal Jeemon, and Dorairaj Prabhakaran. 2013. "Serum Omega-6/Omega-3 Ratio and Risk Markers for Cardiovascular

Disease in an Industrial Population of Delhi." *Food and Nutrition Sciences (Print)* 2013 (9A): 94–97. https://doi.org/10.4236/fns.2013.49a1015; Al-Khudairy, Lena, Louise Hartley, Christine Clar, Nadine Flowers, Lee Hooper, and Karen Rees. 2015. "Omega 6 Fatty Acids for the Primary Prevention of Cardiovascular Disease." *Cochrane Database of Systematic Reviews* 11: CD011094. https://doi.org/10.1002/14651858.cd011094.pub2; Jurado-Fasoli, Lucas, Francisco J. Osuna-Prieto, Wei Yang, Isabelle Kohler, Xinyu Di, Patrick C.N. Rensen, Manuel J. Castillo, Borja Martinez-Tellez, and Francisco J. Amaro-Gahete. 2023. "High Omega-6/Omega-3 Fatty Acid and Oxylipin Ratio in Plasma Is Linked to an Adverse Cardiometabolic Profile in Middle-Aged Adults." *Journal of Nutritional Biochemistry* 117: 109331. https://doi.org/10.1016/j.jnutbio.2023.109331; Li, Na, Min Jia, Qianchun Deng, Zhen Wang, Fenghong Huang, Hanxue Hou, and Tongcheng Xu. 2021. "Effect of Low-Ratio n-6/n-3 PUFA on Blood Lipid Level: A Meta-Analysis." *Hormones* 20 (4): 697–706. https://doi.org/10.1007/s42000-020-00248-0.

p. 178   *A biotin deficiency can cause*   Kuroishi, Toshinobu. 2015. "Regulation of Immunological and Inflammatory Functions by Biotin1." *Canadian Journal of Physiology and Pharmacology* 93 (12): 1091–96. https://doi.org/10.1139/cjpp-2014 -0460; Kuroishi, Toshinobu, Yasuo Endo, Koji Muramoto, and Shunji Sugawara. 2008. "Biotin Deficiency Up-Regulates TNF-α Production in Murine Macrophages." *Journal of Leucocyte Biology* 83 (4): 912–20. https://doi.org/10 .1189/jlb.0607428.

p. 178   *Mice studies have also shown*   Kuroishi, Toshinobu, and Shunji Sugawara. 2020. "Metabolomic Analysis of Liver from Dietary Biotin Deficient Mice." *Journal of Nutritional Science and Vitaminology* 66 (1): 82–85. https://doi.org/10 .3177/jnsv.66.82.

p. 178   *Some studies show that adults and teenagers who*   Stratton, Shawna L., Thomas D. Horvath, Anna Bogusiewicz, Nell I. Matthews, Cindy L. Henrich, Horace J. Spencer, Jeffery H. Moran, and Donald M. Mock. 2010. "Plasma Concentration of 3-Hydroxyisovaleryl Carnitine Is an Early and Sensitive Indicator of Marginal Biotin Deficiency in Humans." *American Journal of Clinical Nutrition* 92 (6): 1399–1405. https://doi.org/10.3945/ajcn.110.002543; Baugh, C. M., J. H. Malone, and C. E. Butterworth. 1968. "Human Biotin Deficiency a Case History of Biotin Deficiency Induced by Raw Egg Consumption in a Cirrhotic Patient." *American Journal of Clinical Nutrition* 21 (2): 173–82. https://doi.org /10.1093/ajcn/21.2.173.

p. 179   *research shows that the only way to completely inactivate avidin*   Zhu, Yao, Jin Wang, Sai Kranthi Vanga, and Vijaya Raghavan. 2021. "Visualizing Structural Changes of Egg Avidin to Thermal and Electric Field Stresses by Molecular Dynamics Simulation." *LWT.* https://doi.org/10.1016/j.lwt.2021 .112139.

p. 179 *there is some evidence that marginal biotin deficiency* Mock, Donald M., Cindy L. Henrich, Nadine Carnell, and Nell I. Mock. 2002. "Indicators of Marginal Biotin Deficiency and Repletion in Humans: Validation of 3-Hydroxyisovaleric Acid Excretion and a Leucine Challenge 1, 2, 3." *American Journal of Clinical Nutrition* 76 (5): 1061–68. https://doi.org/10.1093/ajcn/76.5.1061; Mock, Donald M. 2009. "Marginal Biotin Deficiency Is Common in Normal Human Pregnancy and Is Highly Teratogenic in Mice 1–3." *Journal of Nutrition* 139 (1): 154–57. https://doi.org/10.3945/jn.108.095273; Mock, Donald M. 2017. "Biotin: From Nutrition to Therapeutics." *Journal of Nutrition* 147 (8): 1487–92. https://doi.org/10.3945/jn.116.238956.

Chapter 13

p. 183 *seafood comes close, providing your body with* Mendivil, Carlos O. 2021. "Fish Consumption: A Review of Its Effects on Metabolic and Hormonal Health." *Nutrition and Metabolic Insights* 14: 11786388211022378. https://doi.org/10.1177/11786388211022378.

p. 183 *Researchers recently published a paper showing several studies* Chen, Guo-Chong, Rhonda Arthur, Li-Qiang Qin, Li-Hua Chen, Zhendong Mei, Yan Zheng, Yang Li, Tao Wang, Thomas E. Rohan, and Qibin Qi. 2021. "Association of Oily and Nonoily Fish Consumption and Fish Oil Supplements with Incident Type 2 Diabetes: A Large Population-Based Prospective Study." *Diabetes Care* 44 (3): 672–80. https://doi.org/10.2337/dc20-2328.

p. 184 *MCI can be an early sign of Alzheimer's* Bredesen, Dale E., Edwin C. Amos, Jonathan Canick, Mary Ackerley, Cyrus Raji, Milan Fiala, and Jamila Ahdidan. 2016. "Reversal of Cognitive Decline in Alzheimer's Disease." *Aging (Albany, NY)* 8 (6): 1250–58. https://doi.org/10.18632/aging.100981.

p. 184 *omega-3 fatty acids, which are associated with boosting brain health* Loong, Spencer, Samuel Barnes, Nicole M. Gatto, Shilpy Chowdhury, and Grace J. Lee. 2023. "Omega-3 Fatty Acids, Cognition, and Brain Volume in Older Adults." *Brain Sciences* 13 (9): 1278. https://doi.org/10.3390/brainsci13091278.

p. 184 *Several recent studies have even suggested that people who include fish* Hosomi, Ryota, Munehiro Yoshida, and Kenji Fukunaga. 2012. "Seafood Consumption and Components for Health." *Global Journal of Health Science* 4 (3): 72–86. https://doi.org/10.5539/gjhs.v4n3p72.

p. 184 *Oily fish are a particularly good source* Chamorro, Franklin, Paz Otero, Maria Carpena, Maria Fraga-Corral, Javier Echave, Sepidar Seyyedi-Mansour, Lucia Cassani, and Miguel A. Prieto. 2023. "Health Benefits of Oily Fish: Illustrated with Blue Shark (Prionace Glauca), Shortfin Mako Shark (Isurus Oxyrinchus), and Swordfish (Xiphias Gladius)." *Nutrients* 15 (23): 4919. https://doi.org/10.3390/nu15234919.

p. 184 *Other studies have focused on the connection between eating seafood and* Schweitzer, Guilherme R. B., Isabela N. M. S. Rios, Vivian S. S. Gonçalves, Kelly G. Magalhães, and Nathalia Pizato. 2021. "Effect of N-3 Long-Chain Polyunsaturated Fatty Acid Intake on the Eicosanoid Profile in Individuals with Obesity and Overweight: A Systematic Review and Meta-Analysis of Clinical Trials." *Journal of Nutritional Science* 10: e53. https://doi.org/10.1017/jns.2021.46.

p. 184 *Our bodies can convert only about 1 percent of ALA, so seafood is a much better source* Takic, Marija, Biljana Pokimica, Gordana Petrovic-Oggiano, and Tamara Popovic. 2022. "Effects of Dietary α-Linolenic Acid Treatment and the Efficiency of Its Conversion to Eicosapentaenoic and Docosahexaenoic Acids in Obesity and Related Diseases." *Molecules* 27 (14): 4471. https://doi.org/10.3390/molecules27144471.

p. 185 *Taurine—a sulfur-containing amino acid—is the most abundant* Ripps, Harris, and Wen Shen. 2012. "Review: Taurine: A 'Very Essential' Amino Acid." *Molecular Vision* 18: 2673–86.

p. 185 *taurine is important for . . . powerful antioxidant* Northrop, Alyssa. 2023. "What Is Taurine? Benefits, Side Effects and Supplements." *Forbes Health*, 2023. https://www.forbes.com/health/supplements/taurine/.

p. 186 *Researchers have since demonstrated that this amino acid is a reliable warrior* Surai, Peter F., Katie Earle-Payne, and Michael T. Kidd. 2021. "Taurine as a Natural Antioxidant: From Direct Antioxidant Effects to Protective Action in Various Toxicological Models." *Antioxidants* 10 (12): 1876. https://doi.org/10.3390/antiox10121876.

p. 186 *The longest-living organisms on earth include* Ridgway, Iain D., C. A. Richardson, E. Enos, Z. Ungvari, S. N. Austad, E. E. R. Philipp, and Anna Csiszar. 2011. "New Species Longevity Record for the Northern Quahog (=Hard Clam), Mercenaria Mercenaria." *Journal of Shellfish Research* 30 (1): 35–38. https://doi.org/10.2983/035.030.0106.

p. 186 *researchers recently reported in the journal* Science Singh, P., Gollapalli, K., Mangiola, S., Schranner, D., and et. al. 2023. "Taurine Deficiency as a Driver of Aging." *Science.* https://www.science.org/doi/10.1126/science.abn9257.

p. 186 *Another animal study—this one with mice—showed* Yoshimura, Tomohisa, Chika Manabe, Yuki Inokuchi, Chikako Mutou, Tohru Nagahama, and Shigeru Murakami. 2021. "Protective Effect of Taurine on UVB-Induced Skin Aging in Hairless Mice." *Biomedicine & Pharmacotherapy* 141: 111898. https://doi.org/10.1016/j.biopha.2021.111898.

p. 186 *taurine can help people manage diabetes* Inam-u-llah, Fengyuan Piao, Rana Muhammad Aadil, Raheel Suleman, Kaixin Li, Mengren Zhang, Pingan Wu, Muhammad Shahbaz, and Zulfiqar Ahmed. 2018. "Ameliorative Effects of Taurine Against Diabetes: A Review." *Amino Acids* 50 (5): 487–502. https://doi.org/10.1007/s00726-018-2544-4.

p. 186   *Scientists have also shown that taurine has neuroprotective properties*   Rafiee,
          Zeinab, Alba M. García-Serrano, and João M. N. Duarte. 2022. "Taurine
          Supplementation as a Neuroprotective Strategy upon Brain Dysfunction in
          Metabolic Syndrome and Diabetes." *Nutrients* 14 (6): 1292. https://doi.org/10
          .3390/nu14061292.

p. 187   *this longevity ally can also help us combat the retinal disorders*   Castelli, Vanessa,
          Antonella Paladini, Michele d'Angelo, Marcello Allegretti, Flavio Mantelli,
          Laura Brandolini, Pasquale Cocchiaro, Annamaria Cimini, and Giustino Var-
          rassi. 2021. "Taurine and Oxidative Stress in Retinal Health and Disease."
          CNS Neuroscience & Therapeutics 27 (4): 403–12. https://doi.org/10.1111/cns
          .13610.

p. 187   *there's a form of blindness found in cats fed a plant-based diet*   Hayes, K. C. 1982.
          "Nutritional Problems in Cats: Taurine Deficiency and Vitamin A Excess." *The
          Canadian Veterinary Journal = La Revue Veterinaire Canadienne* 23 (1): 2–5.

p. 187   *there is research showing that they can suffer from neutropenia*   McCarty, Mark F.
          2004. "A Taurine-Supplemented Vegan Diet May Blunt the Contribution of
          Neutrophil Activation to Acute Coronary Events." *Medical Hypotheses* 63 (3):
          419–25. https://doi.org/10.1016/j.mehy.2004.03.040.

p. 192   *one of the most recommended supplements is omega-3 fish oils, and there is plenty of
          research*   Shahidi, Fereidoon, and Priyatharini Ambigaipalan. 2017. "Omega-3
          Polyunsaturated Fatty Acids and Their Health Benefits." *Annual Review of
          Food Science and Technology* 9 (1): 1–37. https://doi.org/10.1146/annurev-food
          -111317-095850.

p. 192   *The typical Western diet has a ratio of around 15:1*   Simopoulos, Artemis P. 2011.
          "Evolutionary Aspects of Diet: The Omega-6/Omega-3 Ratio and the Brain."
          Molecular Neurobiology 44 (2): 203–15. https://doi.org/10.1007/s12035-010
          -8162-0.

Appendix

p. 276   *Table 2: Digestible Indispensable Amino Acid Score (DIAAS) and Essential Amino
          Acid Quantities for Certain Foods*   United States Department of Agriculture,
          FoodData Central database. https://fdc.nal.usda.gov/.

INDEX

ABOUT THE AUTHORS

Dr. Loren Cordain is the founder of The Paleo Diet, a *New York Times* bestselling author, and a professor emeritus in the Department of Health and Exercise Science at Colorado State University. Over his world-renowned, decades-long career, Dr. Cordain has contributed to more than 68 peer-reviewed publications in medical, nutritional, and scientific literature (all available on ResearchGate.net), focusing on the many forms of the ancestral human diet and exploring which modern foods are healthy and which are unhealthy for us. Dr. Cordain is the author or coauthor of seven books, including *The Paleo Diet*, *The Paleo Answer*, *The Paleo Diet for Athletes*, *Real Paleo Fast & Easy*, *The Real Paleo Diet Cookbook*, and *The Paleo Diet Cookbook*, as well as dozens of articles on ThePaleoDiet.com. He lives with his wife, Lorrie, in Colorado.

    Trevor Connor, MS, is the CEO of The Paleo Diet, LLC, which owns and operates the trademarked The Paleo Diet® program, The Paleo Diet website (www.thepaleodiet.com), two industry-leading food certification standards, and a branding and cobranded licensing program. Connor was Dr. Cordain's final graduate student; his research focused on exercise bioenergetics and the impacts of diet on the immune system and autoimmune conditions. A graduate of Cornell University and a former professional cyclist and Canadian National Centre coach, Connor is the cofounder and CEO of Fast Talk Laboratories. He lives in Colorado.

Dr. Mark J. Smith was Dr. Cordain's first graduate student to study Paleolithic nutrition; he has worked with Dr. Cordain in the field since 1990. Dr. Smith holds a master's degree in exercise and sport science and a PhD in physiology from Colorado State University. For over 30 years, Dr. Smith has helped people solve or ease health conditions using the Paleo Diet, making him one of the most experienced Paleolithic nutrition educators in the world. He is a leading expert on supramaximal interval training and maintains an office in California.